Chinese Medicine

Chinese Medicine

Edited by **Patrick Lampard**

hayle
medical

New York

Published by Hayle Medical,
30 West, 37th Street, Suite 612,
New York, NY 10018, USA
www.haylemedical.com

Chinese Medicine
Edited by Patrick Lampard

International Standard Book Number: 978-1-63241-079-5 (Hardback)

Printed in the United States of America.

Contents

Preface

This book introduces the readers to the vast field of Chinese medicine with the help of comprehensive details and information. In the past few years, traditional Chinese medicine (TCM) has drawn the attention of researchers from all over the world. TCM is gradually evolving as a subject area with high potential and a possibility for original innovation. The book gives understanding of the TCM researches by discussing its fundamental theories, latest advances, diagnostic approach, current clinical applications etc. It talks about unrecognized issues which are important such as the theory of TCM property, and how to carry out TCM research in the direction of TCM property theory using modern scientific technology. This book includes contributions of eminent researchers who possess clinical knowledge and have years of experience in this field. It serves the objective of providing deep understanding of the distinct characteristics of Chinese medicine.

This book is the end result of constructive efforts and intensive research done by experts in this field. The aim of this book is to enlighten the readers with recent information in this area of research. The information provided in this profound book would serve as a valuable reference to students and researchers in this field.

At the end, I would like to thank all the authors for devoting their precious time and providing their valuable contribution to this book. I would also like to express my gratitude to my fellow colleagues who encouraged me throughout the process.

Editor

Introductory Chapter

Haixue Kuang

Key Laboratory of Chinese Materia Medica (Heilongjiang University of Chinese Medicine), Ministry of Education, Harbin, China

1. Introduction

The long-term clinical practice of traditional Chinese medicine (TCM) confirms its importance and essential role in the health care system in China, especially in the prevention and treatment of chronic diseases [1]. TCM is not only looked upon as a bright pearl, but also a treasure house in Chinese ancient culture. TCM has made great contribution to the health of Chinese people for thousands of years, and it became an independent medical system in world medical field with its special clinical effect, rational theory system and rich practice experience [2]. TCM is the holistic medicine under the guidance of system theory, emphasizing harmony between human and nature, focusing on equilibrium and balance, and focusing on state of functional system and normal function of the human organism viewing it as the integral entity. TCM is based on the Chinese philosophy of Yin-Yang and Five Elements. The oldest classic of TCM is *Huangdi Neijing* (Inner Canon of Huangdi or the Yellow Emperor's Medicine Classic), which was written around 2300 years ago. The basic theory of TCM includes five-zang organs and six-fu organs, qi (vital energy), blood, and meridians. TCM is based on the holistic principles and emphasizes harmony with the universe. It categorizes the causes of diseases into two groups: external causes and internal causes. It differentiates syndromes according to the eight principles (yin, yang, exterior, interior, cold, heat, deficiency (*xu*) and excess (*shi*)). Besides, the theory of TCM property is also one of the basic theories of the science of TCM. It is the connection between the TCM theory and the clinic. The interpreting of the scientific meaning of TCM property is one of the critical problems for the modernization process of TCM. It mainly includes four properties, five flavors, toxicity, and raising, lowering, floating, and sinking.

Although, TCM at present is based on the phytochemistry and the pharmacology research, this study provides an example for the modernization of TCM with certain research ideas. In fact, it has followed the study of Western medicine research method [3]. Nowadays, though a large number of young researchers are engaged in the study of TCM, some are deviating from unique characteristics of Chinese medicine. With the developing of their research work, people come to realize the importance of TCM characteristics, and begin to lay more emphasis on its special clinical effect, rational theory system and rich practice experience. Otherwise, the essential character of the role of TCM cannot be fully and correctly explained. It is essential to clarify the role of TCM theory, principles of TCM and material basis. In a manner of speaking, this is an effective way to develop TCM industry in the direction of TCM theory with the idea of modern scientific technology. This leads us to conclude that Chinese medicine is the subject area with the most potentiality and the possibility for original innovation. So, it is necessary for discussing practical application, promotion and worldwide spreading of TCM knowledge. Moreover, there is a new chance and challenge for the TCM industry.

2. Discussion

Chinese medicines have been attracting interest and acceptance in many countries. An estimated 1.5 billion people now use these preparations worldwide. This may be primarily because of the general belief that herbal drugs are without any side effect besides being cheap and locally available [4]. The abundant philosophical connotation of TCM, its profound cultural foundation, and its integration with great wisdom of the world are still amazing the world. TCM theories are originated from the profound experiences and understanding of ancient Chinese medicine practitioners. As far as I am concerned, digging TCM theories is able to effectively break through the bottleneck of the development of Chinese medicine. In order to make sufficient use of the advantages of TCM, it is essential to clarify the role of TCM theory, principles of TCM and material basis. In that case, we wrote this book *Recent Advances in Theories and Practice of Chinese Medicine* with 26 chapters. It is divided into four sections, namely, basic theories of TCM, clinical practice, pharmacological experimental research and pharmacodynamic material base research, respectively. Next, we make a briefly introduction of these four sections by several representative chapters, respectively.

2.1 Studies on basic theories of TCM
2.1.1 Metabonomics research of the four properties in TCM based on UPLC-QTOF-MS
The theory of TCM property is an important part of theories of TCM. It is one of the basic theories of the science of TCM, which is composed of multiple contents. It mainly includes four properties(Si Xing), five flavors(Wu Wei), channel tropism (Guijing), toxicity, and raising, lowering, floating and sinking (Sheng Jiang Fu Chen). It is the connection between the TCM theory and the clinic. The interpreting of the scientific meaning of TCM property is one of the critical problems for the modernization process of TCM. In TCM, diagnosis and medication are based on "Syndrome" ("ZHENG" in Chinese Mandarin), which can be regarded as a profile of symptom combination, or clinical phenotypes, such as Cold or Hot Syndrome, and "Hot medication curing Cold Syndrome and Cold medication curing Hot Syndrome" is a standard therapeutic guide line. This classical systems medicine at the macro level has been validated and developed by its repeated clinical practice for thousands of years. Hot and Cold medication are the four properties of Chinese medicinal herbs, precisely including cold, hot, warm and cool, which are also called the four natures or "four xing" in TCM. Cold-cool and warm-hot are two completely opposite categories of natures, whereas cold and cool or hot and warm differ in the degree. Chinese medicinal herbs with cold and cool nature can clear away heat, purge fire and eliminate toxic materials, which are mainly used for heat-syndrome; while with hot and warm nature have the actions of expelling cold, which are mainly used for cold syndrome. The four natures are summarized mainly from the body's response. On the base of syndrome differentiation theory, only distinguish heat or cold nature of disease, and have a good understanding of the cold or hot property of TCM, so selectively apply corresponding medicinal herbs that you could achieve the desired effect.

The theories of TCM are so broad and profound, and considered the civilization treasure of China. The four properties, the essence and important component of TCM theories, the high generalization on the basic property and typical characteristics of TCM, are a significant theoretical foundation for the clinical use of Chinese medicine. In recent 30 years more and more reports on the four natures of TCM have appeared in the literature. To date several aspects of research such as the characteristics of thermodynamics, the changes of nervous system and the endocrine glands, energy metabolism, the systems biology analysis include genome, transcriptome, proteome, and metabolome are all supposed to explored the macro and micro framework on the four properties, among which metabonomics is the most novel tool. It is a rapidly growing area of scientific research, which has been widely used in disease diagnosis, biomarker discovery, and research into the disease mechanisms.

Metabonomics is an emerging subject of the post-genome era, which, together with genomics, transcriptomics and proteomics, jointly constitutes the 'Systems Biology'. Metabonomics is the branch of science concerned with the quantitative understandings of the metabolite component of integrated living systems and its dynamic responses to the changes of both endogenous factors (such as physiology and development) and exogenous factors (such as environmental factors and xenobiotics). Recently, as a novel systemic approach to study metabolic profile and accelerate the course of drug development, metabonomics has achieved great growth, which is attracting more and more concerns from the academic community [5]. Metabolite or metabolic profiling, the compositional analysis of low molecular-weight (MW) species in biological samples (urine, plasma and serum), has been in existence for at least 35 years and has traditionally used mass spectrometry (MS) coupled to some modern separation technique such as ultra-performance liquid chromatography (UPLC) and gas chromatography (GC) for resolution and detection [6]. Integrity of metabonomic processes includes sample collection and pretreatment, data collection and analysis, and metabolic variation interpretation.

In this study, UPLC-QTOF-MS techniques coupled to metabonomics methods were used to prove the existence of the four properties in TCM, to illustrate its multi-component, multi-target, multi-channel and the complex mechanism. Metabonomics aims to assess metabolic changes in a comprehensive and global manner in order to infer biological functions and provide the detailed biochemical responses of cellular systems. We successfully established predict models based on cold and hot medicines as references. To estimate the predictive ability of our model, we used herb-Flos Datura to cross-validation, and excellent separation among the TCM varieties obtained by OPLS-DA, which a hot medication belonging to the hot medication group, are presented in terms of recognition and prediction abilities. It represented the percentage of the samples correctly classified during model training and cross-validation, respectively, while the prediction ability was only qualitative rather than quantitative.

This chapter is aimed at guiding researchers to understand a new way of drug discovery based on the theory of TCM property. More commonly, some researchers focused on traditional chemical constituents and ignore many other effective ones in TCM so that the characteristics of TCM were seriously lost. Also, it could be applied to explore Western medicine properties to effectively guide the clinical application. Considering the encouraging results obtained in this study, it seems to be very promising approach to apply metabonomics for further study on theory of TCM property.

2.1.2 An approach to the nature of Qi in TCM-Qi and bioenergy

TCM has been practiced for more than five thousand years, is a complete ancient medical system that takes a deep understanding of the laws and patterns of nature and applies them to the human body. TCM believes that the human body is a microcosm of the Universal macrocosm. Therefore, humans must follow the laws of the Universe to achieve harmony and total health. Even today TCM practitioners use these essential theories to understand, diagnose and treat health problems. In TCM, "harmony" is the ultimate goal. So, when nature's Qi undergoes change as it does seasonally, a person's internal Qi will respond automatically. If, for any reason, it can't make a smooth transition to the energy of the next season, TCM understands that illness will result. Often Western Complementary and Alternative Medicine (CAM) practitioners and their patients or clients derive their understanding of TCM from acupuncture. However, acupuncture is only one of the major treatment modalities of this comprehensive medical system based on the understanding of Qi or vital energy. These major treatment modalities are Qigong, herbal therapy, acupuncture, foods for healing and Chinese psychology.

Meridians, or channels, are invisible pathways through which Qi flows that form an energy network that connects all parts of the body, and the body to the universe. The ancient medical text 'The Yellow Emperor's Inner Canon (Nei Jing)' states: "The function of the channel (meridian) is to transport the Qi and blood, and circulate yin and yang to nourish the body". The energy practice of Qigong, with its postures and movements, also affects the flow of Qi. The energy pathways and the Organ Systems they link provide TCM with a framework for identifying the root cause of health problems and the diagnoses to heal them. Meridians work by regulating the energy functions of the body and keeping it in harmony. If Qi stagnates for too long in any meridian, it can become blocked and eventually turn into matter, setting the stage for conditions that can create a physical mass. TCM Meridian Theory states: "As long as Qi flows freely through the meridians and the Organs work in harmony, the body can avoid disease".

The study of Qi phenomena in this Chapter may help bridge some of the apparent difference between Western and Eastern culture. This chapter covered the nature of Qi as well as its philosophical aspects and the significance in the modern civilization because the true foundation of TCM is Qi.

2.1.3 A geomedical approach to Chinese medicine: The origin of the yin-yang symbol

This chapter shows how to compute Yin and Yang for different latitudes so traditional Chinese herbalists can quantify the efficacy of herbal drugs. Based on daylight hours, the chapter provides a simple formula that allows computation of Yin and Yang for each day of the year. Moreover, using daily Yin and Yang values, the chapter shows how to render the Yin-Yang symbol properly in accordance with its original meaning. Considering the importance of Yin and Yang in TCM, the rendering method presented in this chapter provides evidence that TCM, in its origin, is a geomedical science.

Herbal medicines collected from different geographic locations can significantly differ in their therapeutic efficacy. The concentration of bioactive substances varies depending on many local factors, such as sunshine hours or chemical and physical properties of the soil. To guarantee the optimal composition of herbal drugs, Chinese herbalists use "geo-authentic" herbs from recognized locations. However, it is often difficult to confirm geographical authenticity. The lack of formal models for Yin and Yang, and herbal efficacy in general, complicates objective comparisons and evaluations. Herbalists and practitioners of TCM need a better formal understanding of the Yin-Yang composition of each herb. This chapter contributes to the solution to this problem by providing a formal description of Yin and Yang. It shows in a mathematical way how Yin and Yang vary depending on latitude. The latitude of a herb's location determines the number of daylight hours and sunshine the herb is exposed to during the year. The number of daylight hours is one of the components affecting the concentration and composition of bioactive substances and therefore the efficacy of the herb. To standardize herbal preparation and administration, rigorous mathematical methods are essential to measure the Yin-Yang composition of herbs quantitatively. The work presented in this chapter is a first step towards such standardization.

2.2 Clinical practice of TCM
2.2.1 A comparison study on arterial blood pressure and pulse data of condenser microphone

As a pilot study to investigate the relationship between Chinese and modern medicines with microphone pressure sensor, we conduct a cross analysis of pulse data measured by microphone sensor and intra-arterial catheter, and Electrical CardiaoGram (ECG.). Unlike the ABP and ECG data, which are widely applied in most modern hospitals, the microphone data acquisition system is noninvasive and is easy to construct. It uses the commercial microphone, the software and hardware built in a personal or notebook computer and the data analysis of time series data. The measuring point of the microphone data should have prominent feeling of pulse when one touches his forefinger's tip to the wrist skin. Then, one just firmly presses the front head of the small microphone to the point. Since a commercial electret condenser microphone is generally very sensitive, the time series data can be successfully picked up. This measuring technique is closely related to the ancient Chinese diagnostic technique via three fingers.

As to the post processing, a fast and diffusive filter is first used to remove the trend of all the data. The remaining part is just the Fourier spectrum of the periodic part of the time series because the fast filter is carried out on the spectral domain. By imposing a Gaussian window, the band-pass- limited spectra are obtained and the corresponding results of applying the inverse Fast Fourier Transforms (FFT) is the real part of the wavelet coefficient. Then, using the Hilbert transform, the energy or amplitude of the spectral bands is evaluated. The cross correlation coefficients of the real part between the ECG, ABP, and microphone data are separately calculated with the spectral center of the Gaussian window scans over the range of 0.1 to 10 Hz which are corresponding to several organ-meridian modes. Six test cases in an intensive care unit were examined. Most numerical results show that the microphone data is related to ABP data in the real part correlation in the spectral region around the heart rate mode. The similarity between two spectrograms is considered to have the partial energy correlation. It seems that all the test cases are not in critical situations because ABP to ECG or microphone data to ECG are either correlated or partially correlated and all of them still alive. Although the sample size does not achieve a reasonable statistical level, these limited cases show that the Chinese and modern medicines are closely related to each other.

In this Chapter, the ECG signals were obtained from the three-lead ECG recording device. The ABP signals were conveyed from an invasive arterial-line system which involves an insertion of an arterial catheter connecting to a conducting tube filled with properly pressured fluid. The mechanical signals were then transformed to the electrical ones with a midway pressure transducer. Both ECG and ABP data were transferred back to the Philips MP60 module which was the physiological signal monitoring system used in our study. The analog signals were output to the data acquisition card where they would be converted to the digital signals with a sampling rate of 500Hz and then forwarded to the portable computer for further analysis.

If we can prove that the microphone arterial signal's heart rate mode can be used to provide the index, the preventive medicine would become a practical issue for the general population. Moreover, the connection between the ancient Chinese and modern medicines will become more solid in near future.

2.2.2 Hyperspectral imaging technology used in tongue diagnosis

Among the four diagnostic processes of TCM: inspection, auscultation and olfaction, inquiry, and pulse feeling and palpation, the examination of tongue is one of the most important approaches for getting significant evidences in diagnosing the patient's health conditions. However, owing to its drawbacks in quantification and standardization, the development of tongue diagnosis is stagnated. Computerized methods for TCM allow researchers to identify required information more efficiently, discover new relationships which are obscured by merely focusing on Western medicine, and bridge the gaps between Western Medicine and TCM. Therefore, getting the overall information about tongue surface is very important for computerized tongue diagnosis system. In this chapter, an an acousto-optic tunable filter (AOTF) based hyperspectral tongue imaging system (THIS) which can capture hyperspectral images of human tongue at a series of wavelengths is developed and used in tongue diagnosis. The basic principles and instrumental systems of the new system, the data pre-processing method as well as some applications are presented. Compared with the pushbroom hyperspectral tongue imager used in our previous works, this new type of hyperspectral tongue imaging system has the advantage of having no moving parts and can be scanned at very high rates. As the hyperspectral tongue images can provide more information than the traditional charge coupled device CCD based images, we can find some successful applications in computerized tongue diagnosis such as tongue body segmentation, tongue colour analysis and discrimination, tongue cracks extraction and classification, sublingual veins analysis, etc. Preliminary experiments show that the AOTF-based hyperspectral tongue imaging system is superior to the traditional CCD based methods because the hyperspectral images can provide more information about the tongue surface. In future studies, we will extract the quantitative features of the tongue surface and find some methods to model the relationship between these features and certain diseases.

The new system can capture image scenes in contiguous but narrow spectral bands under the control of the AOTF controller. The hyperspectral tongue images provided by the instrument can be visualized as a 3D cube because of its intrinsic structure, where the cube face is a function of the spatial coordinates and the depth is a function of wavelength. In this case, each spatial point on the face is characterized by its own spectrum (often called spectral signature). This spectrum is directly corresponds to the amount of energy that the tongue represented, as hyperspectral sensors commonly utilize the simple fact that a tongue can emits light in certain frequency bands. Consequently, the hyperspectral tongue image data provides a wealth of information about an image scene which is potentially very helpful to tongue diagnosis.

2.2.3 Advances in Chinese medicine diagnosis: From traditional methods to computational models

Although Chinese and Western physicians were not distinct in their conceptual framework, their respective medical practices evolved on different cultures and historical contexts. Therefore, it is expected that the advances on medical knowledge represent this cultural divergence.

Many efforts have been made to integrate the ancient, traditional knowledge of Chinese medicine into contemporary, Eastern medical practice. Diagnosis is the key element in this integration of medical systems since it links the patient's needs to the available therapeutic resources. The art of Chinese medicine diagnosis was enriched throughout history but it main traditional aspect remains unchanged: the exclusive use of information available to the naked senses. Clinical information provided by vision, hearing, smelling, and touching is interpreted in a framework of Chinese medicine theories of physiology. No equipment or instrument was developed with specific diagnostic purposes or based on Chinese medicine theories. However, advances in computation and biomedical instruments allowed more powerful analysis of clinical data and quantification of parameters otherwise assessed only in a qualitative fashion. As a consequence, computer models for diagnosis in Chinese medicine were developed and tested in the last few decades and are promising tools in the clinical environment.

This chapter introduces the traditional methods of diagnosis in Chinese medicine and introduces their evolution into computational models. Current methods for validation of computational model by the assessment of their diagnostic accuracy and possible sources of errors are also presented. Finally, perspectives on the issue of computational diagnosis are discussed.

2.3 Pharmacological experimental research
2.3.1 Effects of vasoactive Chinese herbs on the endothelial NO system

Nitric oxide (NO) produced by the endothelial NO synthase (eNOS) plays a protective role in the vasculature. It is a potent vasodilator and protects blood vessels from thrombosis by inhibiting platelet aggregation and adhesion. In addition, endothelial NO possesses multiple anti-atherosclerotic properties. Interestingly, the purported effects of "circulation-improving" herbs used in TCM show striking similarities with the vascular actions of eNOS-derived NO. Therefore, we hypothesized that part of the pharmacological effects of such TCM herbs may be mediated by NO.

This Chapter studied the effects of 17 Chinese herbs with potential effects on the vasculature, and have identified *Salviae miltiorrhizae radix*, *Zizyphi spinosae semen* and *Prunella vulgaris* L. as potent eNOS-upregulating agents. In cultured human endothelial cells, aqueous extracts of these herbs increased eNOS promoter activity, eNOS mRNA and protein expression, as well as NO production in a concentration- and time-dependent manner. In addition, we have studied the constituents from the abovementioned Chinese herbs and have found that ursolic acid and betulinic acid are capable of enhancing eNOS gene expression. More recently, we have found that betulinic acid also stimulated NO production through post-translational mechanisms. By enhancing eNOS phosphorylation at serine 1177 and dephosphorylation at threonine 495, betulinic acid also increases eNOS enzymatic activity. In summary, we have described the pharmacological effects of Chinese herbs on endothelial NO system and have identified some active compounds from these plants. By performing modern pharmacological studies, we have provided some molecular mechanisms that may partially explain the therapeutic effects described in TCM.

2.3.2 Traditional Chinese herbal medicine – East meets West in validation and therapeutic application

The holistic views of TCM generally have no conflicts with the western medicine, perhaps they were just expressed in different terms. Western medicine is usually more concrete in diagnosis and judgment. Treatment is often quicker, particularly in acute cases, and surgery is its strength. Its weak points are that it sees disease as something to be measured and quantified and often ignores the psychological, social and behavioral factors involved in illness. Chinese medicine, on the other hand, can be too flexible and too general where diagnosis and judgment are concerned, and sometimes relies too heavily on the individual practitioner's experiences. Its strong points are its highly flexible approach, which enabling treatments to be changed as the patient improve, and its emphasis on preventive medicine. The Chinese way tends to treat the whole body rather than to try to isolate a particular infected area. And, finally, the herbs themselves, compared with chemically produced medicines, are relatively cheap and easy to use. They have minimal side-effects, and most have been tried and tested for over many thousand years. Western medicine focuses more on symptomatic management, whereas TCM focuses more on cause and effect. Western medicine is more useful for first-aid and surgical interventions, whereas TCM is more useful in treating internal and chronic illnesses. An ideal health care system should be established to concern people's physical and mental health, to deal with all personal problems, and to improve people's quality of life. A new model of health care should be composed by a different medical system to provide a holistic approach. TCM, today as an alternative and complementary medicine should be included into the conventional medicine to form the new modern medicine. This is in line with the aim of the WHO to promote recognition of traditional medicine and to support its integration into the mainstream health service. There is space of integration for TCM and modern medicine. A new paradigm for developing medicine is needed, and Chinese medicine could make a significant contribution in this field. To achieve such integration, modern science and technology had to be used to study the action, efficacy and toxicity of Chinese medicines. Although, there are many issues to concern, especially safe and effectiveness, some compromise and agreement are needed.

Thus botanicals should be defined, authenticated and documented as to their source and conditions of cultivation using modern methodology. Manufacturing and preparation processes of Chinese medicine should be carefully monitored and standardized. Claims for Chinese medicine should be verified from rigorous controlled trials. Interaction between Western and Chinese medicines should be better studied and information obtained centralized into accessible databases. This would be an enormous undertaking requiring international collaboration and participation of governments worldwide. In fact, the feasibility of herbal validation by using Western methods is well-illustrated. In particular, concerns about identity authentication, quality control, evidences of efficacy and safety of herbal remedies, are being addressed with the modern science and technology, and ultimately allow the gathering of information necessarily to support clinical trials. Along with this route, efforts being played will return with the transition of TCM into a recognized science specialty to fill up the gaps between Eastern and Western medical approaches. In this perspective, it may not be necessary to isolate the active ingredients from herbal remedies or purity them to finally become chemical drugs. To promote the effectiveness, Chinese herbal medicine can remain in formulae but standardizations are needed. Meanwhile, both Chinese and western practitioners should come together and sort out the best treatment they can offer to patients, which very often may be the combination of the modern and Chinese medicine, instead of favoring one over the other. Conventional Western medicine and Chinese medicine should be seen as complementary to each other, rather than as alternatives. Both types of medicine have their advantages and drawbacks, which is why they need to work hand in hand for optimal results. Together, Chinese and Western medicine could form the most effective disease treatment the world has ever known.

2.3.3 Targeting effect of traditional Chinese medicine

Meridian guide drug had the effect of synery and attenuation, and this effect based on concentrated drug at target-site. Meridian guide effect had an close relatiship with drug transporters and metabolism enzyme. Differnert components had different affinity to transporters or enzymes, and meridian guide effect is the combination of all components in meridian guide drug. Therefore, it is necessary to investigate the exact effect of main components of meridian guide drug on transporters and metabolism enzyme, establish the relationship between its dose and its effect as well as effects in kinds of diseases. As we known more about the relatiship among components in meridian guide drug, kinds of transporters and metabolism enzymes, activity in nomal and disease state, we could design target delivery system freely as we like.

2.4 Pharmacodynamic material base research

2.4.1 Therapeutic effects of lignans isolated from schisandra chinesis on hepatic carcinoma

The development of novel therapeutic drugs for hepatic carcinoma is a very important objective in the field of pharmacological research. Among the variety of approaches thus far pursued to develop novel drugs, identification and screening of natural compounds from medical herbs has proven a very effective one — not least, because this method saves a great deal of time and cost. Recently, many institutes and companies in advanced countries have focused on an approach to novel drugs for hepatic carcinoma via the use of various lignins isolated from S. chinensis. This chapter introduces three lignans and one blend which may prove valuable in efforts to combat hepatic carcinoma. Gomisin A at high concentration was found to significantly induce anti-proliferative and pro-apoptotic effects in hepatic carcinoma. Schizandrin A markedly increased vincristine-induced hepatic carcinoma apoptosis and anti-tumor activity. Additionally, tigloygomisin H induced the death of hepatic carcinoma cells and inhibited quinone reductase activity. Furthermore, KY88 was a blend composed of 10 herbal extracts and effects a dose-dependent inhibition of hepatocellular carcinoma cellular proliferation. Collectively, the results of this chapter demonstrated that these lignins and the blend from S. chinensis were regarded as an anti-cancer drug candidate capable of inducing apoptosis and inhibiting the cell proliferation of hepatocellular carcinoma via a variety of mechanisms.

2.4.2 Separation and quantification of component monosaccharides of polysaccharide extracts from ephedra sinica by MECC with photodiode array detector

TCM polysaccharides with multiple pharmacological activities have recently stimulated the interest of academia and the pharmaceutical industries. In fact, the roles of water-soluble polysaccharides from traditional Chinese medicines in biological processes have been studied with increasing attention over the past recent years because of their broad spectrum of therapeutic properties and relatively low toxicity. Indeed, immunomodulation, anti-tumour, antivirus, anticoagulant, hypoglycaemic, anti-complementary, anti-inflammatory and antioxidation bioactivities have been presented by many polysaccharides extracted from medicinal fungi and plants.

The Ephedra plant, or "Mahuang" of traditional Chinese medicine, is one of the oldest medicinal plants known to mankind. More than 45 species of Ephedra plants exist and are indigenous to regions of Asia, North, Central and South America and Europe. Mahuang contains ephedrine alkaloids as their principal components, which are primarily localized in the aerial parts of the plant. In recent years, many herbs used in popular medicine have been reported to contain polysaccharides with a great variety of biological activities and the water-soluble Mahuang polysaccharides are also demonstrated to be one of the main bioactive constituents of *Ephedra* plant except for a series of ephedrine alkaloids. For these reasons, great interest arose on the reliable analytical methods of the Mahuang polysaccharides, which can be used for exploring the new functional products with polysaccharides due to its pharmacological importance and application in the pharmaceutical industry. Immunosuppressive effects of acidic polysaccharides from the stems of *E. sinica* have been demonstrated by carbon clearance test, delayed type hypersensitivity reaction and humoral immune response *in vivo*.

In this chapter, a rapid and sensitive method was optimized and validated for the separation and quantification of derivatized monosaccharides in cold water-soluble polysaccharide extract from the stems of *E. sinica* using 1-phenyl-3-methyl-5 -pyrazolone (PMP) as precolumn derivatization reagent by micellar electrokinetic capillary chromatography (MECC) with photodiode array detector. The separation was carried out on a on an unmodified fused silica capillary and UV detection at 250 nm, and the 8 PMP derivatives of mannose, rhamnose, glucuronic acid, galacturonic acid, glucose, xylose, galactose and arabinose were baseline separated within 12 min.

3. Conclusion

This book may help our readers gain a deeper understanding of unique characteristics of TCM and will bridge the gap between the methods of Chinese medicine and modern biomedicine through the discussion of TCM with advanced instrumental methods. Also, it will be providing cutting-edge information about TCM research including its basic theories, diagnostic approach, current clinical applications, latest advances, and so on. Hopefully, it could play a very important role in disseminating TCM knowledge, promoting TCM influence in the world and accelerating the modernization of TCM.

4. References

[1] Jiang, M., Zhang, C., Cao, H., Chan, K., & Lu, A. The Role of Chinese Medicine in the Treatment of Chronic Diseases in China. *Planta Medica*, 2011, 77, 873-881.

[2] David, M., Eisenberg, Eric, S. J., Harris, Bruce, A. Littlefield, et al. (2011). Developing a library of authenticated Traditional Chinese Medicinal (TCM) plants for systematic biological evaluation -Rationale, methods and preliminary results from a Sino-American collaboration. *Fitoterapia*, 82, 17–33.

[3] Dou,S.S., Liu, R.H., Jiang, P., *et al*. System biology and its application in compound recipe of traditional Chinese medicine study. *Mode Tradit Chin Med Mater Med*, 2008, 10, 116-121.

[4] Li, S.P., Zhao, J., Yang, B. Strategies for quality control of Chinese medicines. *Journal of Pharmaceutical and Biomedical Analysis* 2011, 55, 802-809.

[5] Lao, Y.M., Jiang, J.G., and Yan L. Application of metabonomic analytical techniques in the modernization and toxicology research of traditional Chinese medicine. *British Journal of Pharmacology*, 2009, 157, 1128-1141.

[6] Keun, H.C. Metabonomic modeling of drug toxicity. *Pharmacology & Therapeutics*, 2006, 109, 92-106

Part 1

Basic Theories of TCM

A Geomedical Approach to Chinese Medicine: The Origin of the Yin-Yang Symbol

Stefan Jaeger
*National Library of Medicine**
United States

1. Introduction

This chapter shows how to compute Yin and Yang for different latitudes so traditional Chinese herbalists can quantify the efficacy of herbal drugs. Based on daylight hours, the chapter provides a simple formula that allows computation of Yin and Yang for each day of the year. Moreover, using daily Yin and Yang values, the chapter shows how to render the Yin-Yang symbol properly in accordance with its original meaning. Considering the importance of Yin and Yang in traditional Chinese medicine (TCM), the rendering method presented in this chapter provides evidence that TCM, in its origin, is a geomedical science.

Herbal medicines collected from different geographic locations can significantly differ in their therapeutic efficacy. The concentration of bioactive substances varies depending on many local factors, such as sunshine hours or chemical and physical properties of the soil. To guarantee the optimal composition of herbal drugs, Chinese herbalists use "geo-authentic" herbs from recognized locations. However, it is often difficult to confirm geographical authenticity. The lack of formal models for Yin and Yang, and herbal efficacy in general, complicates objective comparisons and evaluations. Herbalists and practitioners of TCM need a better formal understanding of the Yin-Yang composition of each herb. This chapter contributes to the solution to this problem by providing a formal description of Yin and Yang. It shows in a mathematical way how Yin and Yang vary depending on latitude. The latitude of a herb's location determines the number of daylight hours and sunshine the herb is exposed to during the year. The number of daylight hours is one of the components affecting the concentration and composition of bioactive substances and therefore the efficacy of the herb. To standardize herbal preparation and administration, rigorous mathematical methods are essential to measure the Yin-Yang composition of herbs quantitatively. The work presented in this chapter is a first step toward such standardization.

The chapter structure is as follows: Section 2 discusses the main ideas of the philosophical Yin-Yang concept. Section 3 shows today's most common Yin-Yang symbol and discusses its typical shape. Then, Section 4 presents the origin of the Yin-Yang symbol and introduces a daylight model that allows computation of Yin and Yang depending on the daylight hours for each geographic latitude. Using the computed values for Yin and Yang, the section will show how to render the Yin-Yang symbol properly, and in accordance with its original meaning. The chapter concludes with a discussion of the consequences of the results for researchers in TCM and herbal medicine. Finally, the appendix contains examples of Yin-Yang symbols computed for different latitudes in the northern and southern hemispheres.

---
*Work on this study began while the author was affiliated with the Chinese Academy of Sciences.

2. Yin and Yang

Yin-Yang has become a universal philosophical concept that many people readily embrace to their advantage. The concept of Yin and Yang is deeply rooted in Chinese philosophy (Miller, 2003; Watts, 1999). Its origin dates back at least 2500 years, probably much earlier, playing a crucial role in the formation of the Chinese ancient civilization. Chinese thinkers have attached great importance to Yin and Yang ever since. In Asia's search for a universal formula describing balance and harmony, Yin-Yang today appeals to fields as different as medicine, arts, religion, sports, or politics.

According to the Chinese philosophical concept, there are two opposing forces in the world, namely Yin and Yang, which are constantly trying to gain the upper hand over each other. However, neither one will ever succeed in doing so, though one force may temporarily dominate the other one. Both forces cannot exist without each other; it is rather the constant struggle between both forces that defines our world and produces the rhythm of life. Yin and Yang are not only believed to be the foundation of our universe, but also to flow through and affect every being. For example, typical Yin-Yang opposites are night/day, cold/hot, rest/activity.

Chinese philosophy does not confine itself to a mere description of Yin and Yang; it also provides guidelines on how to live in accordance with Yin and Yang. The central statement is that Yin and Yang need to be in harmony. Any imbalance of an economical, biological, physical, or chemical system can be directly attributed to a distorted equilibrium between Yin and Yang. For example, an illness accompanied by fever is the result of Yang being too strong and dominating Yin. On the other hand, for example, dominance of Yin could result in a body shivering with cold. The optimal state every being, or system, should strive for is therefore the state of equilibrium between Yin and Yang. It is this state of equilibrium between Yin and Yang that Chinese philosophy considers the most powerful and stable state a system can assume.

Yin and Yang already carry the seed of their opposites: A dominating Yin becomes susceptible to Yang and will eventually turn into its opposite. On the other hand, a dominating Yang gives rise to Yin and will turn into Yin over time. This defines the perennial alternating cycle of Yin or Yang dominance. Only the equilibrium between Yin and Yang is able to overcome this cycle.

3. Yin-Yang symbol

Figure 1 shows the well-known black-and-white symbol of Yin and Yang. This Yin-Yang

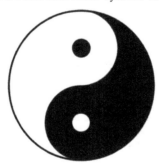

Fig. 1. A common Yin-Yang symbol.

symbol, also known under the name Tai Chi symbol, is arguably one of the most flamboyant symbols today. It stands on the same level as the Christian cross and other mainstream religious symbols. We can see the intertwining spiral-like curves in Figure 1, which are actually semicircles, separating the Yin and Yang area. The small spots of different color in each area indicate the above mentioned conception that both Yin and Yang carry the seed of their opposites; Yin cannot exist without Yang, and Yang cannot exist without Yin. These spots will play no role in this chapter. Neither will the assignment of black and white to Yin and Yang have any significance here, though Yin is typically associated with black and Yang with white.

Spiral-like curves are a common occurrence in nature. They appear in various forms in a wide range of living beings and processes; e.g., mollusk shells, hurricanes, or galaxies (Cook, 1979; Séquin, 1999). Depending on the form of these curves, the Yin-Yang symbol can take on different shapes. It is therefore necessary to define a standard rendering method before plotting the Yin-Yang symbol. For example, Figure 2 shows two versions of the South Korean Flag.

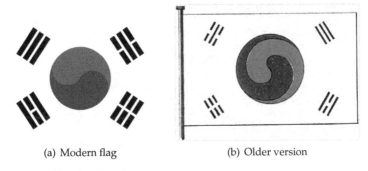

(a) Modern flag   (b) Older version

Fig. 2. Flag of South Korea (Wikipedia).

The South Korean flag's modern version is on the left-hand side of Figure 2. On the right-hand side is an older version of the flag. Both versions feature the Yin-Yang symbol prominently in their center, which is again testimony of the importance of the Yin-Yang concept for Asian countries. However, the shapes of the Yin-Yang spirals are clearly different for both flags. To agree on a common flag, it is necessary to define a standard construction scheme for rendering the Yin-Yang symbol. Figure 3 shows the standard construction sheet for the modern South Korean flag. However, the next section shows that the rendering method in Figure 3 does not reflect the original meaning of the Yin-Yang symbol.

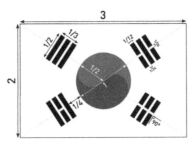

Fig. 3. Construction sheet for the South Korean flag (Wikipedia).

Contemporary literature has been mostly neglecting the plotting of the Yin-Yang symbol, paying more attention to philosophical questions. However, a mathematical formalization of the Yin-Yang symbol is desirable to open hitherto mathematically inaccessible fields, such as Chinese traditional medicine, for rigorous scientific research.

4. The origin of the Yin-Yang symbol

Despite its presence in everyday life, it is fair to say that only a few people know about the origin of the Yin-Yang symbol. Very often, even the most devoted practitioners have to pass on the question about its origin. Contrary to what one would expect, literature dealing with the origin of the Yin-Yang symbol is rare. Contemporary books and articles typically deal in detail with the philosophical facets of Yin and Yang, but do not address the origin of the Yin-Yang symbol. It turns out that the original Yin-Yang symbol is more complex than its modern representation as two semicircles suggests (Browne, 2007; Graf, 1994).

The Yin-Yang symbol has its origin in the I-Ching; one of the oldest and most fundamental books in Chinese philosophy. The I-Ching, which is typically translated as "The Book of Changes", deals with natural phenomena and their seasonal cycles. From the constant changes and transformations in nature, the I-Ching tries to derive the unchanging rules governing our cosmos and our very existence. The observation of celestial phenomena is therefore of central importance to the I-Ching (Hardaker, 2001). It is here, where one finds the roots of the Yin-Yang symbol (Tian & Tian, 2004).

For example, by observing the shadow of the sun and recording the positions of the Big Dipper at night throughout the year, the ancient Chinese determined the four points of the compass: The sun rises in the east and sets in the west. The direction of the shortest shadow measured on a given day reveals south (www.chinesefortunecalendar.com/yinyang.htm). At night, the Pole Star indicates North.

4.1 Shadow model

The Yin-Yang symbol is tightly connected with the annual cycle of the earth around the sun, and the four seasons resulting from it. To investigate this cycle, the ancient Chinese used a pole that they put up orthogonally to the ground, as shown in Figure 4. With this setup, the

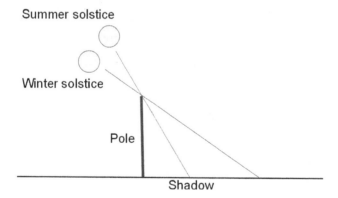

Fig. 4. Shadow model.

ancient Chinese were able to record precisely the positions of the sun's shadow and divide the year into different sections. They found the length of a year to be about 365.25 days.

Furthermore, they divided the circle of the year into segments, including the vernal equinox, autumnal equinox, summer solstice, and winter solstice. In addition, they used concentric circles around the pole, helping them to record the length of the sun's shadow every day. As a result, they measured the shortest shadow during the summer solstice, and measured the longest shadow during the winter solstice. After connecting the measured points and dimming the part that reaches from summer solstice to winter solstice (Yin), they arrived at a chart like the one in Figure 5. The resemblance between this chart and the modern Yin-Yang

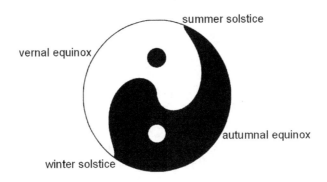

Fig. 5. Yin-Yang symbol for Latitude $L = 68°$ (near polar circle) with equinoxes and solstices.

symbol in Figure 1 is striking. Figure 5 provides visual evidence that the original Yin-Yang symbol describes the change of a pole's shadow length during a year. In fact, by rotating the chart and positioning the winter solstice at the bottom, the Yin-Yang chart of the ancient Chinese becomes very similar to the modern Yin-Yang symbol depicted in Figure 1.

The white area of the Yin-Yang symbol is typically called Yang. It begins at the winter solstice and indicates a beginning dominance of daylight over darkness, which is the reason why the ancient Chinese associated it with the sun (or male). Accordingly, the dark area of the Yin-Yang symbol represents Yin, which begins with the summer solstice. Yin indicates a beginning dominance of darkness over daylight. The ancient Chinese therefore associated it with the moon (or female).

Note that the shape of the Yin-Yang symbol also depends on the ecliptic angle of the earth. The ecliptic affects the angle between the white Yang area, or black Yin area, and the outer circle of the Yin-Yang symbol. The ecliptic is the sun's apparent path around the earth. It is tilted relative to the earth's equator. As a result, one can observe four different seasons throughout the year. In the year 2000, the obliquity of the ecliptic was about $23°26'19''$. The ecliptic's obliquity is not stable and can change during the millennia. This is due to the different forces exerted by the bodies in the solar system on the earth. The obliquity varies between about $21°55'$ and $24°18'$ within a period of $40,000$ years (Wikipedia, March 2008). For example, in the year $3,000$ BC, the ecliptic was about $24°1.6'$. Therefore, the ancient Yin-Yang symbol looks slightly different than the modern Yin-Yang symbol when rendered based on the shadow model.

4.2 Daylight model

This section presents a rendering method for the Yin-Yang symbol based on daylight hours, which are connected with shadow lengths. A long day has the sun standing high on the horizon at noon, casting a short shadow. On the other hand, a short day is the result of the sun standing low on the horizon at noon, which in turn produces a long shadow. For computing the daylight time for a given day in the year, this section uses the formula given in (Forsythe et al., 1995). The formula takes many different factors into account, most notably the refraction of the earth's atmosphere. The daylight model presented here is therefore an accurate description of the actual daylight measurement of an observer on the ground. A detailed investigation of the formula is beyond the scope of this paper, though.

The formula requires two input parameters, namely the day of the year J and the latitude L of the observer's location. It consists of two parts. The first part computes an intermediate result P, which is the input to the second part. The equation for the first part is as follows:

$$P = \arcsin[0.39795 * \cos(0.2163108 + 2 * \arctan\{0.9671396 * \tan[0.00860(J - 186)]\})] \quad (1)$$

Given P, the second part then computes the actual day length D in terms of sunshine hours:

$$D = 24 - \left(\frac{24}{\pi}\right) * \arccos\left\{\frac{\sin\left(\frac{0.8333*\pi}{180}\right) + \sin\left(\frac{L*\pi}{180}\right) * \sin(P)}{\cos\left(\frac{L*\pi}{180}\right) * \cos(P)}\right\} \quad (2)$$

Using Equation 2, Figure 6 shows the daylight time for each day of the year and a latitude of $68°$. This latitude is close to the polar circle, or Arctic Circle, in the northern hemisphere. The

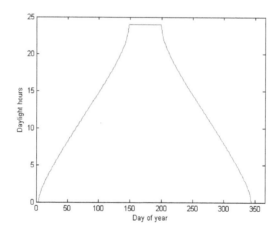

Fig. 6. Daylight hours for Latitude $L = 68°$ (near polar circle).

equivalent latitude in the southern hemisphere is the Antarctic Circle. The Arctic Circle marks the southernmost latitude in the northern hemisphere where the sun shines for 24 hours at least once per year (midnight sun) and does not shine at all at least once per year. Theoretically, the Arctic Circle marks the area where these events occur exactly once per year, namely during the summer and winter solstices. However, due to atmospheric refractions and because the sun is a disk rather than a point, the actual observation at the Arctic Circle is different. For example, the midnight sun can be seen south of the Arctic Circle during the summer solstice. According to Figure 6, the midnight sun shines for about 50 days at latitudes around $68°$.

Figure 7 shows the daylight hours in Figure 6 as a polar plot. In this polar plot, the distance to the origin stands for the daily sunshine hours. One full turn of $360°$ corresponds to one year. There is another important difference to Figure 6, though. For the second half of the

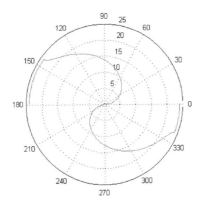

Fig. 7. Polar daylight plot for Latitude $L = 68°$ (near polar circle).

year, Figure 7 shows the hours of darkness instead of the daylight hours. The number of hours with darkness is simply the number of daylight hours subtracted from 24. Drawing the daylight hours in such a way produces the two spirals depicted in Figure 7. Coloring the areas delimited by both spirals and the outer circle in black and white then produces a rotated version of the Yin-Yang symbol in Figure 5. Note that this symbol is not quite symmetrical. This is correct because spring and fall are not completely symmetrical in terms of the solar cycle; a fact not discussed further in this chapter. For latitudes around the polar circle, the spirals in Figure 7 originate either directly in the origin of the polar plot or in a point close to it. This is because there will be at least one day with no sunshine.

Figure 8 shows the daylight hours and polar plots generated in the same way for different latitudes L, according to Equations 1 and 2. In particular, Figure 8 shows plots for $L = 40°$ (near Beijing), $L = 0°$ (Equator), and $L = 88°$ (near North Pole). For Latitude $L = 40°$, which is about the latitude of Beijing, the daylight curve is flatter compared to the daylight curve for $L = 68°$ in Figure 6. The reason for the flatter shape is that each day of the year has sunshine as well as darkness at $L = 40°$. For this latitude, the shapes of the spirals in the polar plot are approaching semicircles. Their starting points are relatively far from the center of the polar plot. This degeneration into semicircles continues with decreasing latitude. It reaches its extreme at the equator, with $L = 0°$. Here, each day has the same number of sunshine hours, namely exactly 12 hours. Consequently, the Yin and Yang spirals complement each other to form a perfect cycle for observers on the equator.

The last example in Figure 8 shows the daylight hours and polar plot when the observer's location is close to one of the earth's poles. For $L = 88°$, which is close to the North Pole, the year is split into two halves. For one half, the sun shines continuously for 24 hours on each day. For days in the other half, the sun does not shine at all. The transition from one half to the other happens very quickly. Due to this rapid transition between day and night, each of the Yin and Yang spirals in Figure 8 covers a sector in the polar plot. Both spirals together describe an almost vertical axis.

5. Conclusion

The chapter shows that the origin of the Yin-Yang symbol lies in the graphical representation of the daily change of a pole's shadow length. This length varies for each day, when measured

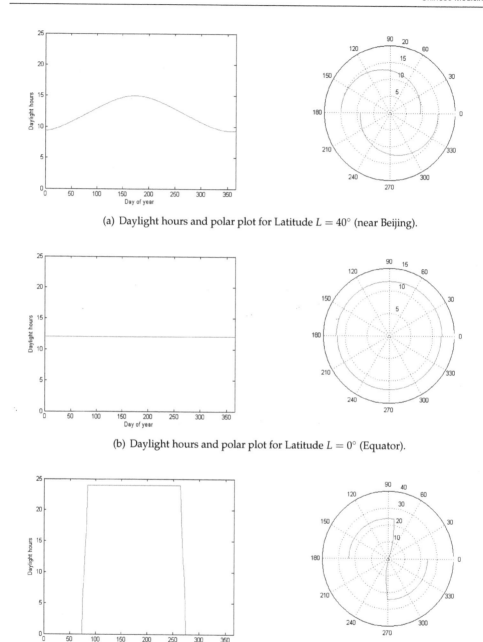

(a) Daylight hours and polar plot for Latitude $L = 40°$ (near Beijing).

(b) Daylight hours and polar plot for Latitude $L = 0°$ (Equator).

(c) Daylight hours and polar plot for Latitude $L = 88°$ (near North Pole).

Fig. 8. Daylight hours and polar plots for different latitudes.

at the same time, and depends on the geographic latitude of the observer. Given the significant role the Yin-Yang symbol plays in TCM, ancient herbalists and practitioners of TCM must have attached great importance to geographic location from the outset. It is reasonable to assume that they considered geographical aspects for both drug preparation as well as administration. To ensure an authentic TCM treatment, modern practitioners of TCM need to take geographic location into account not only when preparing drugs but also during the treatment of their patients. They must be aware of the geomedical origin of TCM. Latitude is one important factor in finding geo-authentic herbs. A mathematical formalization of this factor is a first step toward a well-defined and standardized TCM; a TCM that has the same scientific foundation as western medicine. This chapter equips herbalists with a means to compute Yin and Yang for different locations. They can now begin formalizing their daily work routine, such as herb evaluation, with the results presented here. The mathematical formalization of other factors determining the geo-authenticity of herbs, such as the physical and chemical soil properties, is a goal of future research. With a formalization of all these factors, herbalists can compute the overall Yin-Yang composition of herbs and herb combinations.

To render the Yin-Yang symbol, the chapter presents a daylight model to compute daylight hours for each day and latitude. However, the rendered Yin-Yang symbols differ from the common Yin-Yang symbol shown in Figure 1. The common symbol is an oversimplification. It represents Yin and Yang as two semicircles, which is a rough approximation at best. Therefore, the most popular Yin-Yang symbol is not in accordance with the original meaning of the Yin-Yang symbol. In fact, none of the symmetrical symbols existing today can coincide with any of the asymmetric symbols generated by the rendering method presented in Section 4. In particular, all symbols presented in the appendix of this chapter are asymmetric. This raises the question whether the common Yin-Yang symbol should be replaced by a symbol closer to the original meaning. In principle, any of the Yin-Yang symbols presented here could replace the common symbol and serve as a new standard. A particular good candidate would be the Yin-Yang symbol of the Arctic Circle, shown in Figure 5, because it looks very similar to the common symbol. Whatever the choice, there is yet another problem. Due to the cyclic change of the earth's ecliptic, any chosen Yin-Yang symbol is only a snapshot in time. It will eventually become less accurate. To avoid this problem, one could simply continue using the old Yin-Yang symbol or design a new symbol that does not feature these defects. Anyway, the choice of the standard Yin-Yang symbol depends on many factors, including personal taste. The ultimate answer to this question is therefore beyond the scope of this chapter.

6. Appendix

On the following six pages, the appendix shows examples of Yin-Yang symbols computed for different latitudes in the northern and southern hemispheres. All examples are polar plots of the output of Equations 1 and 2 for different input latitudes. All polar plots are rotated counter-clockwise by $45°$ so the x-axis is vertical. A closer inspection shows that none of the symbols is symmetrical. The symbols of the southern hemisphere are mirrored versions of the corresponding symbols in the northern hemisphere, apart from some numerical inaccuracies close to the polar circles and poles. Several popular variants of the Yin-Yang symbol are visible north of the Arctic Circle and south of the Antarctic Circle. Both spots in each Yin-Yang symbol lie on the vertical axis, plotted halfway between the polar plot's origin and the outer circle.

Note that for latitudes L with $|L| \leq 68°$, the Yin-Yang symbol will look similar to the symbols observed at the polar circles when plotted as a polar plot in the following way: Instead of the daylight hours, the polar plot shows the daylight hours minus the minimum day length. Furthermore, instead of the number of hours with darkness, the polar plot shows the difference between the maximum day length and the number of daylight hours.

6.1 Yin-Yang symbols for the northern hemisphere

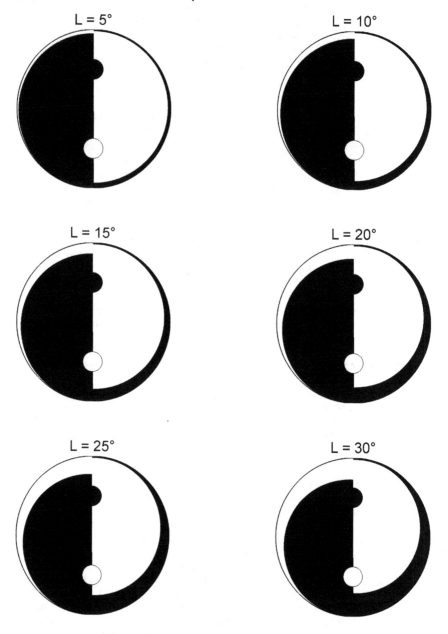

Fig. 9. Yin-Yang symbols for $L = 5°, 10°, 15°, 20°, 25°, 30°$.

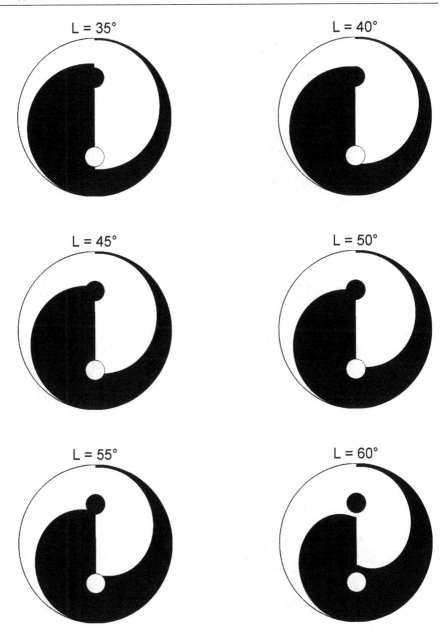

Fig. 10. Yin-Yang symbols for $L = 35°, 40°, 45°, 50°, 55°, 60°$.

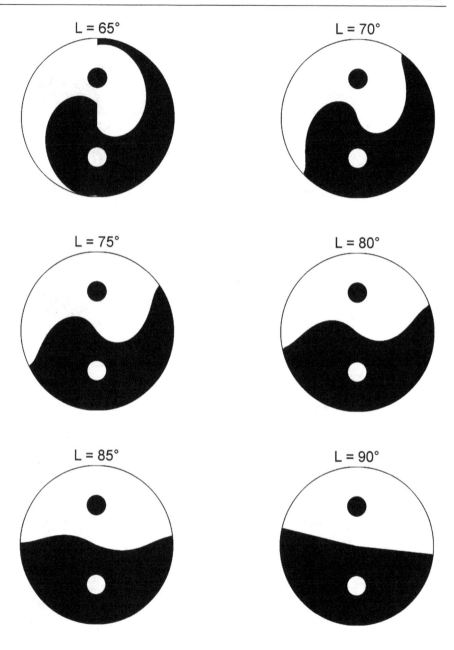

Fig. 11. Yin-Yang symbols for $L = 65°, 70°, 75°, 80°, 85°, 90°$.

6.2 Yin-Yang symbols for the southern hemisphere

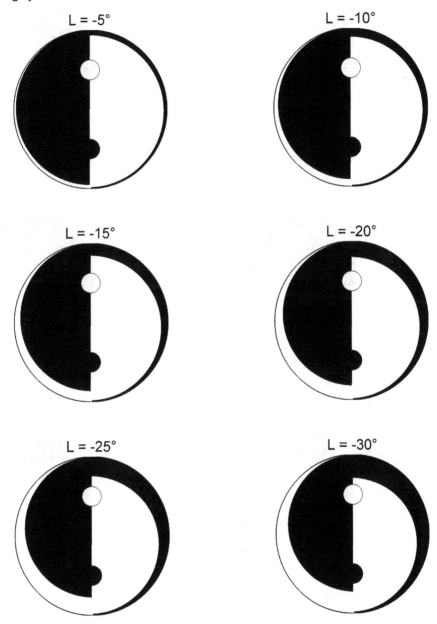

Fig. 12. Yin-Yang symbols for $L = -5°, -10°, -15°, -20°, -25°, -30°$.

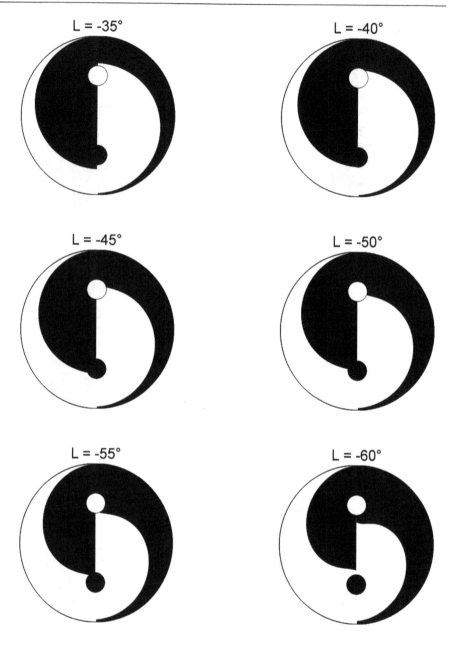

Fig. 13. Yin-Yang symbols for $L = -35°, -40°, -45°, -50°, -55°, -60°$.

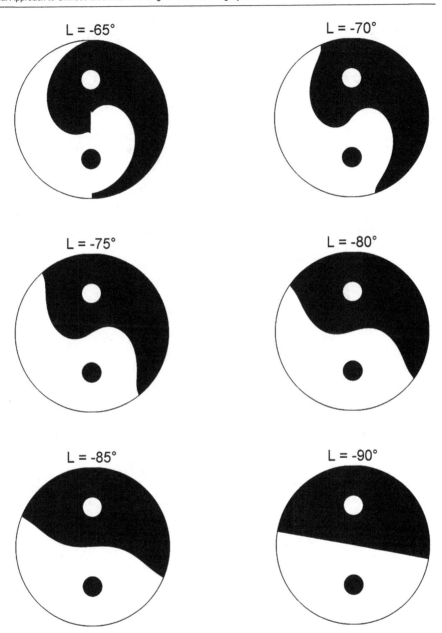

Fig. 14. Yin-Yang symbols for $L = -65°, -70°, -75°, -80°, -85°, -90°$.

7. References

Browne, C. (2007). Taiji variations: Yin and Yang in multiple dimensions, *Computers & Graphics* 31(1): 142–146.

Cook, T. (1979). *The Curves of Life*, Dover Publications.

Forsythe, W., Rykiel, E., Stahl, R., Wu, H.-I. & Schoolfield, R. (1995). A model comparison for daylength as a function of latitude and day of year, *Ecological Modelling* 80(1): 87–95.

Graf, K.-D. (1994). Mathematics and Informatics in old symbols: Tai Chi symbol and hexagrams from the I Ging, *K. Yokochi and H. Okamori (Eds): Proceedings of the Fifth Five Nations Conference on Mathematics Education*, Osaka, Japan, pp. 15–21.

Hardaker, C. (2001). The hexagon, the solstice and the kiva, *Symmetry: Culture and Science* 12(1-2): 167–183.

Miller, J. (2003). *Daoism: A Short Introduction*, Oneworld Publications.

Séquin, C. H. (1999). Analogies from 2D to 3D, exercises in disciplined creativity, *BRIDGES - Mathematical Connections in Art, Music, and Science*, Winfield KS.

Tian, H. & Tian, F. (2004). *The true origin of Zhou Yi (in Chinese)*, Shanxi Science and Technology Publishing House.

Watts, A. (1999). *The Way of Zen*, Vintage.

2

Metabonomics Research of the Four Properties in Traditional Chinese Medicine Based on UPLC-QTOF-MS System

Haixue Kuang, Yanyan Wang, Qiuhong Wang,
Bingyou Yang and Yonggang Xia

*Key Laboratory of Chinese Materia Medica (Heilongjiang University of Chinese Medicine),
Ministry of Education, Harbin,
China*

1. Introduction

TCM has long been practised as an empirical system and retrieved tens of millions of lives from historically to currently [1]. It is considered as an ancient and classical paradigm of systems biology. In TCM, diagnosis and medication are based on "Syndrome" ("ZHENG" in Chinese Mandarin), which can be regarded as a profile of symptom combination, or clinical phenotypes, such as Cold or Hot Syndrome, and "Hot medication curing Cold Syndrome and Cold medication curing Hot Syndrome" is a standard therapeutic guide line. This classical systems medicine at the macro level has been validated and developed by its repeated clinical practice for thousands of years [2]. Hot and Cold medication are the four properties of Chinese medicinal herbs, precisely including cold, hot, warm and cool, which are also called the four natures or "four xing" in TCM. Cold-cool and warm-hot are two completely opposite categories of natures, whereas cold and cool or hot and warm differ in the degree. Chinese medicinal herbs with cold and cool nature can clear away heat, purge fire and eliminate toxic materials, which are mainly used for heat-syndrome; while with hot and warm nature have the actions of expelling cold, which are mainly used for cold-syndrome. The four natures are summarized mainly from the body's response. On the base of syndrome differentiation theory, only distinguish heat or cold nature of disease, and have a good understanding of the cold or hot property of TCM, so selectively apply corresponding medicinal herbs that you could achieve the desired effect.

Herbal medicine has attracted much attention as a means of alternative therapy along with the orthodox medical system [3, 4]. In recent 30 years more and more reports on the four natures of TCM have appeared in the literature. To date several aspects of research such as the characteristics of thermodynamics, the changes of nervous system and the endocrine glands, energy metabolism, the systems biology analysis include genome, transcriptome, proteome, and metabolome are all supposed to explored the macro and micro framework on the four properties, among which metabonomics is the most novel tool [5]. It is a rapidly growing area of scientific research, which has been widely used in disease diagnosis, biomarker discovery, and research into the disease mechanisms [6-10]. Metabonomics aims at comparing the pattern of endogenous metabolites under defined temporal conditions as comprehensively as possible. In the past few years, widely used analytical techniques in metabonomics were nuclear magnetic resonance spectroscopy (NMR) [11], mass spectrometry in combination with gas chromatography (GC-MS) [12], capillary electrophoresis (CE-MS) [13] and especially liquid chromatography (LC-MS) [14]. Because of the advantages of robust operation and usability, separation with a reversed-phase column is a routine in LC-MS based metabonomic analysis. Advances in mass spectrometric techniques, particularly when linked to liquid chromatography, have resulted in the development of robust methods for low molecular mass organic molecules in biological matrices [15, 16]. Indeed in a preliminary study the potential for LC-MS to detect differences in the composition of urine from control and dosed animals in a properties study of TCM has been demonstrated. Here we describe preliminary studies on the variety of the endogenous metabolite of different herbs.

Metabonomic strategies produces complex data sets, and therefore, the uses of appropriate multivariate statistical and visualization tools are mandatory keys that include efficient and robust methods to model, analyze, and interpret the complex chemical and biological data [21]. In metabonomics studies chemometrics analysis techniques including PCA and OPLS-DA are often used to classify the samples[17]. Loading plots and Variable importance in the Project (VIP) value are commonly used for biomarker selection. Besides, the S-plot also plays an important role in screening for statistically significant compounds. It is a scatter plot which combines the covariance and correlation in loading results.

In this work, we employed a metabonomics strategy based on UPLC-QTOF-MS to discriminate the global urine profiles, and PCA was performed to detect the perturbation metabolites as many as possible. Furthermore, the potential biomarkers were screened out, which might be the target components in the future pathogenesis research, as well as predicted model was builded up using OPLS-DA. One of the intentions is to discuss whether this model is suitable for other herbs. The other purpose is to find potential criterion to evaluate the properties in TCM.

2. Experimental

2.1 Reagents and materials

Acetonitrile (HPLC grade) was purchased from Fisher Scientific (Loughborough, UK); formic acid (HPLC grade) used as mobile phase additives (each of purity ≥ 99%), were supplied by Sigma-Aldrich (MO, USA); the distilled water was purified by a Milli-Q system (Millipore, MA, USA); Pentobarbital sodium was purchased from the Shanghai Chemical Agent Company of China Medicine Clique (Shanghai, China); Leucine-enkephalin was obtained from Sigma-Aldrich (MO, USA).

The six crude drugs, Rhizoma Coptidis, Radix Scutellariae, Cortex Phellodendri, Radix Aconiti Lateralis Preparata, Rhizoma Zingiberis Pricklyash Peel and Flos Datura were purchased from the Harbin Tongrentang Drugstore and were authenticated by Professor Zhenyue Wang of the Department of Pharmacognosy, Heilongjiang University of Chinese Medicine. The crude drugs were refluxed extraction with distilled water two times for an hour each time. The extracts of the six herbs were filtered and concentrated, their concentrations were shown in Table 1, and stored in 4°C for animal experimental usage.

2.2 Animals and dosing

Male Sprague-Dawley rats (n = 8 per group), approx. 220 g in weight, were allowed to acclimatize in metabolism cages for 5 days prior to treatment. Food and water was provided ad libitum. The whole procedure of administration for each group was shown in Table 1. Urine was collected every other day (7:00 pm-7:00 am) from metabolism cages at ambient temperature throughout the whole procedure and centrifuged at 12,000 rpm at 4°C for 10 min, and then the supernatants were aliquot into eppendorf tubes with 1.5 mL urine in each stored at -20°C until analysis. In the exploratory study, in order to improve the matching rate of subjects, all groups were male. And there were no diet while drink free in the sample collection.

No.	Groups	Concentrations of crude drugs (g/ml)	Administration dosage (g/kg)
1	control	-	-
2	Rhizoma Coptidis	0.35	7.0
3	Radix Scutellariae	0.30	6.0
4	Cortex Phellodendri	0.42	8.4
5	Radix Aconiti Lateralis Preparata	0.525	10.5
6	Rhizoma Zingiberis	0.42	8.4
7	Pricklyash Peel	0.20	4.0

Table 1. The whole procedure of administration for each group, mean±SD, n = 8.

2.3 UPLC-QTOF-MS
2.3.1 Reversed-phase liquid chromatography
Urine samples were centrifuged again at 12,000 rpm for 10 min at 4°C, the supernatants were transferred to autosampler vials for analysis. The autosampler was maintained at a temperature of 4°C for the duration of the analysis. The UPLC-MS analysis was performed on a Waters ACQUITY™ UPLC system (Waters Corporation, MA, USA). Separation was achieved on an ACQUITY UPLC™ BEH C_{18} column (50 mm×2.1 mm, i.d., 1.7 μm) maintained at 40 °C. The column was eluted with a linear gradient of 2-40 % B over 0-8.0 min, 40-98 % B over 8.0-10.0 min, 98-2 % B over 10.0-12.0 min and kept at 2% B for 2 min, the composition was held at a flow rate of 600 μl/min, where mobile phase A consisted of 0.1% formic acid in demonized water and mobile phase B consisted of 0.1% formic acid in acetonitrile. The injection volume was 2 μl and the gradient duration was 14 min. A blank was analyzed between every five samples to wash the column.

2.3.2 Mass spectrometry
A Waters Xevo quadrupole time-of-flight Mass Spectrometer (Manchester, UK) equipped with an electrospray ionization (ESI) source was used to collect metabolic profiling. Mass spectrometry was operated in the positive ion mode, according to our preliminary experiments for determination of system, the optimal conditions were as follows: capillary voltage of 3.0 kV, cone voltage of 40 V, source temperature of 120°C and desolvation temperature of 400°C. Nitrogen was used as the desolvation and cone gas with the flow rate of

800 and 50 L/h, respectively. The data acquisition rate was set to 0.2 s with a 0.02 s interscan delay. The scan range was from 100 to 1000 m/z. All analyses were acquired by using the lock spray to ensure accuracy and reproducibility, leucine-enkephalin was used as the lock mass at a concentration of 400 pg/ml in acetonitrile (0.1% formic acid): H_2O (0.1% formic acid) for the positive ion mode ($[M+H]^+$ = 556.2771). Data were collected in pareto mode, the lock spray frequency was set at 1 s and the lock mass data were averaged over 10 scans for correction. A "purge-wash-purge" cycle was employed on the autosampler with 90% aqueous formic acid used for the wash solvent and 0.1% aqueous formic acid used as the purge solvent.

For the further identification of potential markers, a mass spectrometric data were collected in full scan auto mode from 0 to 14 min in positive ion mode. In the MS/MS experiments, the conditions were the same as above except the collision energy was set from 15 to 30 eV for each analyte.

2.4 Data processing and statistical analysis

UPLC-MS data were analyzed with the MassLynx software version V4.1 (Waters Corporation, Milford, USA). Before multivariate statistical analysis, the data of each sample was normalized to total area to correct for the MS response shift from the first injection to the last injection due to the long duration, overnight or longer, of an LC-MS analysis in metabonomics studies. The main parameters were set as follows: retention time range 1-9 min, mass range 100-1000, mass tolerance 0.05, mass window 0.05, retention time window 0.20, noise elimination level 6. the MarkerLynx Application Manager (Waters Corporation, Milford, USA) was used for the peak detection and the EZinfo software was used for PCA and OPLS-DA. Pareto scaling was used in all the models to avoid chemical noise. Potential biomarkers were selected according to Variable importance in the Project (VIP) value, the loading plot and the S-plot. For the identification of potential markers, the following databases have been used: HMDB (http://www.hmdb.ca/), METLIN (http://metlin.scripps.edu/), Massbank (http://www.massbank.jp), PubChem (http://ncbi.nim.nih.gov/) and KEGG (http://www.kegg.com/).

3. Results

3.1 UPLC-QTOF-MS method development

In this study, non-targeted analyses of Urine samples metabolic components were performed. As there was no specific group of target analyses, some generic settings had to be applied both to LC separation and MS detection during the method development, in order to obtain urine metabolic profiling containing as many compounds as possible. UPLC employs smaller stationary phase particle size column, generating high efficiency to the separation, which concurrently increases resolution and sensitivity. All urine metabolites were eluted in 14 min and full scan was set in the positive ion mode because it gave more information rich data than negative ion mode. For LC-MS-based metabonomics, the stability of analytical system is one of the most important factors to obtain the valid data. Extracted ion chromatographic peaks of seven ions (m/z 105.04, 154.02, 267.08, 271.08, 338.04, 340.03 and 675.13 in positive ion mode) were selected for method validation. Method repeatability was evaluated by five replicate analysis of a urine sample. The relative standard deviations (R.S.D.s%) of peak areas and retention times were estimated to be 1.14-3.52% and 0.445-1.36%, respectively. The stability of sample was tested by analyzing a sample left at autosampler (maintained at 4 °C) for 4, 8, 12 and 24 h. The R.S.D.s% of peak areas were from

4.58% to 7.54%. These results demonstrated the excellent stability and reproducibility of chromatographic separation and mass measurement during the whole sequence [18].

3.2 Chemometric analysis
3.2.1 Metabolic profiling analysis

The positive ion base peak intensity (BPI) chromatograms of urine samples collected from representative rats for each of the different groups are presented in Fig. 1 Urine samples on the 30th day from each group were used for UPLC-MS analysis. Some differences could be visually noted among these chromatograms.

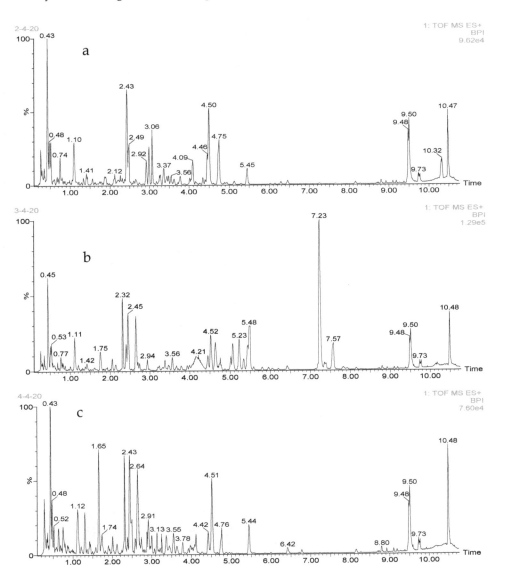

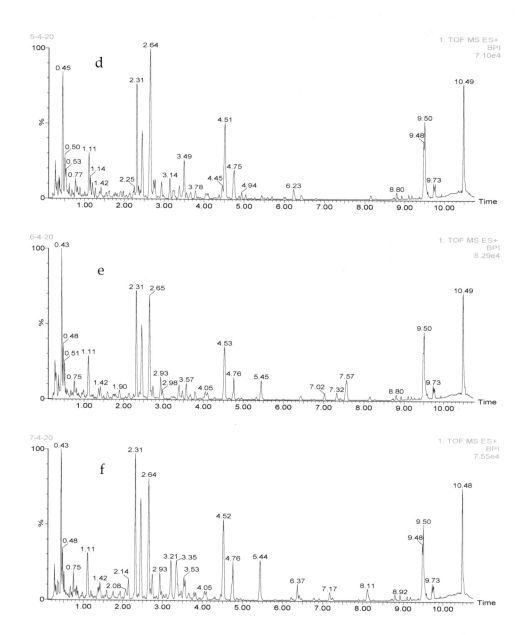

Fig. 1. BPI chromatograms of (a) Rhizoma Coptidis, (b) Radix Scutellariae, (c) Cortex Phellodendri, (d) Radix Aconiti Lateralis Preparata (e) Rhizoma Zingiberis (f) Rhizoma Zingiberis and Pricklyash Peel groups urine samples on the last day analyzed by UPLC-MS in positive ESI mode.

3.2.2 PCA analysis

In order to clearly differentiate among groups, unsupervised pattern recognition PCA was used for analyzing the chromatographic data. PCA is a bilinear decomposition method that allows original data to be reduced to a few principal components while retaining the features that contribute most to the variance. It does not require any prior knowledge of class membership and was used here to detect any inherent trends within the data and to identify potential markers. The urinary data was subjected to EZinfo software, PCA score plots separated urine samples into different blocks, and samples with the same treatment were located on the same trajectory, indicating that treatments have greatly disturbed the normal urine metabolic profiles of rats (Fig. 2). Urine from the 2-4 groups were further from control group, suggesting the metabolic profiles have significantly changed as a result of Cold-cool medication administration. Rats in 5-7 groups were administrated with warm-hot medication for 24 consecutive days, the results were separated from the control group, demonstrating that the endogenous metabolic disorders occured after stimulus from warm-hot medication, nevertheless, the perturbation of metabolic profiles are different from Cold medication group even with opposite trend. It was consistent with the clinical report that the four natures cold and hot are summarized mainly from the body's response after taking Chinese medicinal herbs are taken. Following the above data pre-treatment, PCA was employed in the first phase of chemometric analysis for positive data to evaluate urine sample clustering according to the character of the herbs variety, which is the most suitable for discrimination among the sample classes.

3.2.3 OPLS-DA analysis

In order to obtain better discrimination between different characteristic herbs and find the significant change of endogenous metabolites (i.e. potential biomarkers), an OPLS-DA model was constructed. OPLS-DA score plots separated urine samples of control group and Chinese medicinal herbs with cold nature groups as well as hot nature groups into two blocks, respectively, especially in the component P1 direction, and component P2 properly explained individual variation in each group (Fig. 3), which indicates biochemical changes happened in the urinary of male rats after the treatment of different property herbs. Loadings for component P1 indicated the content of each ion in the control and herbs groups; the Y+ axis represented the herbs group; the Y-axis represented the control group; the X-axis represented the number of detected ions. To exhibit the responsibility of each ion for these variations more intuitively, S-plots and VIP-value plots were shown (Fig. 4). In the S-plot, most of the ions were clustered around the origin point; only a few of them scattered in the margin region, and just these few ions contributed to the clustering observed in the score plot and were also the differentiating metabolites. The VIP-value plot represents the value of each ion. The farther away from the origin, the higher the VIP value of the ions was. As illustrated in Fig. 3, Urine of the six herbs-treated groups were analyzed by OPLS-DA, the result of score plots indicating Cold and hot medication could separated well from each other, Rhizoma Coptidis, Radix Scutellariae and Cortex Phellodendri-treated groups have similar metabolic profiles were located the same quadrant, Similarly to Radix Aconiti Lateralis Preparata, Rhizoma Zingiberis and Pricklyash Peel-treated groups. The analysis of the chromatographic data identified the Cold and hot medication-treated rats based on the differences in their metabolic profiles, demonstrating that the classic herbs showed significant intervened effects on the normal rats, which was consistent with the theory of clinical medicine.

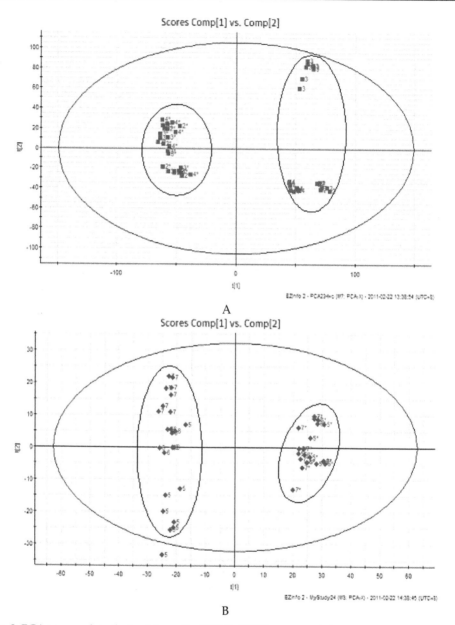

Fig. 2. PCA scores plots derived from the UPLC-QTOF spectra of the urine in positive mode. (A) 2-4 groups originated from Rhizoma Coptidis, Radix Scutellariae and Cortex Phellodendri, belong to cold medication 2*-4* groups originated from control groups. (B) 5-7 groups originated from Radix Aconiti Lateralis Preparata, Rhizoma Zingiberis and Rhizoma Zingiberis and Pricklyash Peel groups, belong to hot medication groups and 5*-7* groups originated from control groups.

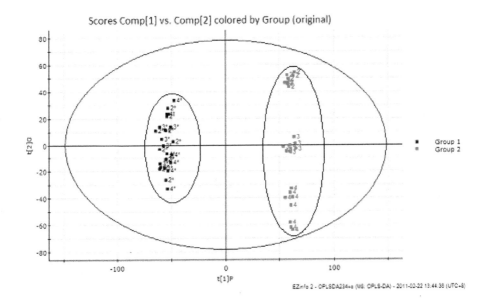

A

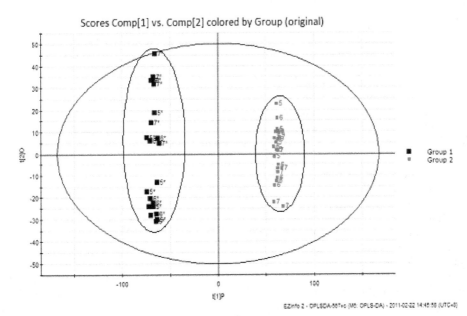

B

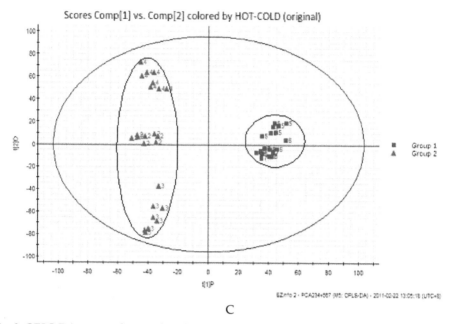

C

Fig. 3. OPLS-DA scores plots to classification the six groups of cold and hot medication. A, (■) Group 1 is cold medication group and (■) group 2 is control group. B, (■) Group 1 is hot medication group and (■)group 2 is control group. C, (■) Group 1 is hot medication group and (▲) group 2 is cold medication group.

For demonstration of the discrimination potential offered by the above data, OPLS-DA, a widely used supervised pattern recognition method capable of sample class prediction, was used to construct and validate a statistical model for traditional Chinese medicine classification. To estimate the predictive ability of our model, we used another herb-Flos Datura to cross-validation, and excellent separation among the TCM varieties obtained by OPLS-DA is shown in Fig. 5, which a hot medication belonging to the hot medication group, are presented in terms of recognition and prediction abilities. It represented the percentage of the samples correctly classified during model training and cross-validation, respectively, while the prediction ability was only qualitative rather than quantitative.

3.2.4 Biomarker identification

According to the VIP values of independent test (Table 2), these ions show significant differences between the controls and TCM groups. The same trend ions of three cold-cool or warm-hot medication groups were found, they may be biomarker candidates to reflect metabolic differences on the four properties of TCM. All the detected ions were arranged in descending order according to VIP values, and the highest VIP value was 20.75 in the positive mode. Combining the results of the OPLS analysis with the amount variation of ions in each group, 9 ions with VIP values exceeding two were selected preliminary identified in the Cold medication groups. At the same time, the highest VIP value was 12.73 in the positive mode, and 9 ions with VIP values exceeding two were selected and preliminary identified. The UPLC-MS segregation analysis platform provided the retention

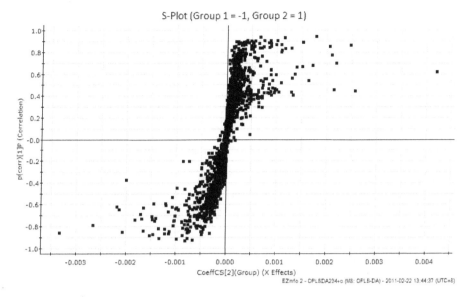

A

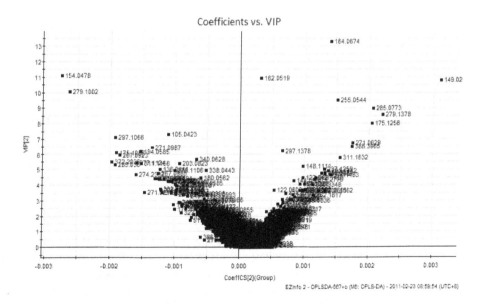

B

Fig. 4. S-plot and VIP values in positive ESI mode. A, S-plot of Cold medication group(Gruop 1 originated from cold medication, and group 2 originated from control ones). B, VIP values plot of Hot medication group.

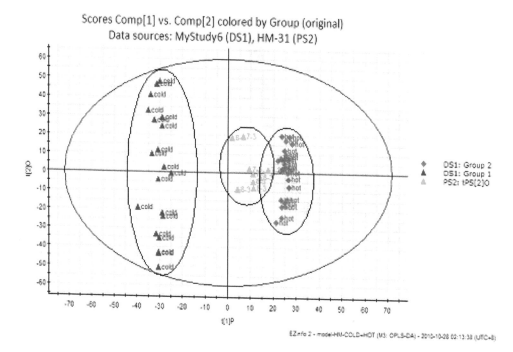

Fig. 5. Another hot medication-Flos Datura was used to verify the reliability of the forecasting model of OPLD-DA. (▲) cold medication group, (♦) hot medication group. (▲) Flos Datura.

time, precise molecular mass and MS/MS data for the structural identification of biomarkers. The precise molecular mass was determined within measurement errors (<5 ppm) by Q-TOF, and meanwhile, the potential elemental composition and fractional isotope abundance of compounds were obtained. The presumed molecular formula was searched in METLIN Database and other databases to identify the possible chemical constitutions, and MS/MS data were screened to determine the potential structures of the ions. Taking two ions as examples, the identification procedure was as follows. Taking two ions as examples, the identification procedure was as follows. In the positive mode, the ion at Rt = 5.46 and $[M+H]^+$ = 146 has a high VIP value. This ion might contain an odd number of nitrogen atoms because its precise molecular weight was 145.0739, and its molecular formula was speculated as $C_6H_{11}NO_3$ from the analysis of its elemental composition and fractional isotope abundance. The main fragment ions analyzed by MS/MS screening were m/z 128 and 101, which could be the $[M+H]^+$ of lost -NH_4, and -C_2H_7N, respectively. Finally, it was speculated as (S)-5-Amino-3-oxohexanoic acid, the ion at Rt = 4.26 and $[M+H]^+$ = 162 has a high VIP value, and the main fragment ions were m/z 145, 144 and 117, which could be the $[M+H]^+$ of lost -NH_4, -NH_3 and -NO_2, respectively. Finally, it was speculated as L-2-Aminoadipic acid.

NO.	VIP values	Rt-M+	Actual M	Proposed compound	Trend	MS/MS	Losses	Proposed structure
1	2.70	5.25_134.0986	133.0375	Aspartic Acid $C_4H_7NO_4$	Hot↑	118 103	O HNO	
2	3.00	3.64_190.041	189.0637	N-Acetyl-L-glutamate $C_7H_{11}NO_5$	Cold↓	172 146 133	CH_6 C_2H_4O C_2H_3NO	
3	2.71	3.94_135.0962	134.0215	L-Apple acid $C_4H_6O_5$	Cold↓	104	NO	
4	2.13	4.73_233.0837	232.1212	Melatonin $C_{13}H_{16}N_2O_2$	Cold↓	191 174	C_2H_2O C_2H_5NO	
5	3.25	2.62_137.0683	136.0385	Hypoxanthine $C_5H_4N_4O$	Cold↑	120	HO	
6	5.84	2.7_180.0886	179.0582	Acetylisoniazid $C_8H_9N_3O_2$	Cold↑	135	CHO_2	
7	2.20	6.25_285.0773	284.0757	Xanthosine $C_{10}H_{12}N_4O_6$	Cold↑	267 228	H_2O CHN_2O	
8	7.76	2.81_300.1645	299.0770	D-4'-Phosphopantothenate $C_9H_{18}NO_8P$	Cold↑	242 187 114	$C_2H_2O_2$ H_2O_5P $C_3H_9NO_6$ P	
9	2.91	3.26_308.0929	307.0838	Glutathione $C_{10}H_{17}N_3O_6S$	Cold↑	262 179 147	CH_2S $C_5H_7NO_3$ $C_5H_7NO_3$ S	
10	2.25	3.04_133.0853	132.0535	L-Asparagine $C_4H_8N_2O_3$	Hot↓	118	HN	

NO.	VIP values	Rt-M+	Actual M	Proposed compound	Trend	MS/ MS	Losses	Proposed structure
11	5.02	4.14_146.0618	145.0739	(S)-5-Amino-3-oxohexanoic acid $C_6H_{11}NO_3$	Hot↓	128 101	H_4N C_2H_7N	
12	3.23	3.5_178.0469	177.046	N-Formyl-L-methionine $C_6H_{11}NO_3S$	Hot↓	148 132 104	CH_2O CH_2S C_2H_2OS	
13	4.31	9.57_301.1442	300.2089	Vitamin A acid $C_{20}H_{28}O_2$	Hot↓	284 175	HO C_9H_{18}	
14	5.13	4.1_289.1075	288.0246	2-Dehydro-3-deoxy-D-arabino-heptonate 7-phosphate (DAHP) $C_7H_{13}O_{10}P$	Hot↑	242 158	CH_3O_2 H_4O_6P	
15	2.78	4.05_151.0389	150.1045	Myrtenal $C_{10}H_{14}O$	Hot↑	123 108	C_2H_4 C_3H_7	
16	12.73	4.26_162.0519	161.0688	L-2-Aminoadipic acid $C_6H_{11}NO_4$	Hot↑	145 144 117	NH_3 NH_4 NO_2	
17	2.04	3.89_319.1289	318.2195	Leukotriene A4 $C_{20}H_{30}O_3$	Hot↑	273 259 162	C_3H_{10} C_4H_{12} $C_8H_{13}O_3$	
18	20.75	4.48_164.0674	163.0633	3-Methyldioxyindole $C_9H_9NO_2$	Cold↓	146 122	$-H2O$ $-CNO$	

Table 2. Potential biomarkers identified in positive ESI mode.

4. Discussion

Metabonomics aims to assess metabolic changes in a comprehensive and global manner in order to infer biological functions and provide the detailed biochemical responses of cellular systems [19]. In this study the successful discrimination and classification of the four properties in TCM was made. Multivariate statistical analysis was used to find the most characteristic markers in complex records. This demonstrates the potential of UPLC-QTOF-MS combined with metabonomics to determine the four properties of TCM. It should be noted that for this particular purpose, the molecular identification of these marker compounds is not necessary, some different chemometric tools, such as PCA and OPLS-DA have been proposed as powerful tools for the four properties classification [20]. However, the benefit of obtaining MS/MS accurate mass spectra of marker compounds (metabolites) were shown to provide a high level of confidence for the identification process. Even with this data, the identification of true unknowns is a rather difficult task. Biological Interpretation of several biomarkers: L-Apple acid is a tart-tasting organic dicarboxylic acid that plays a role in many sour or tart foods. In its ionized form it is malate, an intermediate of the TCA cycle along with fumarate. It can also be formed from pyruvate as one of the anaplerotic reactions. It is a key intermediate in energy metabolism and the change indicated that energy metabolism was perturbation by Chinese herbs.

5. Conclusion

The four properties, the essence and important component of TCM theories, the high generalization on the basic property and typical characteristics of TCM, are a significant theoretical foundation for the clinical use of Chinese medicine. In this study, UPLC-QTOF-MS techniques coupled to metabonomics methods were used to prove the existence of the four properties, to illustrate its multi-component, multi-target, multi-channel and the complex mechanism. All the work are aimed at guiding researchers to carry out new drug develop work with the theory of Chinese medicine, simultaneously, eliminating too much emphasis the effective chemical composition while ignore the many other ones, result in the loss of characteristics of Chinese herbs and even highlights the toxicity and side effects. This theory also could apply to explore Western medicine properties to effectively guide the clinical application. Considering the encouraging results obtained in this study, the application of metabonomics for authentication and other purposes in TCM seems to be very promising approach [22].

6. Acknowledgements

Our work was supported by the Major State Basic Research Development Program of China (973 Program 2006CB504708) the National Natural Science Foundation of China (No. 30371736, 30672633) and Special Fund Project of National Excellent Doctoral Dissertation of China (200980).

7. References

[1] C. Auffray, Z. Chen, L. Hood, Genome Med.1 (2009) 1-2.
[2] T. Ma, C.g. Tan, H. Zhang, M.Q. Wang, W. J. Ding, S. Li, Mol. BioSyst. 6 (2010) 613-619.
[3] A.P. Lu, H.W. Jia, C. Xiao, Q.P. Lu.. World J Gastroenterol 13 (2004) 1854-1856.
[4] D. Normile. Science 299(2003) 188-190.
[5] J. Lindon, J. Nicholson, E. Holmes, Elsevier, Amsterdam, (2007) 279-287.

[6] J. Chen,W.Z.Wang, S. Lv, P. Y. Yin, X. J. Zhao, X. Lu, F. X. Zhang, G.W. Xu, Analytica Chimica Acta 650 (2009) 3-9.

[7] D.M. Drexler, J.H.M. Feyen, M. Sanders, Drug Discov. Today Technol. 1 (2004) 17-23.

[8] J.C. Lindon, E. Holmes, M.E. Bollard, E.G. Stanley, J.K. Nicholson, Biomarkers 9 (2004) 1-31.

[9] D.G. Robertson, M.D. Reily, J.D. Baker, J. Proteome Res. 6 (2007) 526-539.

[10] I.D. Wilson, R. Plumb, J. Granger, H.Major, R.Williams, E.M. Lenz, J. Chromatogr. B 817 (2005) 67-76.

[11] E. Holmes, P.J.D. Foxall, M. Spraul, R.D. Farrant, J.K. Nicholson, J.C. Lindon, J. Pharm. Biomed. Anal. 15 (1997) 1647-1659.

[12] C. Wang, H.W. Kong, Y.F. Guan, J. Yang, J.R. Gu, S.L. Yang, G.W. Xu, Anal. Chem. 77 (2005) 4108-4116.

[13] F. Benavente, R. van der Heijden, U.R. Tjaden, J. van der Greef, T. Hankemeier, Electrophoresis 27 (2006) 4570-4584.

[14] J. Zhang, L. J. Yan, W. G. Chen, L. Lin, X. Y. Song, X. M. Yan,W. Hang, B. l. Huang, Analytica Chimica Acta 650 (2009) 16-22.

[15] R.S. Plumb, J.H. Granger, C.L. Stumpf, K.A. Johnson, B.W. Smith, S. Gaulitz, I.D. Wilson, J. Castro-Perez, Analyst 130 (2005) 844-849.

[16] J.H. Granger, R. Williams, E.M. Lenz, R.S. Plumb, C.L. Stumpf, I.D. Wilson, Rapid Commun. Mass Spectrom. 21 (2007) 2039-2045.

[17] R. Madsen, T. Lundstedt, J. Trygg, Analytica Chimica Acta 659 (2010) 23-33.

[18] P. Wang, H. Sun, H.T. Lv, W. J. Sun, Y. Yuan, Y. Han, D. W. Wang, A. H. Zhang, X. J. Wang, J. Pharm. Biomed. Anal. 53 (2010) 631-645.

[19] O. Fiehn;, B. Kristal, B. van Ommen, L. W. Sumner, S. A. Sansone, C. Taylor, N. Hardy, R. Kaddurah-Daouk, OMICS, 10 (2006), 158-63.

[20]L. Rafael, U. S. Mireia, J.Olga, M.Maria, A. L. Cristina, Journal of Proteome Research, 8(2009), 5060-5068.

[21] S.Wiklund, E. Johansson, L. Sjostrom, E. J. Mellerowicz, U. Edlund, J. P. Shockcor, J. Gottfries, T. Moritz, J. Trygg, Anal. Chem., 80 (2008), 115-22.

[22] F. Y. Du, Y. Bai, Y. Bai, H.W. Liu, Anal. Chem. 82 (2010), 9374-9383.

3

Application of "Five Elements Theory" for Treating Diseases

Yasuyo Hijikata
Toyodo Hijikata Clinic
Japan

1. Introduction

The ancients thought that there were five indispensable qualities for living. These are Wood, Fire, Earth, Metal and Water, and they are otherwise known as the five phases. They each possess different characteristics, and all phenomena and substances within the universe belong to one of these five phases.

The idea which has developed into the five-phase theory is that all phenomena and substances in the universe are the products of the movement and mutation of these five phases. The five-phase theory, as described in the Neijing, is a philosophical theory of medical practice in ancient China.

This theory has served as the guiding ideology and methodology of physiology, pathology, clinical diagnosis and treatment. The characteristics of each phase in this theory have been derived from the observations of countless generations over the millennia, and they are reflected in clinical experiences. As will be mentioned, among these phases both engendering and restraining patterns exist. In the case of the excess of one phase, engendering becomes overwhelming, and restraint becomes rebellion.

However, in five-phase theory, not every situation is well-defined because there are some contradictions and cross-overs in the signs of various physiological features. In both Yin Yang theory and five-phase theory, not all notions are necessarily clear. Nonetheless, despite such a lack of clarity, intractable diseases are sometimes cured or else ameliorated by applications of five-phase theory.

More details about five-phase theory will be described below.

2. Characteristics and categorization

Wood signifies both bending and straightening, and has the characteristics of growth, up-bearing and effusion. It refers to the state of the growing tree. All things which are characteristic of growth, development and elongation belong to Wood.

Fire flares upwards, and has the characteristic of blazing heat. Things which have the characteristics of heat and rising belong to Fire.

Earth is the source of everything, and it represents the characteristics of sowing, reaping and engendering transformation. Things which form and grow, or are sown, raised, and reaped belong to Earth.

Metal is the working of change, and it has the characteristics of purification, elimination and malleability. Things which are constantly changing or are involved in purification and elimination belong to Metal.

Water is the moistening and descending element. It has the characteristics of moistening, downward movement and coldness. Things which are cold, cool, humid and move downwards belong to Water.

3. The relation between the five phases and the five viscera

The five viscera (Liver, Heart, Spleen, Lung, and Kidney: the first capital letter means Viscus in TCM) are related to the five phases according to their own properties. The physiological characteristic of Liver is to govern free-coursing, to thrive by orderly reaching, to rise and to move. As it is likened to spring - when plants grow - and since of the five elements spring relates to Wood, Liver is attributed to Wood. As Liver controls the sinew, and the eyes express the function of Liver, these also belong to Wood.

The function of Heart is to control blood vessels and to warm the whole body by propelling qi and blood. It is likened to the summer heat. As the summer is attributed to Fire, Heart belongs to Fire. As pulse is caused by blood flow and Heart meridian leads to the tongue, they also belong to Fire.

Spleen controls the transportation and transformation of the essence of food, and it is the origin of the engendering transformation of qi and blood. It is likened to the late summer and humid weather - when all things grow - and to Earth which brings up all things. As late summer corresponds to Spleen, Spleen belongs to Earth. Since the condition of Spleen is expressed in muscle and lips, they belong to Earth as well.

Lung pertains to purification and down-sending. It is likened to the cool, crisp air of autumn - a quiet time when everything contracts. As autumn corresponds to Metal, Lung belongs to Metal. Equally, as the condition of Lung is expressed in body hair and the surface of the skin, as well as the nose, these also belong to Metal.

The function of Kidney is to store essence and fluid. It is likened to the winter, when all things are stored and the bitter cold exists. As winter corresponds to Water, Kidney belongs to Water. Kidney opens into bone, ears and two yins. Accordingly, they belong to Water. Other correspondences between the natural world and the human body are shown in Table 1.

Elements	Viscera	Bowels	Color	Flavor	Emotions	Senses	Climate	Season	Tissues	Direction
Wood	Liver	Gall-bladder	Green	Sour	Anger	Eyes	Wind	Spring	Tendon	East
Fire	Heart	Small Intestine	Red	Bitter	Joy	Tong	Heat	Summer	Vessels	South
Earth	Spleen	Stomach	Yellow	Sweet	Pre-occupation	Mouth	Damp	Late summer	Muscle	Center
Metal	Lung	Large Intestine	White	Pun-gent	Sorrow	Nose	Dryness	Autumn	Skin & Body Hair	West
Water	Kidney	Urinary Bladder	Black	Salty	Fear	Ears	Cold	Winter	Bones	North

Table 1. Categorization of objects and phenomina based on Five Phase theory.

4. Engendering and restraining in the five elements and the five viscera

The five phases of engendering and restraining are seen in Wood, Fire, Earth, Metal and Water. Engendering denotes the principle whereby each of the phases nurtures, produces and benefits another specific element or phase. Restraining denotes the principle by which each of the phases constrains another phase. Arranged in cyclic form, the engendering cycle is shown below:

Wood→Fire→Earth→Metal→Water→Wood

The restraining cycle is shown as follows:

Wood→Earth→Water→Fire→Metal→Wood

Applied to the viscera, these cycles are:

Engendering: Liver→Heart→Spleen→Lung→Kidney→Liver

Restraining: Liver→Spleen→Kidney→Heart→Lung→Liver

According to the *Lei-jing*, Nature requires both engendering and restraining forces. Without engendering nothing will arise. Without restraining, things will become powerful without limitation and will therefore become harmful. Thus, the successful functioning of the united whole is considered to be based on the existence of mutual engendering and restraining. Concerning this fact, two key maxims are advanced: "In engendering, restraint exists" and "With restraining, things work". Accordingly, within the movement and changes in nature, engendering and restraining exist. Interestingly, Si-sheng-xin-yuan instead describes the engendering and restraining work through qi transformation rather than through change of quality.

Relationships of engendering among the various viscera are well-defined by the five-phase theory. Kidney stores essence and Liver stores and controls the blood, and Kidney essence forms the liver blood (Kidney engenders Liver). The ability of Liver in blood storing and free-coursing engenders the heart to control blood vessels (Liver engenders Heart). Heat produced by Heart warms Spleen yang. Spleen controls the transportation, transformation and the origin of the engendering transformation of qi and blood, and so controls the blood. Accordingly, Heart supports the ability of Spleen to control the blood (Heart engenders Spleen). Spleen engenders transformation of food to qi and blood, and carries them to Lung and so supports Lung in working efficiently (Spleen engenders Lung). Kidney controls Water, stores essences and absorbs qi. If Lung qi works smoothly, Lung can regulate the waterway and supports Kidney in controlling Water (Lung engenders Kidney).[Ref 1]

Relations of restraining among the viscera are also well defined. The characteristic of Lung function is purification and down-sending. Accordingly, it can restrain the ascending Liver qi and the ascendant hyperactivity of Liver yang (Lung restrains Liver). As Liver has the ability of free-coursing, it can dissipate stagnated Spleen qi (Liver restrains Spleen). Spleen's function of transportation and transformation supports Kidney in controlling the water and also protects the overflow of water moisture (Spleen restrains Kidney). The moistening action of Kidney restrains the progression of Heart "Fire" (Kidney restrains Heart). The yang heat of Heart restrains the excessive purification and down-sending of Lung (Heart restrains Lung).

Engendering and restraining among the five viscera keeps the body in balance. Wherever a viscus is functionally suppressed by the restraining viscus, it is simultaneously engendered so that it doesn't become deficient or damaged. Likewise, where a viscus is supported by its engendering viscus, it is also restrained by its restraining viscus, so that it maintains a sound state, without acceleration.[Ref 2]

5. Overwhelm and rebellion amongst the five phases

When the normal restraining element gets excessive power, so-called overwhelm occurs. Overwhelm is an abnormal, excessive restraint. This happens in two cases. First, it may occur when one phase becomes excessively powerful and so overwhelms the corresponding viscera. Second, it may also arise when the restrained viscera becomes too weak and hence is overwhelmed by its restraining viscera Ref 3.

Conversely, when the restraining viscera becomes too weak, or the restrained viscera becomes excessively powerful, the opposite of restraining occurs. This is called rebellion. For example, Metal naturally restrains Wood. However, when Wood gets too much power, Metal can't, not only restrain Wood, but it is also injured by Wood's excessive rebellion against Metal.

Similarly, and in applying this concept to the viscera, Lung normally restrains Liver. Nonetheless, when Liver becomes excessively powerful, Lung is not only unable to restrain Liver, but it is injured by Liver's reaction to Lung. Again, this is called Rebellion.

In Zhong-yi-bing-yin-bing-ji-xue,Ref 4 engendering and restraining concern the mutual relations among human viscera. Overwhelm and rebellion relate to a pathological idea concerning the mutual influences and actions among viscera. For example, when Fire (Heart) gets excessive power, Water (Kidney) cannot ordinarily restrain Fire and so Fire overwhelms Metal to the point of damage; at this stage, inferior Water is boiled down by Fire qi (rebellion). In this way - in illness - overwhelm and rebellion always appear at the same time."

6. The physiological function and condition of the five viscera

Liver lies on the right side, beneath the diaphragm, whilst Gallbladder sticks to the under-surface of the right hepatic lobe. Liver is connected to Gallbladder with channels. Liver is an "exterior" organ and Gallbladder is an "interior" organ.

Liver controls free-coursing, blood storage and the sinews. Free-coursing relates to the regulation of qi movement, psychological and emotional activity, and bile secretion etc. Blood storage means that it controls the blood in circulation as well. Controlling the sinews implies that Liver works to maintain the normal movement of the muscles and joints of the whole body. Liver channel starts from the great toe, climbing the leg and passing through the genitals and the lower abdomen, and then goes up through the costal region to the eyes and the vertex of the head. When pathological changes appear along Liver channel, they are described as Liver diseases.

Dysfunction of the free-coursing causes change to Liver qi depression[*1], stagnated Liver qi transforming into fire, damage to Liver yin, yin deficiency, ascendant hyperactivity of Liver yang[*2], and further progresses to" Liver wind[*3]. On the contrary, dysfunction of storing blood[*4] is caused by blood deficiency as has been mentioned, "Liver yang and Liver qi exist always in excess and Liver yin and Liver blood exist always in insufficiency."[Ref 5, Ref 6]

The treatment for dysfunction of free-coursing is to smooth Liver and regulate the qi, and to apply drugs to pacify Liver and purge Fire. The treatment for dysfunction of blood storage is to tonify Blood and emolliate Liver, enrich Liver and tonify Kidney and so on.[Ref 7]

(Symptoms of *1 include depression, chest and side pain, and digestive symptoms; of *2, nervousness, surliness, headache, vertigo, tinnitus, insomnia, and lumbago; of *3, severe dizziness, headache, stiffness in the neck, tingling in the limbs, trembling lips and fingers, convulsive spasms and inhibited speech; and of *4, dizziness, insomnia, excessive dreams, flowery vision, inhibited sinew–vascular movement, lustreless nails, and reduced menstrual flow).

Heart is in the chest and is covered by the pericardium. Heart controls the blood vessels and the spirit. Heart opens at the tongue. Heart meridian is entangled with the meridian of Small Intestine, which is the corresponding interior viscus.

Pathologies based on Heart qi deficiency[*1], Heart yang deficiency[*2], Heart blood deficiency[*3] and Heart yin deficiency[*4] involve diseases of the blood vessels, including arrhythmia, some psychological diseases and ulceration and/or pain of the tip of the tongue.[Ref 8] Treatment is based on the pathology of the Heart [Ref 9].

(Each of [*1,*2,*3,] and [*4] show symptoms of a dull pale complexion, palpitations, dyspnea and arrhythmia. Symptoms of *1 also include hyperhidrosis and a weak, fine and slow pulse; of *2, a dark grey, cyan or purple complexion, inversion frigidity of the limbs, and cold sweats; of *3, dizziness, insomnia, excessive dreams, a fine pulse, and palpitation; and of *4, vexing heat in the chest, the palms and the soles, and night sweats including the symptoms of *3).

The digestive system is composed mainly of Spleen, Stomach, Large Intestine and Small Intestine, of which Spleen and Stomach are the most important. The meridian of Spleen is external and that of Stomach is internal, and they communicate closely with each other.

Spleen controls the transportation and transformation of water and food, whilst Stomach controls the acceptance of food. Spleen controls upbearing and Stomach controls downbearing. Both Spleen and Stomach are the origin of food digestion and transport, and they enable the transformation of the fine essences and the engendering and transformation of qi and Blood (in this manner it is called the postnatal root). The meridians of Small Intestine and Large Intestine are entangled with Heart and Lung. The function of the separation of clear and turbid substances of Small Intestine and the function of carrying and transforming the food waste of Large Intestine are each a part of digestive power and they have a strong connection with the function of both Spleen and Stomach respectively.

Disorders of Spleen include Spleen qi deficiency, Spleen yang deficiency[*1], centre qi deficiency[*2], blood management failure[*3], Stomach yang deficiency, Stomach yin deficiency[*4], the counter-flow ascent of Stomach qi, persistent diarrhoea, and incontinence and constipation. Clinically, we recognize these as abnormal functions of digestion, absorption, and the carrying and distribution of essence and excretion.[Ref 10, Ref 11]

(Symptoms of *1 and *2 include white complexion and spiritual fatigue; of *1, abdominal pain relieved by warmth and pressure; of *3, bleeding such as hemafecia and metrorrhagia; and of *4, dry mouth, mirror tongue and constipation).

Lung is situated in the chest, connected with the throat, and opens at the nose. As it is the highest location among the viscera, it is called the canopy. The channel of the Lung connects to that of Large intestine; the former is interior and the latter is exterior. Its main function is to dominate the qi and control respiration. Lung qi faces the hundred blood vessels and channels, regulates the water passage, disperses essence externally to the skin and downy hair, and controls the surface defence qi of the whole body. In other words, Lung works as a respiratory system, but it also controls fluid regulation, the movement of qi and blood, and the defence system of whole body.

Abnormalities of Lung include the non-diffusion of Lung qi, impaired depurative downbearing of Lung qi, Lung qi vacuity, and Lung yin vacuity[*1]. Clinically, they appear mostly as dysfunction of the respiratory system, a part of the pathology of fluid metabolism and blood circulation (edema, urination abnormality), external contraction with superficial pathogens and some skin diseases like atopic dermatitis. They are treated based on the lung pathology. [Ref 12, Ref 13]

(*1 shows a dry cough with little phlegm)

The Kidney is located in the lower back on either side of the spinal column and opens into the ear and the two yins (the perineal ante-tract and post-tract). Its condition is reflected in the hair of the head. The meridian of Kidney (interior organ) connects to Bladder (exterior organ). The main function of Kidney is to store essential qi which is the basis of growth, development, reproduction and the maintenance of the physiological activity of all the viscera.

The function of Kidney of controlling the water and bone through the production of marrow is based on both Kidney essence and qi. Kidney yin and yang give yin and yang to all the viscera, which is called innate qi.[Ref 14] As the vacuity of the yin and yang of the other viscera influences Kidney, long-term disease is said to influence Kidney.

Kidney yang has a strong correlation with Spleen yang, as implied by the occurrence of Spleen–Kidney yang deficiency; similarly, Kidney yin has a strong correlation with Liver yin, as implied by the occurrence of "Liver–Kidney yin deficiency." It has been said that Kidney and Liver have the same source. Accordingly, when we coordinate Kidney yin and Kidney yang, we must take care to pay attention to the fact that Kidney yin and yang closely cooperate. The physiological function of Kidney includes the urogenital system, the reproductive system, internal secretion and partial cerebral function. Although the function of Bladder is to store and excrete urine properly, urinary retention, incontinence and enuresis are considered to be diseases of Kidney because of the strong correlation of Kidney yang and qi transformation.

Dysfunctions of Kidney include Kidney yin deficiency[*1], Liver–Kidney yin deficiency[*2], Heart–Kidney yin deficiency[*3], Lung–Kidney yin deficiency[*4], Kidney yang deficiency[*5], Spleen–Kidney yang deficiency[*6], the failure of Kidney to receive qi[*7], Heart–Kidney yang deficiency[*8], yang deficiency with water flood[*9], insufficiency of Kidney essence[*10] and insecurity of Kidney qi[*11]. We must treat these diseases based on their pathology. [Ref 15, Ref 16]

(Symptoms of *1,*2,*3 and *4 include feverishness, dizziness, tinnitus, dry pharynx and/or mouth, and lumbago; those of *3 are palpitation, insomnia, and excessive dreaming; of *4, dry cough and night sweats; of *5, *6, *8 and *9, dizziness, tinnitus, sensitivity to the cold, cold limbs and pale complexion with weak knees and lumbar region; of *10,deficient reproductive function, hair and tooth loss; of *11, enursis, polyurea and low back pain)

7. Transmutation among the five phases and viscera

The mutual influences among diseases of the viscera are called transmutation. This is based on the engendering relation, the "mother and child relation," and restraint-based overwhelm and rebellion[Ref 2].

7.1 Transmutation based on engendering

One case is where the mother's disease is transmitted to the child. Another case is where the child's disease is transmitted to the mother.

The former case is shown through the symptoms of lumbar vertebrae pain or languishing, tinnitus and nocturnal emission in Kidney yin deficiency. It starts to be accompanied by forgetfulness, insomnia, irritation and being easily angered in Liver yin deficiency or ascendant hyperactivity of the Liver yang.

But as nurture exists in the first case, the situation easily improves.

An example of the latter case (child to mother) is shown through Heart–Liver Fire effulgence. That is, Fire symptoms of Liver such as being easily angered, irritation, dizziness and headache, and following Heart fire symptoms such as insomnia, palpitation and inflammation of the mouth and tongue. The mother qi is stronger than that of the child, and so the mother's disease is apt to become aggravated.

7.2 Transmutation based on overwhelm and rebellion

Liver qi depression, with symptoms such as fidgetiness, being easily angered, and pain of the lateral costal region, begins to invade the stomach with symptoms of nausea, vomiting and abdominal fullness. In this case Wood overwhelms Earth. Before long, cough or hemoptysis appears, or Wood invades Metal, whilst in the viscera, Liver rebellions against Lung. As Liver should be restrained by Lung, symptoms are mild. If the viscera are weak, transmutation easily occurs; if not, it rarely occurs. However, in the case of acute disease this mechanism doesn't work.

8. Regulation of win qi and revenge qi among the five phases

In Su-wen, zhi-zhen-yao-da-lun-pian when one phase causes overwhelm to the corresponding phase, it is said to have "win qi". Once this happens, revenge energy to restrain it appears, (which is called revenge qi/Win Revenge). The more win qi there is, the more revenge qi there will be, and vice versa. After all, in the regulation process of win revenge qi, there exists the law of action and reaction, which means the volume of win qi equals that of the revenge qi. This is described in the Fig. 1[Ref 2].

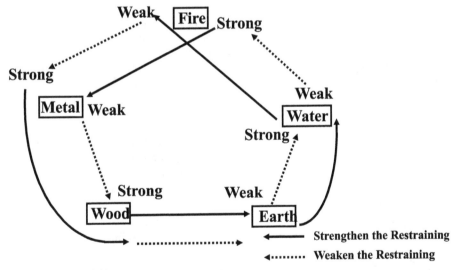

Fig. 1. Win qi and Revenge qi

Explained in terms of Fire in Fig.1, too much Fire qi overwhelms Metal qi → too much decline of Metal qi → Metal qi cannot regulate Wood qi → Wood qi gets excessive win qi → excessive decline of Earth qi → Water qi gets excessive win qi, which restrains Fire → the first excessive Fire qi is normalised. In case of a shortage of Fire qi → Metal gets excessive win qi → Wood qi declines → Earth qi gets excessive win qi → Water qi declines → Fire qi recovers to be normalised. It may be said this mechanism has a kind of feedback system.

When one phase (A) gets excessive qi and the phase which should restrain phase (A) cannot restrain it, the cooperation between these two phases is destroyed and the excessive qi of the phase (A) accumulates more qi while the declined phase is restrained by phase (A) and so declines further. This situation produces an abnormal condition of disorder.

Following Su-wen, in Liu-wei-da-lun-pian: "Once a harmful situation is produced, engendering transformation becomes terribly out of order. In Si-sheng-xin-yuan (wu-xing-sheng-ke-pian), engendering and restraining develop through qi transformation. The quality has no relation with these."

9. Treatments of diseases based on five-phase theory[Ref 2]

9.1 Restrain the transmission of pathological changes of viscera

Diseases develop through dysfunction of viscera, yin-yang and qi-blood.

Dysfunctions of the viscera produce abnormalities of engendering and restraining.

When we treat patients, we must pay attention not only to diseases themselves, but also to the transmission of pathological changes of viscera. We must regulate qi excesses and shortages of viscera based on the law of engendering, restraining, overwhelm and rebellion, by controlling the transmission of pathological changes of viscera and thereby maintaining normal function. For example, when Liver has a disease we must strengthen the function of Spleen and Stomach to protect them from transmission from Liver. Since, by the strengthening of the function of Spleen and Stomach, it is harder for the transmission of pathological change from Liver to Spleen to occur, the disease will be easier to cure.

In Nan-jing.qi-shi-qin-an, it is advanced that once Liver gets a disease, it will transmit it to Spleen. Accordingly, we must give qi to Spleen. The possibility of the transmission of pathological change depends upon the function of viscera. If the viscera qi is in vacuity, the transmission of pathological change will occur; if the viscera qi is in sufficiency, no transmission will occur.

9.2 Treatment rules and treatment methods
9.2.1 Treatment based on the law of engendering

This includes two cases. First there is that of the disease of the mother invading the child. Second, there is that of the disease of the child invading the mother. In Nan-jing (liu-shi-liu nan), it is written that if the child qi is in vacuity, the mother qi must be supplemented (mother qi supplementation), and if the mother qi is sufficient, the child qi must be reduced (child qi reduction).

Mother qi supplementation: In cases where the child qi is insufficient, the mother qi must be supplemented. A dysfunction between mother and child comes from deficiency.

Example

① A shortage of Kidney yin cannot enrich Liver/Wood followed by Liver yin shortage; the ascendant hyperactivity of Liver yang and the so-called Liver qi ascending counterflow will result.

Methods to enrich Water to moisten Wood: this is a therapeutic method to treat Liver yin deficiency by nourishing Kidney yin.

② Methods of engendering Metal-Kidney (enrich Lung and Kidney)

i.   Lung deficiency causes circulation-dysfunction of fluids and humours such that Kidney is not enriched.

ii. Owing to the shortage of Kidney yin, Kidney essence qi can't rise, and this is followed by a failure of purification and the downsending of lung. This situation is characterized, for example, by dry cough, qi counterflow, hemoptysis, bone-steaming tidal fever, night sweat, and nocturnal emission etc.

③ Tonify Spleen to engender Lung qi

Tonify Spleen qi to tonify Lung qi. Usually, a continuing cough with plenty of clears puta, a small quantity of viscous sputa, appetite loss, pale tongue and weak pulse will appear.

Purge Child qi: When mother qi is in excess, the child qi should be purged. The dysfunction between mother and child comes from the existence of excess qi. In the case of a disease of Liver derived from excess qi, such as Liver fire or Liver fire flaming upward, Liver/Wood is the mother and Heart/Fire is the child. The treatment is to purge the Heart Fire and it helps to purge the Liver Fire. When a child's disease is caused by a deficiency, we must not only tonify child qi but also tonify mother qi so as to get engenderment from the mother.

9.2.2 Treatment based on the law of restraining

This refers to the treatment by which the weak phase is recovered either by restraining the strong side or else supporting the weak side. In other words, before the strong side can cause overwhelm, treatment to strengthen the energy of the weak side is started.

I Restraining the strong side is mainly applied to the morbidity in overwhelm and rebellion

A. When Liver overwhelms Spleen, treatment to pacify Liver is applied. In this case, Liver easily causes rebellion to Lung, which means that at one phase, such as overwhelm by Liver, rebellion to Lung easily happens at the same time. When we treat Liver, it means that Spleen and Lung are treated as well. In this case Yi-gan-san-jia-chen-pi-ban-xia (in Japanese :Yokukansankachinpihange) is often applied.

B. Depressed Spleen and Stomach qi → Rebellion from Spleen to Liver occur → Liver cannot do free-coursing and ordered reach, for which treatment to move Spleen-Stomach qi is applied.

II Supporting the weak side because of the shortage of restraining energy

① Method to soothe Liver and fortify Spleen

In Liver deficiency, when Spleen-Stomach transmission and transformation doesn't work, Liver is supplemented and pacified and the Spleen is fortified.

In Liver depression and Spleen deficiency, this method is used. Symptoms include an oppressive feeling in the chest, hypochondria and a distended feeling including pain, appetite loss, abdominal distension, loose passage, belching and gas. (Depressed Liver qi can't give proper restraining to Spleen).

② Method to cultivate Earth and suppress Water

In Spleen, with an abnormal function like weak restraining to Kidney, warming Spleen yang moves the qi and fortifies it to improve the controlling water of Kidney (Spleen restrains for Kidney so as not to get water flood; in other words, fortify Spleen yang in order to warm Kidney). Clinically, this is applied to Spleen deficiency, Spleen-Kidney yang deficiency and water flooding the body tissues with edema, distension and fullness. To this symptom Ren-shen-tan (in Japanese: ninjinto) and fu-zi (in Japanese: bushi) are applied.

③ Method to support Metal to restrain Wood (weak restrain to Liver by Lung). In other words, a method to purge Liver and clear Lung, or else regulate Lung to purify. and downsending to restrain Liver. Hypochondriac pain, a bitter taste in the mouth, nervousness, agony and a string-like, rapid pulse and a cough with hemoptysis are often observed.

④ Method to purge Fire and fortify Water

This means purging Heart Fire and fortifying Kidney water; in other words, to purge south and fortify north, or to nourish yin to move Fire down. With the combination of a shortage of Kidney yin and hyperactive Heart yang, so-called non-interaction between the Heart and Kidney occurs. Lumbago, nervousness, insomnia, nocturnal emission, palpitation, exhausting fever and night sweats are often observed. We must note the fact that Kidney belongs to Water and Fire (Kidney controls yin and belongs to Water, and the life gate that belongs to Kidney controls yang and belongs to Fire).

Kidney yin deficiency causes hyperactive fire, blind movement and functional acceleration, such as nocturnal emission, tinnitus, throat pain and dryness. These phenomena are the result of Kidney yin deficiency or yang hyperactivity of Kidney itself, but they have no relation to the fact that Water cannot restrain Fire.

However, when Kidney is weak to restrain Heart, tonify Kidney with yin and purge heart Fire which will support Kidney to restrain Heart.

We can use the law of the relations of engendering and restraining among viscera as a mental therapy. Sorrow is the emotion of Lung and belongs to Metal. Anger is the emotion of Liver and belongs to Wood. As Metal conquers Wood, sorrow conquers anger. Fright is the emotion of Kidney and belongs to Water. Joy is the emotion of Fire. As Water conquers Fire, fright conquers joy. Anger is the emotion of Liver and belongs to Wood. Thought is the emotion of Spleen and belongs to Earth. As Earth can conquer Water, thought defeats fright.

The modern cognition about the study with five-phase theory

In TCM theory, the core of health exists in the dynamic balance between the body and its circumstances; the destruction of this balance is the real cause of disease.

Accordingly, the main theme of the research and study of TCM is the pursuit of methods and remedies to restore degraded physical conditions to a balanced state.

The basic rule of treatment within TCM lies in the regulating of yin and yang, the reforming of tendencies and defects and the recovery of general physical balances.

In recent years, many monographs in cybernetics theory have been published which elucidate TCM theory. For instance, inhibition and the generation of the law of engendering and restraining within the five-phase theory reflect the self-control principle in the human body. With this law, the concept of feedback is included. The five-phase theory, which reflects the transformation law in the cause-and-effect rule, contains the programmatic control concept from cybernetics theory. Further, the method of classification in five-phase theory through the comparison of shapes is similar to the same class-system concept in cybernetics theory.

The five systems in five-phase theory have many routes and form a closed system, with feedback regulations at numerous levels, and thereby maintains the stability of a self-controlled system.

Further, the regulation of inhibition and the generation and regulation of win qi and revenge qi in five-phase theory exemplify the function of the five-phase system in performing automatic regulations.

Applying the five-phase theory to disease in modern medicines

① Examples of mother-child transmission in five-phase theory

- Between Kidney and Liver
- Prolonged dysfunction of Liver is often followed by Kidney dysfunction (Liver Kidney depletion)

- Several monographs have reported that human bone marrow cells, which belong to Kidney, are related to the improvement or progress of liver cell fibrosis. This pattern has been recognised in mice as well.[Ref 17, Ref 18]
- Between Kidney and Lung
  Goodpasture syndrome shows hemoptysis followed by acute glomerulonephritis, which means that the mother's disease (Lung) is transmitted to the child (Kidney) based on mother-child transmission.
- Between Liver and Heart
  In cardiac liver cirrhosis, liver cirrhosis is often derived from right heart failure. This is another case of transmission from the child to the mother.

② Examples of overwhelm and rebellion

- Between Liver and Spleen
  Nervous gastritis and functional gastrointestinal disorder are caused by stress (Liver qi abnormalities).
- Between Kidney and Heart
  In chronic heart disease, an important deteriorating cause is complication arising from Kidney disease; most likely, this will be accumulated Kidney evil resulting from Kidney disease, which will overwhelm Heart. In chronic Kidney disease, an important cause of death is the complication of Heart disease. This may be said to be a kind of rebellion from Heart to Kidney.
- Between Liver and Lung
  Hepatopulmonary syndrome: in chronic liver disease, like liver cirrhosis, telangiectasis or telangiectasia is often observed in the lung, followed by dyspnea. This may be rebellion from Liver to Lung.

Finally, various modern diseases, including incurable disease, have been recognised by five-phase theory and they have sometimes been successfully treated. Therefore, if five-phase theory is properly applied, chronic intractable diseases are sometimes successfully treated.

In particular, in routine life, we have many stresses that we can't avoid and which inflict pain on us. When we consider that those stresses make liver qi abnormalities, we can obtain clues to their improvement, as shown below.

In this chapter, I have applied the lecture Lu-Gan-Fu gave to his son Lu-xi*a, namely that "The evil qi accumulation in one viscus can overwhelm to the restraining viscus. If yang deficiency aggravated in a viscus, the evil qi equals cold pathogen, if heat accumulated enormously, the evil qi equals heat pathogen.

(*a:13th and 14th generation of Lu family noted for wen-bin in China. Their work appeared in the title "Traditional Chinese Medicines Improve the Course of Refractory Leukemic Lymphoblastic Lymphoma and Acute Lymphocytic Leukaemia." Am.J.Chin.Med, Vol XXIII, No. 2,pp195-211. 1995)

On applying five-phase theory to treatment, the most important point is to identify the viscera causing the various symptoms. Next is the decision of the order of appearance of the symptoms. Usually by this means we can speculate upon which viscus is at the root of the patient's disease. Next by comparing the various symptoms, we can speculate upon the existence of engendering, restraining, overwhelming, and rebellion among the viscera.[Ref 19] The "Organ pattern identification Table" is very useful and convenient[Ref 16] in this regard.

Below, eleven cases are discussed in detail and in terms of the correlations of medical diagnoses with TCM theory using five-phase theory. The formulas prescribed are shown in

"Chinese Herbal Medicine. FORMULAS & STRATAGIES (Bensky Balolet: published by East Land 1990)." Herbs are shown in *CHINESE HERBAL MEDICINE Materia Medica* 3rd Ed.: published by East Land 2004. To save space, their identification in TCM is described after the symptoms in parenthesis. Numerals in circles refer to the numerals in the respective figures. With Liver, ①, Heart,②, Spleen,③, Lung, ④ and Kidney,⑤are used. Peculiar Japanese prescriptions are explained in this text.

Susceptibility to common cold caused by Kidney deficiency

Case 1 A 60-year-old Japanese female

Chief complaint: Recent susceptibility to catching common colds

Present illness: She found herself prone to catching colds. She had been sensitive to the cold and suffers from frequent urination (Kidney yang deficiency). She has had a weak constitution (Spleen qi deficiency) since childhood. Two years ago, a feeling of throat stuffiness continued. A close examination revealed as the cause a benign thyroid tumour, which was left untreated. Upon her visit to my clinic, she reported that every time she felt tired, she caught a cold (Lung qi deficiency), which was unusual for her. Intake of ge-gen-tang (in Japanese Kakkonto) released the exterior muscle layer and exorcised the common cold within a few days, but she soon caught a cold again. She had looked after her mother at her home and paid much attention to both her husband and mother, which induced a great deal of stress (Liver qi depression) until two years ago when her mother died. In spite of the fact that she was freed from her mother's care, since that time she has become even more susceptible to colds and so visited my clinic.

Past history: She has suffered from dysmenorrhoea, for which total extirpation of the uterus was carried out (Liver qi depression with blood stasis). As she does not have enough stamina, she couldn't work hard (qi deficiency) and has been sensitive to the cold.

Present status: Height, 158cm; weight: 48kg; pulse, 74/min, fine, slippery, string-like, tongue body, pale with reddish limbic, tongue fur, whitish with thin centre (yin deficiency); sublingual vessel enlarged (blood stasis)

Identification: Kidney Yang deficiency, Lung qi deficiency

Treatment: Ba-wei-di-huang-wan (tonifies the yang and yin of Kidney, nourishes the blood)

Clinical course: With no change to her lifestyle and working conditions, she did not catch a cold for the 5 months or more since she started taking 30 pills of Ba-wei- di-huang-wan (common dosage: 60 pills/day).

Discussion: Susceptibility to colds indicates qi deficiency of Lung. The fact, especially, that her colds appeared when she had some trouble which caused her stress implies a rebellion of Liver against the Lung. But she felt her stress decreased after her mother's death two years ago. Accordingly, stress does not influence her frequent catching of colds, but the fact that intake of ba-wei-di-huang-wan decreased her frequency of catching colds implies that the qi deficiency of Lung was reversed by giving yang to Kidney, which was transmitted through their engendering relation.

Ulcerative colitis case

Case 2 A 29-year-old Japanese female who works for civil aviation.

Chief complaint: Diarrhoea, abdominal pain, bloody stool, lumbago, stress-induced insomnia

History of present illness: Her bloody stool had continued in spite of the administration of routine remedies including sufficient rest since 24th of Jan, X year. By continuing an adrenocortical hormone for one month, the bloody stool stopped. She visited my clinic in June, X year as she hoped to stop the recurrence of her bloody stools. Nine years earlier, she had been diagnosed with ulcerative colitis, which was brought on by a lot of stress. Since then she had been taking 5-amino salicylate. At the beginning she suffered from only bloody stools, but more recently she has suffered from lumbago as well. From seven years earlier to the present, the ulcerative colitis had recurred about once a year. This recurrence was usually evoked by stress or working all night (Wood overwhelms Earth). Overwork often led to abdominal pain followed by bloody stools. She reported that she was routinely feeling abdominal fullness and gassy stomach. Overeating or coldness caused diarrhoea (Spleen yang deficiency ③, ③-②). She dislikes meats. Her digestive system easily gets cold (Spleen yang Deficiency. ③-②) when stressful things happen and Spleen qi deficiency occurred with the failure of controlling Blood (Liver overwhelms Spleen ①-②).

During childhood, she suffered from chilblains, disliked the air conditioner during the summer, wore too many clothes in the winter, and had cold limbs (Kidney yang deficiency ⑤). More recently, she became fatigued easily and perspired greatly during the summer (qi defficiency). She has an irregular period (Blood deficiency of Liver and Liver qi stagnation ①-①, ①-③) and menstrual pain (Liver qi stagnation and blood stasis ①-①).

Past history: She suffered from alopecia areata several times between the ages of ten and twenty-five years old

Present state: Height, 160cm; weight, 55kg; Pulse, 56/min, fine, sunken, slippery; teeth-marked tongue (retention of water.③-②) with a thin white fur; Blood Pressure (BP), 98/62 (mmHg).

Identification: Spleen failing to control the blood. Spleen and Kidney Yang deficiency with water flood. Bowels with damp and heat.

Treatment: Tonify Spleen qi to control the blood, spread Liver qi and relieve constraint. When stressors lead to insomnia, nourish the blood and yin and warm the Kidney to promote urination and stop diarrhoea.[Ref 16]

Prescriptions: ①Jia-wei-gui-pi-tang (in Japanese: Kamikihito) benefits the Spleen qi to control the blood. This equals gui-pi-tang supplemented with chai-fu (Bupleuri Radix) which spreads Liver qi to relieve constraint and clear heat; and zhi-zi (Gardeniae Fructus) which drains heat and eliminates irritability, clears heat, and eliminates dampness (decoction).[Ref 14] ② Zhen-wu- tang warms Kidney to promote urination and stop diarrhoea. This prescription was made by TSUMURA & CO (http://www.tsumura.co.jp /english/index.htm) (Tokyo Japan).[Ref 20]

Clinical course: After starting herbal therapy, little by little her diarrhoea improved. Her bloody stools decreased in number as well. When she visited my clinic in May, two months after her first visit, she informed me that she had no diarrhoea and no bloody stool, but she would like to continue 5-mino salicylate to make sure. She continued one month's medicine and then stopped. One year and three months later, she visited my clinic to obtain the same herbal remedies for prevention. She told me she had had no symptoms, including diarrhoea and bloody stools, so far (Fig. 2).

Discussion: As the first bloody stool appeared following a stressful episode, the stressful event induced Liver qi depression which in turn overwhelmed Spleen leading to a failure to control Blood. In Jia-wei- gui-pi-tan, ren-shen, bai-chu, zhi-gan-zao, huan-qi worked to tonify the Spleen qi, to stop diarrhoea and bloody stool. Fu-ling, long-yan-rou and suan-zao-ren tonified and nourished Heart blood so as to tranquilise. The chai-fu worked to disperse stagnated Liver qi so that Liver would not overwhelm Spleen. The recent complication of lumbago may be a result of overwhelm from Spleen with excess coldness pathogen to Kidney. As mentioned already, a method to cultivate Earth and suppress Water, like Zhen-wu-tang, was prescribed. The zhi-zi (Gardeniae Fructus) likely supported the subsidence of the colitis. Zhen-wu-tang warmed the yang of Kidney and Spleen, thereby tonifying Spleen and Kidney, which stopped the progression of her lumbago and bloody stools.

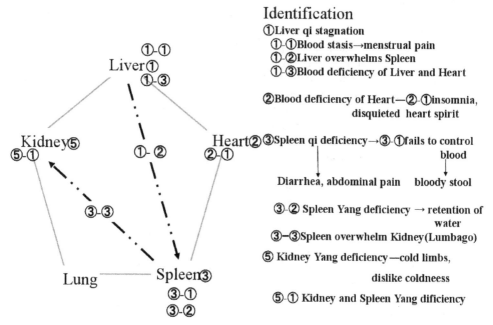

Identification

①Liver qi stagnation
    ①-①Blood stasis→menstrual pain
    ①-②Liver overwhelms Spleen
    ①-③Blood deficiency of Liver and Heart

②Blood deficiency of Heart—②-①insomnia,
                 disquieted heart spirit

③Spleen qi deficiency→③-①fails to control
                                 blood

Diarrhea, abdominal pain   bloody stool

③-② Spleen Yang deficiency → retention of
                               water
③-③Spleen overwhelm Kidney(Lumbago)

⑤ Kidney Yang deficiency—cold limbs,
                dislike coldneess
⑤-① Kidney and Spleen Yang dificiency

Fig. 2. Relations among viscra with five phase theory of Case 2

Great improvement after insertion of intra-cardiac pacemaker

Case 3 A 73-year-old Japanese housewife

Chief complaint (First visit): Dull feeling in Stomach, frequent cystitis, Kidney ptosis with vesical inertia, oversensitivity to the cold

History of present illness: She often had a dull feeling in her stomach. She could not take meats or fatty food. Coldness easily evoked abdominal pain or diarrhoea, and she felt that she easily got colds (Spleen Yang deficiency ③,③ Lung qi deficiency ④-①). She often saw purple spots without any reason. She has serious kidney ptosis and vesical inertia (sunken middle qi ③-①), frequent suffering from cystitis (Kidney yang deficiency ⑤-①), and continuing throat discomfort throughout winter (Lung qi deficiency④-①). She visited my clinic in February of X year to decrease the frequency of cystitis.

Present status: Height 140cm, Weight 41kg, Blood pressure 126/72mmHg, pulse, 70/min, weak

Past history: She reported to have had a weak constitution since childhood and often felt lassitude (qi deficiency). She had been oversensitive to the cold and has suffered from cystitis. Her digestive system was weak. Her throat discomfort had continued throughout the winter and she felt as if she had been catching a cold all winter. Her menopausal symptoms continued for more than ten years with lassitude and perspiration, for which she had to take a tranquiliser.

Identification before insertion of intra-cardiac pacemaker: Spleen and Kidney Yang deficiency, Heart qi deficiency, Lung yang and qi deficiency. Liver overwhelms Spleen

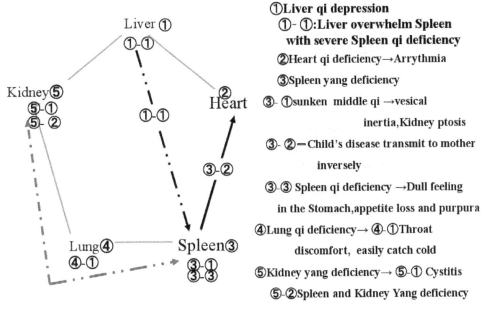

①**Liver qi depression**

①- ①:**Liver overwhelm Spleen with severe Spleen qi deficiency**

②Heart qi deficiency→Arrythmia

③Spleen yang deficiency

③- ①sunken middle qi →vesical inertia,Kidney ptosis

③- ②–Child's disease transmit to mother inversely

③-③ Spleen qi deficiency →Dull feeling in the Stomach,appetite loss and purpura

④Lung qi deficiency→ ④-①Throat discomfort, easily catch cold

⑤Kidney yang deficiency→ ⑤-① Cystitis

⑤-②Spleen and Kidney Yang deficiency

Fig. 3. Relations among viscera with five phase theory of case 3 (Just before insertion of intra-cardiac pacemaker)

Treatments: Warm the Kidney and Spleen yang, tonify Spleen, clear heat and moistness of bladder

Prescriptions:①bu-zhong-yi-qi-tang (in Japanese: Hochuekito) tonifies the qi of the middle burner and raises sunken yang, with fu-zi (Aconiti Radix) reviving and assisting the yang, warming the fire and dispersing cold, ba-wei-di-huang-wan (in Japanese: Hachimijiogan) warms and revives the yang and enriches the yin of Kidney. ③WTTCGE (*Wisteria floribunda* 2g, *Trapa natans* 2g, *Terminalia chebulae* 2g, *Coix lachryma-jobi* 4g, *Ganoderma lucidum* 4g, *Elfuinga applanata* 2g in dry weight/day: effective for herpes genitalis, labialis and chronic herpes viruses infectious diseases to increase the NK cell activity and prevent inflammation). Ref21, Ref22

Clinical Course: I prescribed bu-zhong-yi-qi-tang supplemented with fu-zi for yang deficiency of Kidney, ba-wei-di-huang-wan and hot water extracts of WTTCGE for continuing throat discomfort through the winter. The latter was combined with modified zhu-ling-tang (in Japanese: Chyoreito) in order to promote urination, clear heat, and nourish the yin for frequent cystitis. The cystitis improved but not perfectly. Her digestive system symptoms and purpura remained. Twelve years after her first visit, arrhythmia started -

sometimes 30~40/min - and caused instantaneous unconsciousness. Fourteen years after first visit, the insertion of an intra-cardiac pacemaker was carried out without changing the intake of herbal therapies. After this, her appetite loss and other associated symptoms of digestive system - including purpura - disappeared almost completely and the disease rate of cystitis dramatically decreased and has remained decreased up until the present.

Discussion: On her first visit, she did not have arrhythmia while her yang deficiency of Kidney and Spleen were long-term conditions. Twelve years later she had arrhythmia. This may mean that during the long duration of Spleen yang deficiency, based on the engendering relation between Heart and Spleen, the Spleen may have stolen her Heart qi in the long run. Finally, her arrhythmia continued. Fourteen years later after her first visit, an intra-cardiac pacemaker was inserted and the Heart qi was tonified and followed by the enrichment of Spleen qi. Accordingly, her purpura and digestive symptoms disappeared and her appetite was restored. As Kidney and Heart belong to the same lesser yin, with increasing Heart qi, Kidney qi was increased and Kidney yang was also increased allowing for Bladder to be warmed and being followed by the disappearance of Bladder inflammation. Her nervousness decreased, probably as a result of tonifying Heart.

Male climate period (Severe Autonomic nerve dysfunction syndrome)

Case 4. A 46-year-old Japanese male medicine wholesaler

Chief complaint: Tachycardia, palpitation, hypertension, a hot face and staggering

History of present illness: He began to suffer from a hot face, staggering, insomnia and hypertension (Liver and Kidney yin deficiency ①-①, ②, ⑤-⑤) in April. He had been doing aerobic exercise for a long time without any trouble. However, on September 25 of the same year, tachycardia and palpitation continued for more than one hour after aerobics (non-interaction between Heart and Kidney (②-①). Furthermore, he suffered from tachycardia and palpitation not only after aerobics but also while resting, which led to his giving up aerobics. As he would sit, he felt palpitation and had a pale face and, upon standing up, he felt as though he was losing consciousness.

An intake of psychotropic medications for one week had no beneficial effect. His blood pressure had been high and unstable. On straining during working, his face would get hot and the temples would throb uncomfortably (Ascendant hyperactivity of Liver yang ①-①-①). His stiffness of shoulder, neck and back (Liver qi depression and blood stasis, interruption of meridian and collaterals ①-③) and heaviness of the occipital region (retention of dampness ⑤-②) continued. At his first visit on October 12, he felt something was heaving up from the epigastrium and his BP was 170/100mmHg (Kidney yin deficiency followed by ascendant hyperactivity of deficient fire:⑤-③).

On that day he started taking chai-hu-jia-long-gu-mu-li-tang (in Japanese: Saikokaryukotsuboreito - this unblocks the three yang stages, and sedates and calms the spirit: TSUMURA & CO)[Ref20] which aggravated his hotness of face and palpitations and so was stopped. Generally, his general fatigue was severe, his urination volume was large, and he experienced discomfort on rainy days (retention of dampness:⑤-②). He often had muddy stools (Spleen qi deficiency:③-①) and was irritated, got angry easily, experienced hotness of the face and had night sweats ascendant hyperactivity of Liver yang (①-①-①). When he was tired, his soles were hot with sweat (Kidney yin deficiency ⑤-③). He felt asthenopia, dim eyesight and dry eye (Liver blood deficiency ①-④). (Fig 4).

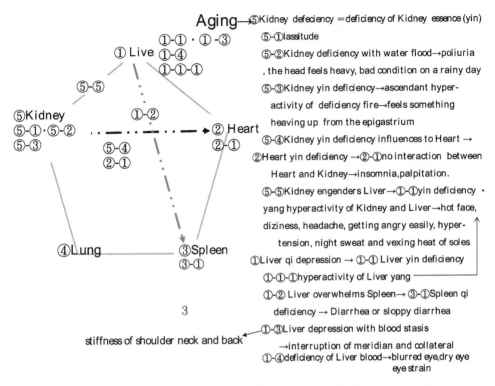

Fig. 4. Relations among viscera with five phase theory of case 4 (before treatment)

On October 25, he began an intake of gui-zhi-fu-ling-wan (in Japanese: Keishibukuryogan - this invigorates the blood and transforms blood stasis: TSUMURA & CO)[Ref 20] but only about 20% of his symptoms decreased. He visited a Kampo clinic and was administered zi-yin-jiang-huo-tang (in Japanese: Jiinkokato[Ref 20, Ref 24] - this tonifies yin:zhi-gan-zao, dang-gu, shao-yao, sheng-di-huang, tian-men-dong, mai-men-dong, bai-shu, chen-pi, huang-bo, zhi-mu, sheng-jiang, da-zao).[Ref.22]

On November 17, tachycardia, palpitation and discomfort started to decrease and his irritation and instances of getting angry decreased by around 50%. No further improvement occurred. On November 24, he visited my clinic and diagnosed as follows.

Identification: Liver qi depression with blood stasis, ascendant hyperactivity of Liver yang (①-①-①), Kidney and Liver yin deficiency(⑤-③,①-①), Kidney deficiency with water flood(⑤-②).

Treatments: Tonify Kidney yin and essence and Liver yin

Prescription: Turtle powder (whole body was treated with heat and dried: 2g/day) was added.

Clinical Course: One week later he had recovered completely. By mid-January of the following year, he could perform aerobics without any trouble, and the intake of all remedies except for turtle powder was stopped. He has been taking turtle powder since then, for several years, because if he stops he starts to feel strange and uncomfortable.

Discussion

During the male climacteric period, the male hormone decreases which means Kidney essence and yin decreases in TCM theory. It is reasonable that the prescription of zi-yin-jiang-huo-tang[Ref 23] caused symptoms to improve by 50%. The reason chai-hu-jia-long-gu-mu-li-tang worsened the situation is because his symptoms originated from the deficiency of Kidney essence and yin rather than by the inhibited three yang stages. This remedy tended to consume yin, which aggravated this situation. Shortage of Kidney yin caused Heart Fire effulgence (⑤-④. ②. ②-①), which means non-interaction between the Heart and Kidney.

My TCM teacher, Lu Xi told me that his father, Lu Gan-fu, taught him that overwhelmingness occurs from viscus with excess evil qi to the corresponding viscus. If this theory is applied to Kidney, it may be said that hyperactive Kidney yang based on Kidney yin deficiency overwhelms Heart. Accordingly, hyperactive Kidney yang and Heart fire can exist together.

Liver yin deficiency by engendering from Kidney (①-①), and ascendant hyperactivity of Liver yang (①-①-①) followed by overwhelm from Liver to Spleen (①-②.③-①), which were almost all resolved by prescribing the turtle powder.

There are many herbs for tonifying Kidney yin or essence, but when they are not effective; it is necessary to try animal-derived material in order to enrich Kidney yin or essence. Animal-derived materials are sometimes very effective for these cases.

Aged female depression after husband's death

Case 5: A 76-year-old Japanese female

Chief complaint: Depression with severe self-reproach, no vitality.

History of present illness: Since two years ago, when her husband died, she had been suffering from impatience, depression with a guilty conscience (Liver qi depression), and insomnia. She could not get to sleep easily and she routinely took tranquilizers. Upon awakening, she felt heavy depression. As her false teeth did not fit, she ate by grinding her food. She had cold forefeet and had difficulty in hearing. Though table tennis had been her hobby, she had stopped due to lack of vitality. Up until her husband's death, she had climbed one mountain (600m height) once a week.

Past history: She had been hospitalized after the great Hanshin earthquake. Menopause occurred at fifty-two years

Family history: Her brothers all died from TB.

Present status: Height, 156cm; weight, 48kg; BP, 138/78mmHg; pulse, 66/min. fine, slippery, sunken, with a weak chi/cubit pulse; tongue body, red; tongue fur, thin (Liver qi depression, Spleen qi deficiency (①, ①-②)

Identification: Qi deficiency, Liver qi depression, Deficiency of Kidney yin and yang

Treatment: Soothe Liver to release depression, tonify Spleen and Kidney

Prescription: ① bu-zhong-yi-qi-tang and ② soft-shelled turtle (tonifies yin and Kidney). Beginning on day thirty-eight nu-shen-san[Ref 24] (in Japanese: Nyoshinsan - dan-gui, chuan-xiong, gui-zhi, bai-chu, mu-xiang, huang-qin, huang-lian, ren-shen, gan-cao, xiang-fu-zi, da-huang, zong-lu-zi, ding-xiang soothes and tonifies Liver, clears heat, and warms the lower body)[*1. Ref 25] was added to her previous prescriptions.

Clinical course: Ten days after starting Kampo medicine (bu-zhong-yi-qi-tang, soft-shelled turtle) her mental irritation - including her depression with guilty conscience - decreased.

However, she still suffered occasionally from extreme depression. She continued with the same medicines. On day thirty-eight, a new prescription, nu-shen-san, was added. Three days after the addition of nu-shen-san, her feelings became more pleasant and her depression improved remarkably. She could go to the theatre and go shopping with a neighbouring housewife. She could not believe how depressed she had been. She continued for another thirty days with the same medicines and quit them all seventy-six days after starting Kampo medicine. She reported that she had completely recovered from her depression and could lead a satisfactory and normal life. Her insomnia disappeared as well.

Discussion: This patient's Kidney yang and yin were rather deficient because her forefoot was cold even in the summer; she felt hot in sole and she had difficulty in hearing. She liked drinking cold cow's milk and had a dry mouth. The body of her tongue was red and her tongue fur was thin (Kidney yin deficiency⑤-③). The soft-shelled-turtle tonifies yin and Kidney. By taking this, Kidney would be enriched. The enriched Kidney may have engendered the Liver, which likely played a role in improving the depression to some extent. Bu-zhong-yi-qi-tang - which tonifies Spleen qi and supports the upbearing of qi - also contributed to improving the depression. It is certain that these two medicines were partly effective in decreasing her depression, but her depression did not disappear completely and the addition of nu-shen-san improved the feeling of loss dramatically. Nu-shen-san soothed Liver and tonified it with other prescriptions, which engendered Heart, and was followed by the improvement of her insomnia and disappearance of her depression.

(*1: This prescription was created by Sohaku Asada during the period between the Meiji and Edo eras, and has been used for any flush and dizziness surrounding childbirth as well as coldness of the lower parts of the body, by soothing Liver, discharging heat, tonifying Liver and warming the lower parts).

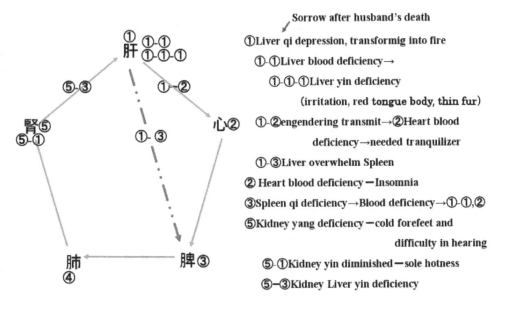

Fig. 5. Relations among viscera with five phase theory of case 5.

Interstitial Pneumonia

Case 6 : A 62-year-old Japanese female

Chief complaint: Cough, dyspnea and palpitation aggravated on motion, cold legs, frequent urination

History of present illness: Her dry cough continued until white sputa was discharged (Lung qi and yin deficiency ④) followed by palpitation. Her cough was aggravated on rainy days (Lung fails in purification and downbearing ④-①). Palpitation and dyspnea were severe (Lung influenced to Heart, Heart qi deficiency ②, ④-④). Recently, even in the summer, her ankles would get cold (the Mother's abnormality is transmitted to the child by way of engendering ④-③). The frequency of urination was more than ten times/day (Kidney yang deficiency: ⑤). In winter, her soles felt hot (yin deficiency ⑤-①). Recently, fatigue has increased (qi deficiency). Since menopause, she has experienced hot flashes and sensitivity to heat (yin deficiency with fire effulgence ①-①,⑤-①,⑤-②). She prefers a cold drink (⑤-②, ①-①). In spite of suffering from cataracts and glaucoma evoked by adrenal cortex hormones, she continues to take 4mg of adrenal cortex hormone (predonine). She had high intraocular pressure (Liver yin deficiency ①,①-①). She has a small gallstone (1 cm). (Liver qi stagnation ①).

Past history: When she was fifty-eight years old, she had such severe dyspnea and palpitation that she was hospitalised for two-and-a-half months. She was diagnosed with interstitial pneumonia and, for three years, adrenal cortex hormones were prescribed. Five years later, dyspnea and palpitation were aggravated again. She visited another doctor and re-started adrenal cortex hormones therapy, which proved ineffective. Various other kinds of treatments have not worked.

Family history: Her grandfather suffered from asthma

Present status: Height, 158cm, weight, 57kg. Pulse, sunken, fine, forceless, 60/min (Heart qi deficiency②); tongue body, pale dark, swollen sublingual collateral vessels (Liver qi stagnation→blood stasis①); BP, 120/78mmHg

Identification: Lung qi and yin deficiency, Heart qi deficiency, Phlegm obstructing the Lung, Kidney yin and yang Deficiency

Treatments: Tonify Lung qi and yin, Tonify Heart qi

Prescriptions: ① zhi-gan-cao-tang(in Japanese: Syakanzoto - this augments the qi, nourishes the blood, enriches the yin and restores the pulse) ② qin-fei-tang[Ref 25] (in Japanese: Seihaito - this clears lung inflammation in order to remove sputa and stop coughs; Wan-bin-gui-chun, written by Gong Ting xian)[*1Ref 24] supplemented with bai-he (Lilli Bulbus - this moistens Lung, clears heat to stop coughs, and enriches Lung yin), zhi-mu (Anemarrhenae Rhizoma - this clears heat and drains Fire and enriches the yin) and pi-pa-ye (Eriobotryae Folium - this transforms phlegm, clears Lung heat and downbears Lung qi).

Clinical course: She first visited my office on August 23, X year. Around seven days after starting herbal therapies, her conditions started to improve, and so she continued with taking them. On November 4 she visited our clinic and reported that she could do some housework, but that if she overworked, asthma occurred. As she felt a dry throat, owing to the side effects of conventional medicines, and I added zi-yin-jiang-huo-tang (in Japanese: Jiinkokato – this tonifies yin)[*2] and ma-xing-gan-shi-tang (in Japanese: Makyokansekito - this facilitates the flow of Lung qi and clears heat)[*3] for her asthma fits. Ma-xing-gan-shi-tang was quick to be effective. On her visit of November 30, she reported she could lead a normal life as a housewife and that her persistent cough and dry throat had disappeared.

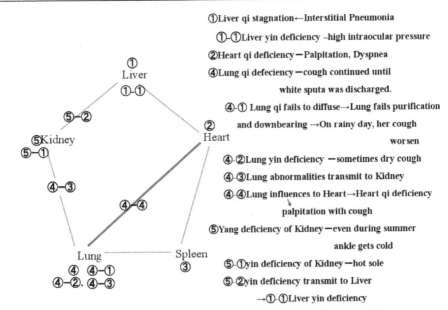

①Liver qi stagnation←Interstitial Pneumonia

①-①Liver yin deficiency –high intraocular pressure

②Heart qi deficiency—Palpitation, Dyspnea

④Lung qi defeciency—cough continued until

white sputa was discharged.

④-① Lung qi fails to diffuse→Lung fails purification

and downbearing →On rainy day, her cough

worsen

④-②Lung yin deficiency —sometimes dry cough

④-③Lung abnormalities transmit to Kidney

④-④Lung influences to Heart→Heart qi deficiency

palpitation with cough

⑤Yang deficiency of Kidney—even during summer

ankle gets cold

⑤-①yin deficiency of Kidney—hot sole

⑤-②yin deficiency transmit to Liver

→①-①Liver yin deficiency

Fig. 6. Relations among viscera with five phase theory of case 6 (Interstitial Pneumonia before treatment)

Discussion: As the patient had not been so oversensitive to the cold in her previous healthy days, the existence of recent cold legs and frequent urination could be the result of the transmission of accumulated Lung abnormalities to Kidney, from Lung, through the engendering route. Her symptom's aggravation on rainy days implies that Lung yang (qi) deficiency leading to retention of moistness. However, Lung yin deficiency also existed, which was the cause of her severe dry cough. Qin-fei-tang and pi-pa-ye cleared the heat and phlegm of the Lung and tonified the yin of Lung along with bai-he and zhi-mu. Enriching the Lung yin strengthened the Lung qi. Zhi-gan-cao-tang tonified the Heart qi, together with Lung qi enrichment, and worked synergistically based upon the close relation between the two viscera. It was likely that this was the reason why she improved so quickly.

Her intraocular high blood pressure may have been due to the Liver yin deficiency transforming into Fire transmitted from the Kidney yin deficiency.

(*1 Qin-fei-tang: fu-lig, dang-gui, mai-men-dong, huang-qin, jie-geng, chen-pi, bei-mu, sang-bai-pi, zhi-zi, tian-men-dong, xing-ren, zhu-ru, da-zao. *1 *2,*3: these are all product of Tsumura Co.)

Pulmonary emphysema

Case 7 A 73-year-old Japanese male.

Chief complaint: Frequent cough with transparent sticky sputa, dyspnea on motion, difficulty in walking with powerless legs, and sensitivity to the cold.

History of present illness: He had serious dyspnea on motion (Lung qi deficiency ④). Taking just one step in walking made him feel like choking (Heart qi deficiency ②,②-①). He complained of powerless legs (Kidney qi deficiency ⑤). During the summer he didn't like air conditioning; instead, he dressed in heavy clothing and used a big futon (⑤-①). He had feet that were cold to numbness (Kidney yang deficiency ⑤-①). He also had a groin hernia. He had been light eater and sometimes he experiences stomach aches (Spleen qi deficiency ④-③,③).

The previous year, he had been diagnosed with serious pulmonary emphysema at a major hospital, but continued to smoke two pieces of cigarettes a day. He generally discharges a lot of transparent sticky sputa (phlegm obstructing the lung (④, ④-①).

Sometimes he discharges yellow sputa (localised inflammation in Lung). He told me that he usually discharges sputa around ten times/day (Lung qi deficiency ④, ④-①). As he easily catches colds during the winter, he rarely goes out.

Present Status: Height, 156 cm; weight, 41 kg; BP, 146/70mmHg, Pulse, 72/min, string-like, slippery, weak (Heart qi deficiency ②), purple-red tongue, white thick fur with spot defoliation (cold damp entering interior, stomach qi and deficiency③).

Past history: Between the ages of nineteen and twenty-four years, he was hospitalised with TB. About four years ago, a fever of more than 39°C continued for around fourteen days, causing him to be hospitalised. Since this time, he has noticed dypnea on motion. His frequent cough and oversensitivity to the cold have been a long-term problem.

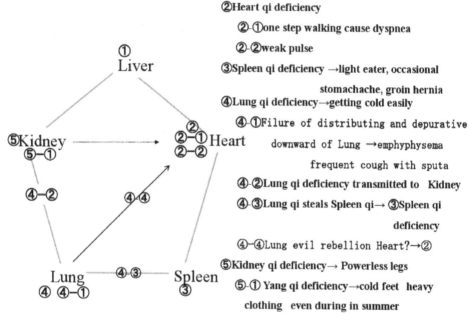

②Heart qi deficiency
②-①one step walking cause dyspnea
②-②weak pulse
③Spleen qi deficiency →light eater, occasional stomachache, groin hernia
④Lung qi deficiency→getting cold easily
④-①Filure of distributing and depurative downward of Lung →emphyphysema frequent cough with sputa
④-②Lung qi deficiency transmitted to Kidney
④-③Lung qi steals Spleen qi→ ③Spleen qi deficiency
④-④Lung evil rebellion Heart?→②
⑤Kidney qi deficiency→ Powerless legs
⑤-① Yang qi deficiency→cold feet heavy clothing even during in summer

Fig. 7. Relations among viscera with five phase theory of case 7 (Pulmonary emphysema before treatment)

Identification: Qi deficiency of Lung and Heart, Failure of Lung in fluid distribution and depurative downbearing. Yang deficiency of Kidney.

Treatments: Tonify Lung and Heart qi.

Prescriptions: ① zhi-gan-cao-tang (TSUMURA & CO.: this augments the qi, nourishes the blood, enriches the yin and restores the pulse).[*1 Ref 24] ② qin-fei-tang[*2] with supplemental bai-he (Lilli Bulbus: this moistens Lung, clears heat to stop coughs and enriches Lung yin)

[*1:]Powder type - a product of Tsumura Co. [*2:same as case 6)]

Clinical course: When the patient visited my clinic on April 11 for the first time, he reported that he had taken preserved zhi-gan-cao-tang for three weeks but that his cough and sputum had not changed, even though he felt slightly better. I added the qin-fei-tang. On his second visit on April 30, he reported that he could walk and move without much trouble. On June 26, he reported that routine movement and walking were much improved, and that the volume of sputa had decreased. He continued taking the same remedies, and around one year later, he could lead a more relaxed life without much trouble. He continues to smoke two cigarettes a day and he plays "go" from time to time. His sensitivity to the cold has improved and he can walk without trouble. He has not caught a cold so far. He has taken only qin-fei-tang for one year, and has done fine on this reduced regimen.

Discussion: The patient suffered from TB during youth and he has continued smoking while playing "go" since then. That may be one of the reasons he suffered from pulmonary emphysema. The heavy abnormalities of Lung (Lung evil qi) were transmitted to Kidney, which depleted the qi further, leading to Kidney yang deficiency. Even in summer he was heavily clothed and used a thick coverlet. His Heart qi deficiency may have derived from Heart–Lung qi deficiency syndrome, or Lung qi abnormalities might have influenced the heart through the rebellion route. Spleen qi deficiency, such as being a light eater, experiencing occasional stomach aches or groin hernia, might have derived from the stealing of Spleen qi by the lung. Once Lung qi was restored, his coldness, stomach aches, groin hernia, and frequency of cough with sputa were remarkably decreased. It is clear that in his case Lung was the main organ that caused and aggravated his various symptoms.

Recurrence of metastatic kidney cancer in bladder

Case 8. A 52-year-old Japanese businessman

Chief complaint: Intractable metastatic kidney cancer, nose dryness

History of present illness: At age 51, the patient had noticed hematuria. Twelve months later, in April, X year, he was diagnosed with cancer of Kidney. A left nephroureterectomy was carried out in a national hospital in May. Partial cancer cell infiltration was recognised, which was resected without gross cancer tissues. Nose dryness has continued (yin deficiency of Lung ④-①).

Past history: He had been a heavy smoker. Since X-6 year, he suffered from hoarseness and pharyngitis (Lung yin deficiency④-①) and choking pressure in the chest (Heart blood obstruction with blood stasis ②-①). In X-4 year palpitations accompanied these symptoms (Heart qi deficiency ②) and his voice would become more hoarse, with a dry mouth and dry lips (Lung yin deficiency④-①). He usually took the drug for angina pectoris.

In spring of the X-3 year, when he looked backwards, dizziness occurred (obstruction with blood stasis, upper orifices interruption①, ②-①), which was much improved with exercise. In June, he again felt tightness of the chest and numbness from right shoulder to the arm (Heart blood stasis ②-①) and sometimes got edema of leg (Kidney qi deficiency, blood stasis ⑤). He occasionally suffered reflex vomiting from too much smoke.

In X-2 year, hematuria was detected. In February of X-1 year, a benign left tonsil tumour was extracted (Blood stasis of Lung meridian ④-②). He stopped smoking after the extraction of this tumour.

Family history: There have been no particular problems in his family regarding cancer or malignant tumours.

Present status: Height, 171cm; weight, 60kg; BP, 146/80mmHg. Right pulse, string-like and slippery; left pulse, string-like; the body colour of the tongue is pale and dark, tooth-marked, and with a slimy yellowish fur (Dampness-heat of Spleen). There were no other particular problems.

Identification: Blood stasis in Kidney, Qi deficiency of Lung and Heart with fluid retention.

Treatments: Activate blood to remove stasis, clean heat, remove moistness and soothe liver, regulate qi.

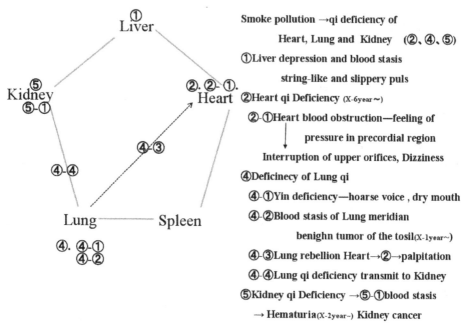

Smoke pollution →qi deficiency of

Heart, Lung and Kidney (②,④,⑤)

①Liver depression and blood stasis

string-like and slippery puls

②Heart qi Deficiency (X-6year~)

②-①Heart blood obstruction—feeling of

pressure in precordial region

Interruption of upper orifices, Dizziness

④Deficinecy of Lung qi

④-①Yin deficiency—hoarse voice , dry mouth

④-②Blood stasis of Lung meridian

benighn tumor of the tosil(X-1year~)

④-③Lung rebellion Heart→②→palpitation

④-④Lung qi deficiency transmit to Kidney

⑤Kidney qi Deficiency →⑤-①blood stasis

→ Hematuria(X-2year~) Kidney cancer

Fig. 8. Relations among viscera with five phase theory of case 8 (Reccurence of metastatic Kidney cancer in bladder)

Prescription: Prescription I composed of: ①Activate blood group: hong-hua (Carthami Flos 3), chuan-xion (Chuanxion Rhizoma 3), dan-shen (Salviae miltiorrhizae Radix 4), yu-jin (Curcumae Radix 3), san-qi (Notoginseng Radix 3, separately taken), she- chong (Eupolyphaga 3.5) and e-shu (Zedoariae Rhizoma 3); ①-②Activate the blood and clean the heat group: mu-tan-pi (Moutan Cortex 3); ② Clean heat and remove dampness group: huang-qin (Scutellariae Radix 3), Huan-bo (Phellodendri Cortex 1); ③ Tonify Spleen qi and drain dampness group: Fu-ling (Poria 5), Bai-shu (Atractylodis Rhizoma 4) and Zhu-ling (Polyporus 3); ④ Spread Liver qi and reduce fever group: chai-hu (Bupleuri Radix 1); ⑤ Tonify the qi, nourish the blood and calm the spirit, augment Heart qi group: ling-zhi (Ganoderma 2); ⑥ Warms and unblocks the channels and collaterals and assists the yang group: gui-zhi (Cinnamomi Ramulus 2) and ⑦ moderate, harmonise and tonify Spleen group: gan-cao (Glycyrrhizae Radix 1.5). The numeral at the end of parenthesis mean the daily used weight. All materials were decocted in hot water with the instrument on the market with the regular method.

Clinical course: From September 28, X year, the patient started the prescription mentioned above and stopped smoking after the operation. During a periodic follow-up at the end of

October, no tumour was detected. On November 25, three small tumours (diameter, 1 mm) and 1 larger tumour (diameter, 5 mm) were found. Until the middle of March of the next year, as intravesical instillation of an anticancer drug was carried out every two weeks(eight times in total) with prescription I . During the periodic follow-up of April 6,X+1 year, only the 5-mm tumor was discovered to have survived and this was excised.

To this situation, Prescription II was added to Prescription I. Prescription II was composed of bai-hua-she-she-cao (Hydyotis diffusae Herba which clears heat and resolves dampness and fire toxicity 4.5), wang-bu-liu-xing(Viccariae Semen which promotes the movement of blood 4.5) and shui-zhi(Hirudo which breaks up and drives out blood stasis and reduces fixed masses 4.5) and continued without any conventional therapies. As a recurrence was not recognised at the periodic check, the moiety of the decoction was halved from October X+1. In April X+2 year, he returned to work and continued to take the same volume of the decoction. From X+11 to X+13year, he reduced his dose at 1/6 of the initial volume, and since X+14 he stopped. Now, more than three years have passed since then and without any recurrence.

Discussion: A therapy of Prescription I with an anticancer infusion every two weeks for four months did not work to eradicate remaining one biggest cancer. Since then, Prescription I combined with Prescription II has been continued for fourteen years. After stopping this, more than three years has passed without a recurrence, so far, which will mean Prescription I and II worked to inhibit the recurrence. The fact that, by stopping smoking in X year before the first visit, the symptoms of Heart and Lung quickly disappeared would imply that these symptoms are all derived from smoking.

In X-6 year, Lung related symptoms (hoarseness and pharyngitis) appeared with Heart related symptoms (a feeling of tightness in chest) appearing in X-4 year; these symptoms have continued and aggravated with palpitations. In X-2 year, hematuria appeared for the first time during a yearly medical check. In X-1 year, benign tonsil tumour was resected. This could mean Lung abnormality rebels Heart when his palpitations started(④-③). Next abnormalities transmitted to Kidney through the engendering route from Lung to Kidney.

By stopping smoking before the first visit, the symptoms of the Heart and Lung had nearly all disappeared, but the abnormal situation of Kidney could not change.

Drugs for activating the blood and moving qi, cleaning the heat and removing dampness, and tonifying the qi, worked synergistically to restore satisfactory function of Kidney such that the cancers would not recur.

A case of depression

Case 9 A 38-year-old Japanese housewife and office worker (48 kg, 155cm)

First visit: On 16th of February in X year

Chief complaints: Depression, spiritlessness, a dull feeling in the stomach, menstrual pain

Clinical history: She began working at age twenty-one, and married at age twenty-five. At thirty-five years, she changed her job because it involved too much stress. She has been suffering from depression, spiritlessness (Liver qi depression and stagnation ①), stiffness of the shoulder and a blocked feeling of the blood vessels in the temple and at the base of the neck (Blood stasis ①-①). Stress creates a dull feeling in the stomach (Wood overwhelms Earth ①-④). Manual therapy improved her condition (freeing the collateral vessels), premenstrual nausea (③-③), and the blood-shot condition and mucus of her right eye

(Liver qi stagnation-transforming into heat ①-②). Other symptoms included a dry feeling of the skin and lip (①-②), coldness of the forefoot, constipation which improved by warming(Kidney yang deficiency ⑤-①). She suffered from profuse dreaming (disquieted heart mind ①-③), hot palms (yin deficiency - fever of three yin meridians of the hand), hay fever with rhinorrhea in fatigue (Spleen–Kidney yang deficiency → water dampness failing in transportation → cold fluid retention in Lung ⑤-②). She smokes ten cigarettes a day (arteriosclerotic progression, impaired viscera).

Past history: During primary school days, she often suffered from convulsions on falling asleep (her yin and yang couldn't copulate successfully). In the past, she has been pale, with a tooth-marked tongue (Spleen yang deficiency with dampness retention ③.③-②), and her sublingual collateral vessels showed blood stasis (Liver qi depression and blood stasis ①-①).

States Present: Height is 162cm; weight is 59kg; pulse is string like, slippery, fine, 72/min; tongue has a pale body and is teeth-marked (retention of water ③-①、③-②) with a thin white fur.

Sublingual blackish vessel is enlarged (blood stasis).

Identification: Liver qi depression and static blood, Liver overwhelms Spleen, Liver causes rebellion in Lung, Spleen–Kidney yang deficiency

Treatment: Soothe Liver. Harmonise Liver and spleen. Warm and free collateral vessels.

Prescriptions and herbs: Si-ni-san[Ref 26] (in Japanese: Shigyakusan*1 - soothes liver, regulates qi, harmonises liver and spleen) [Ref 26] together with xion-gui-tiao-xue-yin[Ref27] (in Japanese: Kyukichoketsuin*2 - this regulates qi, activates blood, tonifies blood/regulates menstruation; this originates from Wan- bin-gui-chun), ban-xia (Rhizoma Pinelliae Ternatae - this dries dampness and transforms phlegm), mahuang (Ephedrae Herba - this induces sweating and releases the exterior) and gui zhi (Cinammomi Ramulus - this releases the exterior and warms yang to unblock the meridian)

(*1: Si-ni-san: chai-fu, shao-yao, zhi-shi, gan-cao

*2: Xion gui tiao xue yin :dan-gui, chun-xiong, sheng-di-huang, bai-chu, fu-ling, chen-pi,

*3: wu-yao, xiang-fu-zi, mu-dan-pi, yi-mu-cao, da-zao, sheng-jiang, gan-cao)

Clinical course: A numerical Rating Scale (NRS) employing the patient's self-report of symptoms in numerals (with the worst condition experienced so far scored as 10 and with no symptoms scored as 0) was used to monitor the course (Fig 9), and the patient's disease situation was described with five-phase theory (Fig 10).

Discussion As shown in Figs. 9 and 10, herbal therapy decreased the NRS. Since I do not prescribe special medicines for Kidney, the improvement of foot coldness was not so successful.

However, other symptoms improved relatively well. Si-ni-san mainly worked to reduce Liver qi stagnation and, with xion-gui-tiao-xue-yin in collaboration, this removed the blood stasis and regulated qi. Furthermore, the rebellion in the lung from Liver must have decreased since, in spite of the absence of treatment for rhinorrhea in fatigue, it disappeared completely (data not shown). The dull feeling in the stomach evoked by stress decreased comparatively well, which means that overwhelm in the stomach disappeared. The simultaneous treatment of every imbalanced viscus often leads to quick recovery because every normalised viscus works simultaneously and synergistically..

The qi movement of each phase will be normalised by this treatment.

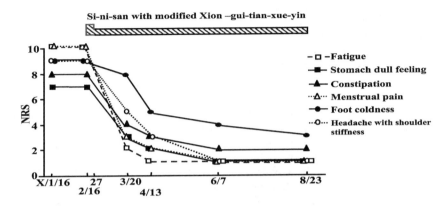

Fig 9 Clinical course of case 9 after taking Si-ni-san with Xion gui tian xue yin

Fig. 9. Clinical course of case 9 after taking Si-ni-san with Xion gui tian zue yin.

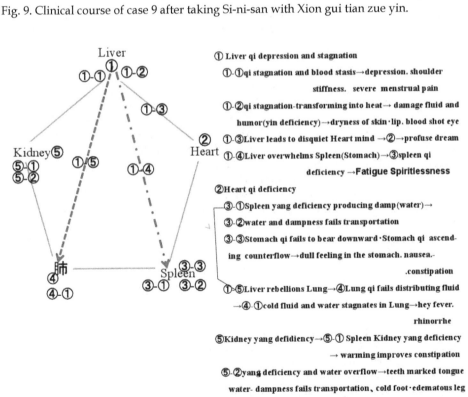

Fig. 10. Relations among viscera with five phase theory of case 9.

Asthma with dyspnea and general fatigue

Case 10   A 50-year-old Japanese female who works for a Japanese pub
Chief complaint: The patient finds it impossible to lie down, due to dyspnea and palpitation (Lung and Heart qi deficiency ②,④). She experiences suffocating dyspnea and general fatigue. Perfumes, cigars, cosmetics and other stimuli cause dyspnea. She has asthma and is sensitive to chemical substances (Lang qi deficiency ④).

History of present illness: For almost a year, beginning in the summer when her stress tremendously increased, she had been suffering from palpitation and suffocating dyspnea (Probably, Liver rebellions Lung, Heart and Lung qi deficiency ①-⑤.②,④), and she could not lie down or maintain a sitting posture with general fatigue (Lung qi deficiency ④). Furthermore, she had cold limbs, sensitivity to coldness, frequent urination during the night, and edema (Kidney Yang deficiency ⑤-①, ⑤-②) and condition worsens on rainy days. She doesn't want to drink water even though she feels thirsty (Kidney yang deficiency with water flood ⑤-①.⑤-②). She often had concentrated urine, her soles are hot during the night (Kidney yin deficiency ⑤-③). She experienced fullness in the abdomen after meals, has many stressors in her life, breast pain, and fullness of the chest around the time of menstruation (Liver depression and qi stagnation ①-①).

Additionally, she has had severe shoulder stiffness, enlargement of the sublingual vessel (blood stasis ①-①), asthenopia, dim eyesight, numbness of limbs (Blood deficiency of liver ①-②), headache, a short temper, facial hotness, and she prefers cold water (ascendant hyperactivity of liver yang ①-③). She cannot sleep easily, having insomnia, profuse dreaming, and a feeling of uneasiness (Heart blood and yin deficiency ②.②-①).

She is sensitive to various chemical substances, such as smoke, dust, insecticide, cosmetics, exhaust gas, and the smell of dishes (Lung qi deficiency ④). The adrenal cortex hormone that she takes causes eye pain, headache, skin irritation and choking (Lung qi deficiency ④). At another clinic, yi-gan-san[Ref 28] (this pacifies liver to extinguish wind)[*1] added with banxia (Rhizoma Pinelliae Ternatae - this dries dampness, transforms phlegm), chen-pi (Citri reticulatae Pericarpium - this regulates qi, dries dampness, transforms phlegm), si ni san[Ref 26], qin-fei-tang[Ref 25] with xing-gan-shi-tang, chai-hu-gui-zhi-tang (in Japanese: Saikokeishito - this releases and harmonises lesser yang-stage disorders and releases the muscle layer and exterior), ban-xia-hou-po-tang (in Japanese: Hangekobokuto - this promotes qi movement, dissipates clumps, directs rebellious qi downward, and transforms phlegm) were prescribed with conventional drugs such as montelukast sodium, salmeterol xinafoate and procaterol, but these were not effective.

(*1 chai-fu, can-zao,dan-gui,bai-chu.fu-ling,diao-teng-gou)

Past history: She had suffered from alopecia areata, which is possibly stress-induced.

Present status: Height 162cm; weight 51.5kg; the tip of the tongue is red (Heart meridian has heat) and there is a fissure in the middle of the body of the tongue (Spleen yin deficiency); the tongue's fur is thin, pale and white; the sublingual vessel is blackish and enlarged (blood stasis).

Pulse: float and weak (Heart blood and yin deficiency)

Identification: Liver qi stagnation with blood stasis ((①-①), Blood deficiency of Liver and Heart ((①-②, ②-①), Liver yin deficiency with ascendant hyperactivity of Liver yang ((①-③). Liver overwhelms Spleen ((①-④), Liver rebellions Lung ((①-⑤). She had to use bronchodilators, such as salmeterol xinafoate and procaterol hydrochloride. She worked for long hours in the air conditioning and her limbs must have been cooled, causing the Kidney yang to decrease, which might be inversely transmitted to Lung and which may be one of the reasons for the aggravation of her asthma.

Treatments: Tonify Lung qi, soothe Liver, regulate qi, tonify Heart qi and blood,tonify qi, yin and yang of Kidney.

Prescriptions: ① zi-yin-zhi-bao-tang[Ref 29] (in Japanese: Jiinshihoto – this soothes Liver, regulates qi, tonifies Spleen and tonifies yin to clear Lung)[*a]; ② zhi-gan-cao-tang; ③ ba-wei-di-huang-wan (the same as in case 3)

([*a]:dang-gui, bai-shao, bai-chu, fu-ling, chen-pi, zhi-mu, bei-mu, xian-fu-zi, di-gu-pi, mai-men-dong bao-he, chai-fu, gan-cao.)

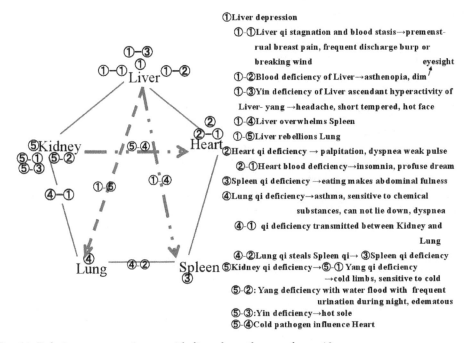

①Liver depression
  ①-①Liver qi stagnation and blood stasis→premenstrual breast pain, frequent discharge burp or breaking wind   eyesight
  ①-②Blood deficiency of Liver→asthenopia, dim
  ①-③Yin deficiency of Liver ascendant hyperactivity of Liver- yang →headache, short tempered, hot face
  ①-④Liver overwhelms Spleen
  ①-⑤Liver rebellions Lung
②Heart qi deficiency → palpitation, dyspnea weak pulse
  ②-①Heart blood deficiency→insomnia, profuse dream
③Spleen qi deficiency →eating makes abdominal fulness
④Lung qi deficiency→asthma, sensitive to chemical substances, can not lie down, dyspnea
  ④-① qi deficiency transmitted between Kidney and Lung
  ④-②Lung qi steals Spleen qi→ ③Spleen qi deficiency
⑤Kidney qi deficiency→⑤-① Yang qi deficiency →cold limbs, sensitive to cold
  ⑤-②: Yang deficiency with water flood with frequent urination during night, edematous
  ⑤-③:Yin deficiency→hot sole
  ⑤-④Cold pathogen influence Heart

Fig. 11. Relations among viscera with five phase theory of case 10.

Clinical course Prescriptions were administered in late April. Ten days later, on May 11, she visited the clinic and reported that, although she was not completely cured, her condition was much improved and that she could resume working. The abnormal sensation of the Lung disappeared. Dyspnea during the day improved, but at night it was still not good. On May 31, she reported that daytime dyspnea had disappeared and that at night her asthma fits decreased and she did not need to use the bronchodilator. She could work without trouble. On June 17, she reported that she had stopped using two of her three bronchodilators and could pursue a routine life as in previous days when she was healthy. Only when she was tired would she use her bronchodilator in order to prevent fits.

Discussion: Her asthma fits began during the summer one year ago, before she visited my clinic. As she experienced much stress through her work, Liver qi stagnation may have played a role in this aggravation. However, many Liver-soothing formulas did not work. I supposed that her asthma was aggravated not only by rebellion from Liver but also from the

Lung qi deficiency brought about from Kidney yang deficiency that was transmitted inversely to Lung. This may be because, during the summer, she worked for long hours in the air conditioning and her limbs must have been cooled, causing Kidney yang to decrease, which was inversely transmitted to Lung. Moreover, she has been - by her nature - sensitive to coldness. Her deficiency of Heart qi may be a result of the mutual relation between the Lung and Heart. Some rebellion from the Kidney of yang deficiency may participate in the Heart qi deficiency. These included zi-yin-zhi-bao-tang for soothing the Liver and regulating qi, tonifying the Spleen and yin to clear the Lung[Ref 30], zhi-gan-cao-tang (Tsumura Co.) for augmenting the qi, nourishing blood, enriching the yin of Heart and restoring the pulse, and Ba-wei-di-huang-wan for warming and tonifying the yang of the Kidney. This means we treat all viscera at the same time. This is the reason she could recover so promptly from her disease and could work again. As a general rule, treating the dysfunction of all viscera to restore their qi at the same time will lead to a quick recovery, based on the smooth circulation of respective qi among viscera with synergy. If one of them were not to have been treated, the recovery would have been slower. (The treatment of this patient was carried out by Dr Shimizu Ishigaki, Director of Yasookodomo Clinic, Shizuoka Prefecture and the author).

Difficulty in walking with staggering for more than 1 year

Case 11: A 67-year-old Japanese housewife 160 cm, 68 kg

Chief complaint: Dizziness, staggering, difficulty in walking (Heart blood and qi deficiency,②-① → interruption of upper orifices), dyspnea, susceptibility to catching colds (Lung qi deficiency ④-①), edema of face and limb (retention of water produced by yang deficiency (③-①-①, ⑤-①), coldness from occipital region to the back (Coldness of Du Meridian: governor vessel), facial flush (stagnated Liver qi transforming into fire → Liver yin deficiency ①-②-①, ③-②), cold forefoot (Kidney yang deficiency ⑤), hand stiffness, numbness and pain on rising (Liver qi deficiency, blood stasis ①).

Clinical history: First visit: February 22 2006. Since more than two years ago, she has often pitched forward and has had a sensation of walking on air in spite of her paying close attention to her gait. Many thorough examinations by brain surgeons, and at several major hospitals, have produced no explanation for these symptoms. She had been suffering from insomnia, profuse dreams and amnesia (Liver, Heart blood deficiency. ①-③, ②-①), a feeling of stool stasis, abdominal fullness (Liver overwhelms Spleen, Spleen qi deficiency, gastric hyperacidity ①-④, ③), edema of face and limbs for several years (Spleen yang deficiency, retention of water and moisture. ③-①-①), low blood pressure on rising, aggravated by warmth, shoulder stiffness (stagnated Liver qi and blood stasis ①,①-①), dry eyes, blood-shot eyes, heat in her palm (Liver depression transforming into fire → Liver yin deficiency ①-②-①), a heavy feeling in her legs (moisture retention by Kidney yang deficiency ⑤-⑤-①), back pain on catching a cold (Lung qi deficiency④, ④-①), and chronic pancreatitis based upon her being a kitchen drinker for the past seventeen years (Spleen dampness–heat ③). She had her menopause at age fifty-six.

Past history: She suffered from rotary dizziness with vomiting between the ages of around forty and fifty (③,③-①). She takes camost mesilate from time to time because of chronic pancreatitis.

Family history: Her older brother died from pancreatic cancer and her younger sister died from lung cancer. She has three children.

Present illness: 72/min, fine, slippery, sunken pulse (Heart qi deficiency ②); a pale red tongue with white fur; over-swelling of dark sublingual collateral vessels (blood stasis). Standing blood pressure 110/80, sitting pressure 140/80.

Identification: Liver depression with blood stasis, fluid retention with yang deficiency of Spleen and Kidney; Deficiency of Heart qi and blood; Interruption to upper orifices

Treatment: Soothe Liver and regulate qi, activate blood, free the collateral vessels, remove moisture and tonify Spleen.

Prescriptions: Bu-yang-huan-wu-tang (BYHWT: tonifies the qi, invigorates the blood, and unblocks the channels)[Ref 30] [a] combined with she-chong-yin (in Japanese: Sesyoin – this activates blood to solve stasis)[Ref 31] [b] included BYHWT, yan-hu-suo (this invigorates the blood and promotes the movement of qi), niu-xi (this invigorates the blood and dispel blood stasis), mu-tan-pi (this clears heat and invigorates and dispels the blood), gui-zhi (this releases the exterior, assists the yang, warms and unblocks the channels and collaterals). Further, gan-cao, wu-yao (this regulates qi, warms the Kidney) , xiang-fu-zi (this spreads and regulates Liver qi, regulates menstruation and alleviates pain), chai-fu(Bupleuri Radix which spreads Liver qi and reduce fever), jie-geng (Platycodi Radix - this opens up and disseminates the Lung qi, pushes out puss and opens up and raises Lung qi) and wu-ling-san (in Japanese: Goreisan - this promotes urination, drains dampness, warms the yang and resolves qi).were added.

([a]: bu-yang-huan-wu-tang:huang-qi, dang-gui, chuan-xion, chi-shao, tao-ren hong-hua and di-long.

[b]: she-chong-yin: tao-ren, dan-gui, mu-tan-pi, chuan-xion, chi-shao, gui-zhi, yan-hu-suo, niu-xi,hong^hua.)

Clinical course: Her constipation disappeared after almost two-and-a-half months. Her dizziness, staggering, pain and the numbness of her hands also improved tremendously within around four months.

Discussion

This patient has had too much stress for a long time, as she became a kitchen drinker with pancreatitis seventeen years ago. Stress made Liver qi depression and blood stagnation - especially in upper orifice - will be the main reason for her dizziness, staggering, and difficulty in walking and probably for her low standing blood pressure (①-①). The excessive over-swelling of her sublingual vessel implies the occurrence of severe blood stagnation. As Liver overwhelmed Spleen, she displayed many symptoms through her digestive system relating to water retention, including pancreatitis. Furthermore, her stress was so enormous that she had dyspnoea, with coldness causing her back pain (Liver rebellions Lung). As she has Kidney yang deficiency, seen through cold feet with a stagger, as well as the retention of moisture (⑤, ⑤-①), this might be caused by overwhelm from Spleen cold evil to Kidney and aging. Enormous Liver abnormalities, transmitted to Heart to cause palpitation, arrhythmia, dizziness with a stagger and blood deficiency (②,②-①). Water or moisture retention may influence her dizziness and staggering to some extent.

I classified herb mixtures (BYHWT+she-chong-yin+others): Gr 1,to activate Blood in order to solve Blood stasis (chuan-xion,chi-shao, tao-ren, hong-hua yan-hu-suo, niu-xi, mu-tan-pi), Gr 2 so as to tonify Blood(dan-gui,chuan-xion); Gr 3 to tonify qi(huang-qi); Gr 4 to regulate Liver qi(chai-fu); Gr 5 to regulate qi(yan-fu-suo, xiang-fu-zi, wu-yao), and Gr 6 including others (gyu-zhi,gan-cao,jie-geng,di-long,wu-ling-san).

Gr-1, Gr-2, Gr-3 and Gr-4 will work to soothe Liver, regulate qi, activate stagnated blood and tonify blood of Liver and Heart. As a result, the transmission of abnormal qi to Heart from Liver, rebellion to Lung from Liver and overwhelm to Spleen from Liver will all decrease. Gr 1, Gr 2, Gr 3, gui-zhi and gan-cao will also operate to tonify Kidney qi and for Spleen and Lung as well. Wu-ling-san would support disappearance of water retention.

As such, each of the five viscus qi is tonified which leads to smooth recovery of her symptoms. Notably, after around two years of taking herbs, she became symptomless and was able to stop two years later without recurrence more than three years.

I suppose main reason of her recovery will be the disappearance of stagnated blood in brain and other parts of the body.

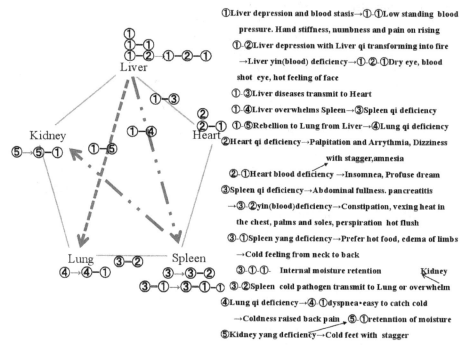

Fig. 12. Relations among viscera with five phase theory of case 11.

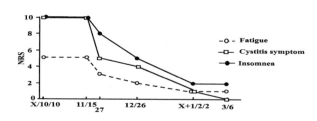

Fig14 Clinical course after taking herbal medecines of case 11

Fig. 13. Clinical course after taking herbal medecines of case 11.

10. Acknowledgement

Dr. Naoki Hirama MD.,Ph.D., director of Japanese Traditional Chinese Medicine and director of Hirama Clinic, for valuable suggestions and advices to this chapter.
Mr Hitoshi Matsunaga working for TSUMURA & CO. for valuable advices.
Xi Lu., lecturer of Traditional Chinese Medicine Foundation of Osaka. Member of Kobe Chuigaku Kenkyukai, for his instructive advices.
Yoko Takahashi, the visiting professor Shanghai University of Traditional Chinese Medicine for her instructive advices.
I am grateful to Dr. Dai Yong Sheng on literaturewhich I failed to include in the work because of failureto get them in time.

11. References

[1] *East Asian Medical Studies Society: Fundamentals Of Chinese Medicine.* Paradigm Publication:1985 p10-22

[2] (xiang-jie)zhong-yi-ji-chu-li-lun: Liu-yan-chi Gong-tian-bin-fu Zhang- rui-fu Jin-lian-rong. Toyogakujyutsusyuppan Kanagawaprefecture 1999 p36-58

[3] (xiang-jie) zhong-yi-ji-chu-li-lun: liu-yan-chi song-tian-bin-fu zhang- rui-fu jin-lian-rong. Toyogakujyutsusyuppan Kanagawaprefecture 1999. p48-50. This book was translated from [Liu-yan-chi"zhong-yi-ji-chu-li-lun-wen-da" Shang-hai-ke-ji-chu-ban-she] 1982.

[4] Song-lu-bing. pian, Chai-qi-ying-zi yi *Zhong-yi-bing-yin-bing-ji-xue* Toyogakujyutsu-syuppan Kanagawa prefecture 1998 p44-49

[5] *East Asian Medical Studies Society: Fundamentals of Chinese Medicine.* Paradigm Publication: 1985:79-84.

[6] *East Asian Medical Studies Society: Fundamentals of Chinese Medici*ne. Paradigm Publication: 1985:p232-243.

[7] *East Asian Medical Studies Society: Fundamentals of Chinese Medicine.* Paradigm Publication: 1985: p233-242

[8] *East Asian Medical Studies Society: Fundamentals of Chinese Medicine.* Paradigm Publication: 1985:p67-72

[9] *East Asian Medical Studies Society: Fundamentals of Chinese Medicine.* Paradigm Publication: 1985:p204-211

[10] *East Asian Medical Studies Society: Fundamentals of Chinese Medicine.* Paradigm Publication: 1985:p74-78

[11] *East Asian Medical Studies Society: Fundamentals of Chinese Medicine.* Paradigm Publication: 1985:p218-232

[12] *East Asian Medical Studies Society: Fundamentals of Chinese Medicine.* Paradigm Publication: 1985:p70-73

[13] *East Asian Medical Studies Society: Fundamentals of Chinese Medicine.* Paradigm Publication: 1985:p211-218

[14] *East Asian Medical Studies Society: Fundamentals of Chinese Medicine.* Paradigm Publication: 1985:p184-187

[15] *East Asian Medical Studies Society: Fundamentals of Chinese Medicine.* Paradigm Publication: 1985:p243-249

[16] *East Asian Medical Studies Society: Fundamentals of Chinese Medicine.* Paradigm Publication: 1985:p250-263

[17] Nikeghbalian S, Pournasr B, Aghdami N et al., Autologous transplantation of bone marrow-derived mononuclear and CD133(+) cells in patients with decompensated cirrhosis. *Arch Iran Med.* 2011 Jan;14(1):p12-17

[18] Takami T, Terai S, Sakaida I, Novel findings for the development of drug therapy for various liver diseases: current state and future prospects for our liver regeneration therapy using autologous bone marrow cells for decompensated liver cirrhosis patients. *J.Pharmacol. Sci.* 2011;115(3):p274-278

[19] *East Asian Medical Studies Society: Fundamentals of Chinese Medicine.* Paradigm Publication: 1985:p203-249

[20] Yasui H, APPENDIX - Composition and Indications of 148 Prescriptions. *The Journal of Kampo, Acupuncture and Integrative Medicine* (KAIM) Volume 1, Special Edition.November 2005 P14

[21] Hijikata Y, Tsukamoto Y, Effect of herbal therapy on herpes labialis and herpes genitalis. *Biotherapy.* 1998;11:p235-240.

[22] Yasuhara A, Yuka Y, Hijikata Y, Effect of herbal therapy on chronic herpes virus infections. *Alternative Therapies in Health and Medicine.* 9(5): 2003 p132-136

[23] Yasui H, APPENDIX-Composition and Indications of 148 Prescriptions. Zi-yin-jiang-huo-tang, *The Journal of Kampo, Acupuncture and Integrative Medicine* (KAIM) Volume 1, Special Edition. November 2005 p101.

[24] Yasui H, APPENDIX-Composition and Indications of 148 Prescriptions. Nu-shen san. *The Journal of Kampo, Acupuncture and Integrative Medicine* (KAIM) Volume 1, Special Edition.November 2005 p92

[25] Yasui H, APPENDIX-Composition and Indications of 148 Prescriptions. Qin-fei-tang. *The Journal of Kampo, Acupuncture and Integrative Medicine* (KAIM) Volume 1, Special Edition.November 2005 p87

[26] Yasui H, APPENDIX-Composition and Indications of 148 Prescriptions. Si-ni-san. *The Journal of Kampo, Acupuncture and Integrative Medicine* (KAIM) Volume 1, Special Edition.November 2005 p89

[27] Yasui H, APPENDIX-Composition and Indications of 148 Prescriptions. Xion gui tiao xue yin *The Journal of Kampo, Acupuncture and Integrative Medicine* (KAIM) Volume 1, Special Edition.November 2005 p99

[28] Yasui H, APPENDIX-Composition and Indications of 148 Prescriptions. Yi-gan-san. *The Journal of Kampo, Acupuncture and Integrative Medicine* (KAIM) Volume 1, Special Edition.November 2005 p93

[29] Yasui H, APPENDIX-Composition and Indications of 148 Prescriptions. Zi-yin-zhi-bao-tang. *The Journal of Kampo, Acupuncture and Integrative Medicine* (KAIM) Volume 1, Special Edition.November 2005 p101

[30] Bensky D, and Barolet R, *Formulas that Warm the Menses and Dispel Blood Statis. Chinese Herbal Medicine - Formulas & Strategies, Eastland Press;* 1990; p320-321

[31] Gagawa Genetsu, *Sanron* (describing the delivery of a baby) Saiseikan 1775

4

An Approach to the Nature of Qi in TCM–Qi and Bioenergy

Xing-Tai Li[1] and Jia Zhao[2]

[1]College of Life Science, Dalian Nationalities University, Dalian
[2]Norman Bethune College of Medicine, Jilin University, Changchun
China

1. Introduction

Traditional Chinese medicine (TCM), has been practiced for more than five thousand years, is a complete ancient medical system that takes a deep understanding of the laws and patterns of nature and applies them to the human body. TCM believes that the human body is a microcosm of the Universal macrocosm. Therefore, humans must follow the laws of the Universe to achieve harmony and total health. Even today TCM practitioners use these essential theories to understand, diagnose and treat health problems. In TCM, "harmony" is the ultimate goal. So, when nature's Qi undergoes change as it does seasonally, a person's internal Qi will respond automatically. If, for any reason, it can't make a smooth transition to the energy of the next season, TCM understands that illness will result. Often Western Complementary and Alternative Medicine (CAM) practitioners and their patients or clients derive their understanding of TCM from acupuncture. However, acupuncture is only one of the major treatment modalities of this comprehensive medical system based on the understanding of Qi or vital energy. These major treatment modalities are Qigong, herbal therapy, acupuncture, foods for healing and Chinese psychology.

Meridians, or channels, are invisible pathways through which Qi flows that form an energy network that connects all parts of the body, and the body to the universe. The ancient medical text 'The Yellow Emperor's Inner Canon (Nei Jing)' states: "The function of the channel (meridian) is to transport the Qi and blood, and circulate yin and yang to nourish the body". The energy practice of Qigong, with its postures and movements, also affects the flow of Qi. The energy pathways and the Organ Systems they link provide TCM with a framework for identifying the root cause of health problems and the diagnoses to heal them. Meridians work by regulating the energy functions of the body and keeping it in harmony. If Qi stagnates for too long in any meridian, it can become blocked and eventually turn into matter, setting the stage for conditions that can create a physical mass. TCM Meridian Theory states: "As long as Qi flows freely through the meridians and the Organs work in harmony, the body can avoid disease".

The study of Qi phenomena may help bridge some of the apparent difference between Western and Eastern culture. Several years ago, I was lucky to notice that some scientists contributed novel experimental works on Qi, and subsequently, the papers by Ohnishi *et al.*(2005) (Ohnishi first attended the school of Nishino Breathing Method in Tokyo over 10 years ago, and 3 years later, the collaboration with Mr Nishino started in order to find a scientific basis for Qi) stimulated the philosophical discussion by Flowers (2006). As Flowers beautifully described, in the Christian West, God was the center of everything as opposed to Qi being the center of everything in the East. Qi may be another name of 'life', Qi may represent the entity of life itself (Ohnishi *et al.*, 2007). Then, the understanding of Qi may shed light on other aspects of biological sciences. These articles prompted us to write this chapter covering the nature of Qi as well as its philosophical aspects and the significance in the modern civilization because the true foundation of TCM is Qi.

2. The history and concept of Qi

2.1 Qi in China

Qi (in Chinese, equivalent to Ki in Japanese) has been used as a healing technique in China for 4000 years. In Japan, Qi has been known to have a healing effect at least for 1500 years (Ohnishi *et al.*, 2007). The origin of the character of Qi was traced back to 3500 years ago. Confucius (who lived approximately 2500 years ago), taught moral and ethical behavior. In his Analects, the character of Qi appeared in four locations. It expressed the concept related to breathe, food and vitality. Taoism, which was founded by Lao-Tze (who was believed to have lived around the time of Confucius or 100 years later), have had more influence on Qi and Qigong. In the book 'Zhuangzi', which compiled the thoughts of Lao-Tze in the third century BC, the character of Qi appeared 39 times. What it explained was: 'Qi exists throughout the universe. When it assembles, it appears as a human life. When it disassembles, the human will dies. Therefore, do not worry about life and death. Live naturally and freely as you are'. The concepts of Qi, Yin/Yang and meridians formed the foundation of Chinese medicine.

A central medical classic, The Yellow Emperor's Inner Canon teaches us: 'It is from, calm, indifference, emptiness, and nondesiring that true Qi arises. If the spirit is harboured inside, whence can illness arise? When the will is at rest and wishes little, when the heart is at peace and fears nothing, when the body labours but does not tire, then Qi flows smoothly from these states, each part follows its desires, and the whole gets everything it seeks'. The Chinese philosopher, Mencius (372–289 BC) described Qi in terms of moral energy, related to human excellence. This reinforces the argument that Qi is contextual, fluid in nature and not a fixed entity.

Qi is pronounced "chee". You may see it spelled "Chi" or even "Ki" in Japanese, but they all carry the same meaning. What is meant by Qi? The concept of Qi is based on the ancient Chinese initial understanding of natural phenomena. That is, Qi is the most basic substance of which the world is comprised. Everything in the universe results from the movements and changes of Qi. Man depends on nature for his production and growth and must observe the common laws of the world. As everything in the world comes from the interaction of Heaven Qi and Earth Qi, man must breathe to absorb Heaven Qi and eat to absorb Earth Qi. Qi was originally a philosophic concept. The ancient Chinese philosophy holds that Qi is the most basic substance constituting the world. This concept was introduced into TCM and became one of its characteristics. Accordingly, TCM also believes that Qi is the most fundamental substance in the construction of the human body and in the maintenance of its life activities. After a comprehensive survey of the statements on Qi in TCM documents, we have come to the conclusion that the meaning of Qi in TCM has two aspects. One refers to the vital substances comprising the human body and maintaining its life activities. The other refers to the physiological functions of viscera and bowels, channels and collaterals. For example, clean Qi, turbid Qi, and the Qi of water and food (food essence) are substantial Qi, while the Qi of the heart, liver, spleen, kidney, stomach, and the Qi of the channels and collaterals are functional Qi. In TCM, Qi is considered to be the force that animates and informs all things. In the human body, Qi flows through meridians, or energy pathways. Qi is the most basic substances that constitute the human body and maintain its functional activities. Generally speaking, Qi is an essential substance that is full of vigor and flows fast. Qi is attributed to Yang, because it is mobile and functions to move and warm. In this sense, Qi is also named Yang Qi.

2.2 Qi in other countries

Qi, that which defies definition, is the key concept in Eastern medicine, Eastern philosophy, as well as in martial arts (Yuasa, 1993). It naturally follows that Qi is an important element in complementary and alternative medicine (CAM). Many authors have presented work on the effects and nature of Qi (Chang, 2003; Lee, 2003; Chen, 2004; Olalde, 2005; Hankey and McCrum, 2006; Shinnick, 2006; Weze et al., 2007; Abbott et al., 2007). For the pre-modern Chinese, Qi comprised both yin and yang, with duality and interdependence in operation. In this thinking, to narrowly define Qi is considered unnecessary. The workings of nature were explained as the workings of Qi. Qi was all encompassing. Humans were subject to the workings of Qi as well as being agents of Qi, every person being so in different ways and at different times. Still, we can not precisely describe Qi. We cannot objectively say 'Look! This is Qi'. When Western people talk about Qi in terms of the healing arts, Qi seems to be understood as 'vitality' or 'life-energy'. For those who are studying Chinese medicine, Qi is presented as being a substance flowing in our body along the 'meridians'. In the view of martial artists, Qi is a source of spiritual strength for winning. When an Eastern philosopher defines Qi, it is a function of life, which permeates through the life of an individual and the life of the universe. Physicists see it as a new kind of 'energy', and still, brain physiologists approach it as 'information' or 'entropy' (Ohnishi and Ohnishi, 2009a). Thermographical studies demonstrated that skin temperature was raised by 3–4°C when exposed to Qi emitted from Qigong healers (Machi, 1993). When Qi was received from Nishino, instructors of his school or from students who practice for many years, a warm sensation was felt. This again supports the idea that Qi has an infrared radiation component (Ohnishi et al., 2007). Depending upon one's profession, discipline and necessity, Qi is understood differently, this looks like reports from many blind persons touching different parts of an elephant.

Qi has energy and entropy aspects. While it is often described in the West as energy, or vital energy, Qi is the energy of the body, of the meridians, of food, of the universe. The term Qi carries a deeper meaning. Qi has two aspects: one is energy, power, or force; the other is conscious intelligence or information. Many believe Qi is an 'energy'. However, it is interesting to note that there is a subtle difference in understanding between the Chinese and the Japanese. The former seems to believe that it is a 'substance' or 'matter' flowing in and through our bodies, and that it can be emitted from the body of a Qigong healer. In contrast, the Japanese considers that it is a form of energy. An interesting concept was published by Shinagawa's group that treats Qi as a form of 'information' (Shinagawa, 1990). Flowers considers Qi as being about 'relationships and patterning'. These concepts are another way of describing 'information'. The most interesting practice in Nishino Breathing Method (NBM) is called the Taiki-practice (a method developed by Kozo Nishino, the founder of the NBM, to develop the level of individual's Qi through the Qi communication between an instructor and a student). Through the study on the Taiki-practice, Ohnishi *et al.* (2006) raised the possibility that Qi-energy may carry information, and that the information is in a form of 'entropy'. If Qi consists of simple energy, then, Qi effects might be mimicked by an instrument. However, if Qi involves entropy, it may be difficult to artificially reproduce the entire Qi effect.

China has, in recent decades, spent an inordinate amount of resources on experiments to determine the existence and nature of Qi. China is easing up on this research for lack of concrete breakthroughs. But the quest to define Qi continues, with there being no breakthroughs that we know of. Whether someone in China or anywhere has the Holy Grail hidden from view I cannot say, but in the report by Ohnishi, it is claimed that the effects of Qi energy can be measured. The question is also posed of what Qi actually is. Qi acts as Subtle Energy? We have still not defined Qi.

3. The formation of Qi

Qi of the human body comes from the combination of three kinds of Qi, Primordial Qi inherited from parents, the fresh air inhaled by the Lung and the refined food Essence transformed by the Spleen. Primordial Qi is derived from the Congenital Essence of the parents and is the primary substance to produce an embryo. So it forms the basis of the human body and its life activities. Without Congenital Essence, there can be no human body. After birth, the congenital Essence is stored in the Kidney to promote development and to control the reproductive activity of the human body. The refined food Essence is generated by the food which is taken in after birth and is distributed all over the body to produce nutrients and Qi and Blood under the action of the Spleen and Stomach. Fresh air is inhaled by the Lung after birth and is the main source of Qi of the human body.

From the process of formation of Qi, we can see that Qi of the human body is closely related to the functional activities of the Kidney, the Spleen and Stomach, and the Lung, in addition to the congenital constitution, food and nutrients, and the environment. Only when these organs function properly can the Qi of the body flourish. Conversely, dysfunction of any of these organs will influence the formation of Qi and the physiological function of Qi. For example, dysfunction of the Lung will weaken respiration, leading to failure of fresh air to be inhaled and the turbid Qi of the body to be exhaled, with the resultant inadequate formation of Qi. The transformation and transportation of the Spleen and Stomach play a particular role in the formation of Qi, for man relies on the nutrients transformed and transported by the Spleen and Stomach for his life after birth. On one hand, the Spleen sends up nutrients to the Lung to be dispersed, on the other hand, it sends down nutrients to the Kidney to supplement Kidney Essence. So, hypofunctioning of the Spleen and Stomach influences all three elementary substances that produce Qi.

4. The functions of Qi

Generally speaking, different kinds of Qi have different functions. Qi of the human body serves several vital functions within the body. When imbalances arise, they are seen as disruptions in the functions of Qi. A prolapse, for example, is seen as a disruption in the ability of Qi to provide the raising and stabilizing function on a particular organ. The main functions of Qi within the body are listed below:

4.1 Promoting function

Qi is a sort of essence full of vitality. It can promote the growth and development of the human body, promote the physiological functions of each viscera, bowel, channel, collateral, tissue and organ and speed up the formation and circulation of blood and the metabolism of body fluid as well. For example, if the above functions are weakened as a result of the deficiency of Qi (vital energy), the following will occur: late and slow growth and development of the human body or senilism; weakened functions of viscera and bowels, channels and collaterals, tissues and other organs; insufficient blood formation or stagnation in blood vessels; and disturbance in the metabolism of body fluid. After birth, the Genuine Qi generated from Kidney Essence determines the growth and development of the human body. After middle age, Genuine Qi gradually declines, so a person grows old. If his Genuine Qi is deficient, a person's development will be poor.

The physiological functions of viscera and bowels and Channels and Collaterals of the human body all depend on the pushing of Qi as well as the nourishing of Blood. The vigor and the ascending, descending, exit and entry movements of Qi play a very important role in promoting the functional activities of viscera and bowels and Channels and Collaterals. Therefore, when Qi is deficient, hypofunctioning of viscera and bowels will ensue. For instance, deficient Lung Qi often leads to feeble breathing, a lower voice, lassitude, weak pulse, etc. Qi also promotes the generation, distribution and discharge of the Blood and Body Fluids. As Yin substances, Blood and Body Fluids depend on Qi's activities to be generated. In other words, generation of these substances relies on the activities of Qi of the Spleen and the Stomach, the Lung and the Kidney. Besides, Qi is a vigorous substance, so it can activate the flow of Blood and Body Fluids, as well as transform them into various secretions and excretions. For this reason, Qi Deficiency often leads to an impeded flow of Blood or stagnation of Blood, or retention of Body Fluids in the body, which, in turn, causes Phlegm or edema.

In TCM theory, blood and Qi are inseparable. Blood is the "mother" of Qi; it carries Qi and also provides nutrients for its movement. In turn, Qi is the "commander" of the blood. This means that Qi is the force that makes blood flow throughout the body. Losing too much blood causes an overall Qi deficiency. When there is a Qi deficiency, the body cannot function properly.

4.2 Warming function

Qi, as a Yang substance, is rich in heat, which can warm viscera and bowels, Channels, skin, and muscles and tendons, to maintain normal body temperature and the normal functional activities of these organs and tissues. Qi helps to control homeostasis and provides warmth for the body. Yellow Emperor's Inner Canon says: "Qi has a warming action". Qi is the main source of the heat needed by the human body. The body keeps its constant temperature mainly through the warming action of its Qi. Motion produces heat, so the heat carried by Qi is in fact, a result of the constant movement of Qi, and the body temperature is maintained by the constant movement of Qi. In addition, Qi's warming function contributes to the movement of Blood and Body Fluids. The warming effect of Qi is an imperative condition for the free flow of Blood and Body Fluids within the body.

Pathologically, disorders of Qi in its warming function are mainly manifested as two kinds: one is a cold manifestation due to Deficiency of Qi, which results mostly from the deficient

Qi failing to produce adequate Heat to warm the body, marked by aversion to cold and a desire for warmth, cold limbs, lower body temperature and sluggish flow of Blood and Body Fluids. A deficiency of Qi can cause lowered body temperature, intolerance to cold and cold limbs. The other is the manifestation of Heat due to stagnation of Qi, which is usually caused by sluggish flow of Qi in a local area.

4.3 Defending function
The defensive ability of the body results from the combined action of a number of physiological functions, of which the function of Qi plays a particularly important role. The defensive effect of Qi mainly indicates that Qi can defend the body from external pathogens. The defending action of Qi is shown in two aspects. One is to guard the surface of the skin against the exopathogen. The other is to combat the invading exopathogen so as to ward it off. Defensive Qi functions to protect the body surface, and control the opening and closing of the pores, so it can prevent the invasion of external pathogens. If the defensive function of Qi is deficient, the resistance of the body against the invasion of these factors will be weakened, and as a result, susceptibility to such diseases as the common cold is likely to occur. When the defending function of Qi is normal, the exopathogen has difficulty in invading the body. When the defending function of Qi becomes weaker, when the ability of the human body to fight the exopathogen is lowered, the body is easily invaded and diseases are caused. And what is more, these diseases are hard to cure.

4.4 Consolidating and governing function
By "consolidating and governing action", we mean that Qi holds organs in their place, keeps Blood in the vessels, governs the removal of fluids. Qi can keep blood flowing within the vessels; control and adjust the secretion and excretion of sweat, urine and saliva, and prevent the body fluid from escaping; consolidate and store sperm and prevent emission and premature ejaculation; hold the organs so as to prevent them from descending. A decrease in the above functions of Qi may cause various kinds of hemorrhage, spontaneous perspiration, polyuria, salivation, spermatorrhea, premature ejaculation, prolapse of the stomach, kidney and uterus. When Qi is deficient, Yin Fluids will be profusely lost. For example, failure of Qi to control Blood will cause various kinds of bleeding; inability of Qi to control Body Fluids will cause spontaneous sweating or profuse sweating, incontinence of urine or profuse urine; and failure of Qi to control emission will cause nocturnal emission, premature ejaculation, or seminal emission. The controlling effect of Qi and the pushing effect of Qi are opposite and supplement each other. On one hand, Qi promotes the distribution and discharge of Blood and Body Fluids; on the other hand, Qi controls the flow of these Yin substances to prevent their unnecessary loss. Only when these two opposite aspects are harmonized can the normal flow and discharge of the Yin substances and the metabolism of Blood and water be maintained.

4.5 Promoting metabolism and transformation
This refers to various conversions occurring along with the movement of Qi. It includes the changes of Qi during its movement and the generation and metabolism of Essence, Blood and Body Fluids and their transformation. "Qi hua" is a specific term in the science of TCM. It refers, in general, to various kinds of changes taking place in the body under the action of Qi. Specifically, it refers to the metabolism of fundamental substances, Qi, blood and body

fluid, and the transformations which can occur between them. For example, Qi, blood and body fluid are formed in the following manner: ingested food is changed into food essence, and food essence is, in turn, transformed into Qi, blood or body fluid, and these can then be changed into any one of the others according to the physiological need of the body. All these are the specific manifestations of the action of the activity of Qi. The dysfunction of Qi in performing its action will affect the whole metabolism of the body. That is to say, it will affect the digestion, absorption, transformation and transportation of food: the formation, movement and transformation of Qi, blood and body fluid; and the excretion of feces, urine and sweat; thus causing various symptoms associated with abnormal metabolism. In short, the process in which Qi performs its functions is the process in which the substances in the body are metabolized, and in which the substances and energy are transformed. Qi assists in the formation and transformations within the body, for example the transformation of food into Qi and Blood. Qi is the foundation of all movement and growth in the body.

Although the above mentioned five functions of Qi differ from each other, they are all based on the basic property of Qi and enjoy close cooperation and mutual support.

5. The movement of Qi

As a whole, Qi in the cosmos takes two patterns of existence, diffused Qi and coagulated Qi. The former is more vigorous, cannot be detected directly and exists everywhere. The latter is manifested as various kinds of things that can be seen or that have certain shapes. In order to survive, coagulated Qi must communicate with diffused Qi and its generation as well as its ending results from movement of the diffused Qi. The movement of Qi is called Mechanism of Qi, which can be generalized as four aspects: ascending, descending, exiting and entering movements, which are based on directions. Ascending refers to the movement from below; descending, from above; exiting, from the interior; and entering from the exterior.

The various functions of Qi are all performed by its movement. The physiological function of viscera and bowels is often reflected on their Qi's ascent, descent, exit and entry movements. Qi flows throughout the whole body because of its strength and vigor. Although the activities of the human body are multiple, they can all be summarized as these four aspects. For example, the dispersing effect of the Lung is a manifestation of the exit and ascent of Qi, while its descending effect is a manifestation of the descending and entering movements of Qi. These movements of Qi are vital to life. Once they stop, life comes to an end. The four movements of Qi have to be kept in harmony. Only in this way can the physiological functions of the human body remain normal in TCM, the physiological state in which the four basic movements of Qi are coordinated and balanced is called "harmonious functional activities of Qi".

Qi has four main states of disharmonies: Qi deficiency, Qi stagnation, sinking Qi and rebellious Qi. These disharmonies may affect many parts of the body at once or within a particular meridian, organ or area. Deficiency of Qi, for example, may affect the Lungs with symptoms of shortness of breath, the Stomach/Spleen with symptoms such as poor appetite and the body in general with symptoms of fatigue and weakness. The ascent, descent, exit and entry movements of Qi are of prime importance in human life. The Kidney Essence, the food Essence transported and transformed by the Spleen and Stomach and the fresh air inhaled by the Lung, will not be distributed over the body to perform their physiological functions if they do not make ascent, descent, entry and exit movements.

6. The classification of Qi

As the most basic substance that constitutes the world, Qi can be used to name everything in the world, so it is hard to classify it. However, Qi mentioned here is something concrete. Qi of the human body also has two patterns of existence. The coagulated Qi is manifested as various visible or structural components of the body, such as viscera, body figure, sense organs, Blood, Body Fluids and Essence; the diffused Qi is manifested as the Qi that flows in the body, but takes no certain form, such as Primordial Qi, Pectoral Qi, Nutritive Qi and Defensive Qi that is classified according to its distribution, origin, and function.

6.1 Primordial Qi (yuan Qi)
Primordial Qi is also called "Inborn Qi", "Primary Qi" or "genuine Qi". It is the most important and fundamental of all, originates from the congenital essence (the innate essence stored in the kidney). But it also depends on the supplement and nourishment of the acquired essence developed in the spleen and stomach. It is received from heaven and combined with food essence to nourish the body. It commences from "the vital gate", the portion between the two kidneys, passes the triple warmer and circulates throughout the body. It goes inward to the five viscera and six bowels and outward to the superficial layer of the body. It goes everywhere and acts on all parts of the body. The primordial Qi has the functions of both activating growth and development and promoting the functional activities of all the viscera and bowels, channels and collaterals, tissues and other organs. Therefore, it is the motivating power of the vital activities of the human body. If Primordial Qi is deficient due to a congenital defect or improper feeding after birth, the functional activities of the whole body will become weakened.

6.2 Pectoral Qi (zong Qi)
Pectoral Qi is also termed Great Qi, it accumulates in the thorax where Qi of the whole body converges. So the thorax is also known as "the sea of Qi". Pectoral Qi is a combination of the fresh air inhaled by the lung and the food essence derived by the spleen and stomach from water and grain. It is stored in the chest and poured into the channels of the heart and lung just as Miraculous Pivot (Lingshu), says: "It goes out of the lung and circulates through the larynx and pharynx. This is the reason why it exits when being exhaled and enters when being inhaled." The book Classified Canon compiled by Zhang Jiebin in 1624 A.D. says: "It goes down to the elixir field to be stored, and fills the Point Qijie of the yangming Channel from which it continues to go downward to the feet." Pectoral Qi has two main functions. One is that it flows through the respiratory tract to promote the respiratory movement of the lung and is involved in the loudness or softness of voice and words. The other is that it fills the heart channel to promote and adjust its beat, and to promote and adjust the circulation of blood and Qi. It also exerts an influence on the warmth and activities of the limbs. In short, it has the function of nourishing the lung and the heart, thus promoting respiration and blood circulation.

Generally speaking, when Pectoral Qi is sufficient, the pulse will be moderate and forceful, and the Heart will beat rhythmically and evenly. If Pectoral Qi is deficient, the pulse will be swift, irregular, feeble or scattered. Pectoral Qi is usually considered a link connecting the functional activities of the Heart and those of the Lung. In the clinic, Deficiency of Pectoral

Qi in most cases indicates Deficiency of Lung Qi leading to Deficiency of Heart Qi and ensuing Blood Stasis. For example, when a patient suffering from chronic bronchitis develops pulmonary Heart disease, which is marked by shortness of breath, a low voice, palpitation, a purplish face, running or intermittent pulse, etc., he or she can be diagnosed as having deficient Pectoral Qi.

6.3 Nutritive Qi (ying Qi)

Nutritive Qi refers to the Qi circulating within the blood vessels and having a nourishing function. As it flows through the vessels with blood, it has such a close relationship with the latter that TCM often mentions them in a combined way "nourishing blood". In TCM, Blood consists mainly of two parts: Nutritive Qi and Body Fluids. Compared with defensive Qi, nourishing Qi belongs to yin, so it is also called "nourishing yin". Nutritive Qi comes mainly from the food essence transformed and transported by the spleen and stomach. After its formation, Nutritive Qi is sent to the Channels to flow in the order of the Twelve Regular Channels. This is why a chapter on Arthralgia-Syndrome of Plain Questions (Suwen) says: "What is nutritive Qi? It is actually the essence Qi transformed from food and water". Nutritive Qi originates from the middle warmer and enters the channels by way of the lung. It circulates throughout the body along one after another of the fourteen channels. The main functions of Nutritive Qi are to generate Blood and to nourish the whole body. That is, it flows into the channels through the lung and becomes a component of blood, and nourish the whole body for the physiological activities of all the viscera and bowels, channels and collaterals, tissues and other organs. Plain Questions says: "Nutritive Qi secretes its fluid, which enters the channels and turns into blood, thus nourishing the four extremities, the five viscera and the six bowels".

6.4 Defensive Qi (wei Qi)

Defensive Qi is the Qi moving outside the conduits and having protective functions. Compared with nourishing Qi, it belongs to yang, so it is also known as "defensive yang", it also comes from the food essence transformed and transported by the spleen and stomach. It is characterized by braveness in defence. That is why a chapter on Arthralgia-Syndrome of Plain Questions says: "Defensive Qi is a brave kind, which is produced by food and water." The distribution of Defensive Qi has two features: the flow following Nutritive Qi and free flow. The former indicates that Defensive Qi also goes along the Twelve Regular Channels, while the latter indicates that Qi is distributed all over the body. Defensive Qi circulates not within but outside the channels. Being vaporized to the diaphragm and scattered in the chest and abdomen, it travels between the skin and flesh. In spite of circulating outside the channels, it still leans against the channels when moving. Defensive Qi has three functions. The first is guarding the surface of the body against exopathogen. The second is keeping a relatively constant body temperature by controlling the opening and closing of the muscular striae and adjusting the excretion of sweat due to its permeation to the muscular striae. The third is nourishing the viscera, bowels, muscles, skin and hair. When defensive Qi is insufficient, the defending function of the human body is weakened, the exopathogen invades the body easily, and the disease is hard to cure. Abnormal circulation of defensive Qi may cause sleep disorders. When defensive Qi is deficient, spontaneous sweating will occur.

Nutritive Qi and defensive Qi have the same source. The former circulates within the channels, has the nourishing function and belongs to yin, whereas the latter circulates outside the channels, has the function of guarding the exterior of the body and belongs to yang. Only when they coordinate with each other can the opening and closing of the pores be kept normal, the body temperature constant, and the defending ability strong.

7. Modern investigations on Qi

In China, Qi has been known for 4000 years. In Japanese literature, the documentation of Qi goes back 1500 years. This is not limited to the East. In the West, Biblical literature suggests that curing sickness by extending a hand was practiced by a gifted individual. Since then, thousands of accounts have been published, and millions of people have talked about Qi-energy. Practical, clinical, philosophical and scientific studies on Qi have been actively reported in journals of complementary and alternative medicine (CAM). However, no reasonable mechanism, which can be examined or refuted from the scientific point of view, has been presented (Ohnishi and Ohnishi, 2009b).

Scientific investigations of Qi started about 30 years ago, but we still know very little and have so much to learn. Flowers (2006) mentioned that the speed of Qi investigation seems to have slowed down in recent years. Now the question comes as to what is the nature of Qi? As to the nature of Qi, Chinese and Japanese scientists have already reported that it involves infrared radiation. It was also reported that other forms of energy may be involved in Qi which include electromagnetic waves, electrostatic energy, magnetic energy, sound waves and so on (Kiang, 1978; Yuasa, 1993; Machi, 1993; Shinagawa, 1990). However, in the study of Qi, one difficult problem encountered. Namely, Qi can't be measured quantitatively with modern technology now (Ohnishi and Ohnishi, 2009a). We do not even know the qualitative nature of Qi yet, not to mention quantitative methods of measuring it. One of the pitfalls in the study on Qi is obviously that there seems to be no 'scientific' objective measure to evaluate its 'quantity'. Thus, the concept of Qi would be as important and effective, and also as difficult to quantify, as the concept of 'stress'.

7.1 The effects of Qi-therapy on health

External Qi-therapy (QT) is a process by which Qi is transmitted from a Qi master to another person for the purpose of preventing and curing disease, as well as protecting and improving health through regulation of mind and body. This may be a very useful intervention. Research studies have shown that QT is effective for relief of pain, relaxation of stress states and increasing immunity (Lee et al., 2001a–c). Several studies attempted to reveal a specific effect of external Qi by modern biochemical and immunological methods (Chien et al., 1991; Fukushima et al., 2001; Lee et al., 2001a and b; Shah et al., 1999). Chien et al. (1991) reported that facilitating Qi from a Qigong masters increased the rate of cell growth and DNA synthesis. Lee et al. (2001a and b) reported psychoneuroimmunological effects of in vivo QT on humans and stimulatory effect on natural killer (NK) cell activity in vitro by emitted Qi. QT has an acute stimulatory effect on neutrophil superoxide generation (Lee, 2003). The studies show that Qi positively affect human innate immunity.

TCM considers chronic fatigue to reflect a disharmony and depletion in the supply of Qi, with blockage, stagnation, imbalance or change in the pattern or organization of Qi resulting in disease (Shin, 2002; Xing, 1987). Disruption to Qi manifests in symptoms such as pain, fatigue and mood disturbances. TCM practitioners consider that chronic fatigue reflects a disharmony and depletion in the supply of Qi in the body. Qigong is one of the traditional complementary interventions used to strengthen Qi through self-practice, and to manage the state of Qi to prevent and cure disease. Qigong seems to improve factors related to chronic fatigue such as sleep, pain, mental attitude and general mobility after 3 and 6 months. Qigong's positive effects indicate that it represents a potentially safe method of treatment for chronic fatigued patients (Mike Craske, 2009).

People attempt to find the mechanism behind the healing effects of Qi. Why do students of NBM continue to attend the class (many of them once a week, but some of them more often) for 10 or even 15 years? Because they feel healthier, or because they have a more youthful feeling than before. Through their study, students were shown to have higher immune activity and lower stress levels (Kimura et al., 2005). Some students overcame cancer themselves by attending the class almost everyday to lift their Qi level. This experience may be related to *in vitro* results that Qi inhibited the growth of cancer cells (Ohnishi et al., 2005). As to the anti-aging effect of NBM, Mr Nishino has long proposed that Qi may stimulate mitochondria to become more active, and thus, to provide more energy to the cells. Ohnishi et al. (2006) demonstrated that in isolated rat liver mitochondria, the respiratory control ratio was protected from deterioration by Qi, and lipid peroxidation was inhibited by Qi. These results suggest that Qi may inhibit apoptosis of the cells in our body, thereby inhibiting aging. Some students were shown to have higher bone density than their age- and gender-matched contemporaries who do not practice NBM (Nishino, 2006). Through *in vitro* tests, Ohnishi et al. found that Qi may be beneficial in preventing osteoporosis (Ohnishi et al., 2007). They are accumulating data on health-related benefits of NBM, and also, trying to correlate this with the molecular and cellular mechanisms of Qi effects.

7.2 The effects of Bu-Zhong-Yi-Qi-Tang on health

TCM, with its long history of clinical practice, occupies an important place among the "alternative medicine" that has been gaining attention in recent years. Because of the general mildness in nature and the emphasis on relief, balance and harmonization rather than forceful suppression, a good many Chinese medicines are particularly suited for the frail, the elderly, the very young and those already weakened by diseases. Bu-Zhong-Yi-Qi-Tang, a basic prescription as an Qi tonic (Chinese medical concept: Bu-Qi) and a general health tonic, also one of the typical formulae in Japanese Kampo which is prescribed for people with the Qi deficient conditions in order to enhance their Qi (Terasawa, 2004; Li, 1992; Kawakita and Nomoto, 1998), composed of Astragali radix, Ginseng radix, Atractyloidis rhizoma, Glycyrrhizae radix, Angelicae sinensis, Aurantii pericarpium, Cimicifugae rhizoma and Bupleurum radix, has been prescribed for the alleviation of fatigue and depressed vitality as well as the improvement of gastroenteric circulation (Shih et al., 2000). It has been reported to possess anti-tumor (Ito and Shimura, 1985), anti-bacterial (Li et al., 1992), anti-nociceptive and anti-depressive activities (Koshikawa et al., 1998), and to have some effects on impairment of hematopoietic organs (Ikeda et al., 1990), stress incontinence (Murakami, 1988) and male infertility (Ishikawa et al., 1992), to reduce the extent of radiation-induced apoptosis and protect the jejunal crypt (Chai et al., 2009) and improve health status in general but slows down or partially reverses aging in particular (Shih et al., 2000).

7.3 The effects of Qi on health

Qi is the concept of the state of the mind/body as a whole. It is thus not a 'subjective' state, which can only be known introspectively. From the clinical experience, the Qi deficiency state is diagnosed very 'objectively': those with 'Qi deficiency' are weak in voice, have no 'strength' in their eyes and their posture is poor. In this sense, Qi is a very objective entity. It is not an abstract and subjective entity like soul or spirit. Practitioners of TCM can judge a patient's Qi state by just glancing at their skin condition. Those people healthy in mind-body, or with good Qi, have bright and 'full' skin. Though difficult to quantify, these are 'objective'. Qi can be approached 'objectively'. There is thus a definite possibility that we can elaborate on the concept of Qi as an objective 'scientific' term. It is a basic East Asian 'philosophy' of health/disease that those with a good Qi state are highly immune to diseases (Kobayashi and Ishii, 2005). It is very nice to see that Western clinical researchers such as Irwin have undertaken the challenge to tackle this difficult problem of Qi or mind-body unity. Now is an exciting era, when for the first time it has became possible for a western psychiatrist and an Eastern dermatologist to work together towards reconciling this fundamental difference between the medicines of the East and the West.

In Asia, the use of Qi in enhancing one's vitality and improving health is employed even today. For example, Qigong therapies are popular in China as Qi-therapies are in Japan. More recently, similar healing techniques were known in Europe as the working of mesmerism or hypnosis. Unfortunately, these techniques are not well accepted as a branch of today's main-stream sciences, especially in the Western hemisphere. Many people consider them as folk medicine. Some people believe that they are 'supernatural' and 'para-psychological' phenomena. In fact, Qi is neither a paranormal nor para-psychological phenomenon but is a normal phenomenon. Since it is a normal phenomenon, Qi can be studied by modern scientific methodology. Only a limited number of investigators have been studying them as the object of scientific, medical investigation for the past 30 years.

In the past 30 years, many Chinese scientists regarded 'Qi' as a real substance flowing in our body, which can be represented by mass. On the contrary, most Japanese scientists treated 'Qi' as energy, except for Shinagawa who considered it to be information. Although neither Qi itself nor the mechanism of its effects is understandable or explicable within any paradigm of modern medical science, its effects on the human body are apparent and some studies have been tried to find the underlying mechanism with laboratory experiments (Ohnishi, 2007).

Ohnishi et al. are demonstrating that so-called 'Qi-energy' is a natural phenomenon, and therefore, it can be analyzed by rigorous scientific and objective investigations. A 'breathing method' was developed by a Japanese leading Qi-expert, Kozo Nishino, Since 'breathing' is directly related to oxygen respiration, he has long proposed that mitochondria may play a key role in maintaining vitality and health (Nishino, 1997;2004). This led them to undertake the project to explore a possible relationship between Qi-energy and mitochondrial function (Ohnishi et al., 2006). Kozo Nishino has hypothesized for many years that the breathing method would increase oxygen delivery in the body, activate cell metabolism including mitochondrial function, thereby bringing us tangible health benefits (Kimura et al., 2005; Ohnishi et al., 2005). Recently, Ohnishi et al. found that his Qi protected isolated rat liver mitochondria from heat-induced deterioration, possibly by reducing the production of reactive oxygen species (ROS). The protection of mitochondria and the reduction of ROS generation would produce more energy from the nutrients and would result in healthier cells and organs. The protection of mitochondria from adverse effects of ROS would reduce the likelihood of premature apoptosis, and therefore would contribute to the longevity of the practitioners. His prediction that mitochondria would play key roles in maintaining health and longevity seems to be supported by these experiments (Ohnishi *et al.*, 2006).

Isolated rat liver mitochondria are a well-established model for studying biophysical and biochemical aspects of energy metabolism. The simplest marker for the integrity and intactness of mitochondria is a respiratory control ratio (RCR, which is the ratio between State-3 and State-4 respiration) (Chance and Williams, 1955). Ohnishi *et al.* measured the RCR and analyzed the degree of lipid peroxidation in the mitochondria by measuring the amount of TBARS (thiobarbituric acid reactive substances). Using this model, they found that a heat treatment (incubation at 39°C for 10 min) decreased the RCR by about 60%. While the Qi-energy emitted from the fingers of Nishino could inhibit the decrease. They also attempted to find the mechanism for the Qi-effect. After the early work by Boveris and Cadenas (1975), ROS has been recognized as an important factor to damage mitochondrial functions. In order to test whether Qi-energy could reduce the ROS production, they measured the amount of mitochondrial lipid peroxidation after the heat treatment using a well-known assay technique for TBARS. Lipid peroxidation was increased during the heat deterioration, suggesting that mitochondria were exposed to oxidative stress. Lipid peroxidation is known to damage the mitochondrial membrane. However, lipid peroxidation was inhibited by Qi-energy, and the mitochondrial integrity was preserved.

From the standpoint of health and longevity, their results may have the following significance: (i) Qi-energy may protect mitochondria from oxidative injury. If the same reaction takes place in the practitioners' body, then mitochondria may produce more energy, and therefore, it has beneficial effects on cellular metabolism. (ii) Mitochondria are known to play key roles in apoptosis of many cell types. If cytochrome c and other apoptosis-inducing factors (AIF) are released from mitochondria, they activate a series of cascade reactions to cause apoptotic cell death (Green and Reed, 1998; Narita *et al.*,1998; Susin *et al.*, 1999; Lorenzo *et al.*, 1999; Shimizu *et al.*, 1999). Although apoptosis is a fundamental feature of almost all animal cells and it is indispensable for the normal development of tissues, organs and immune systems (Jacobson *et al.*, 1997), excessive apoptosis could cause diseases (Thompson, 1995). Therefore, protecting mitochondrial integrity would help prevent cytochrome c release, thereby inhibiting inappropriate apoptosis from taking place. In conclusion, Qi-energy maintains mitochondrial membrane integrity during the heat deterioration process. Mitochondria are constantly exposed to the danger of ROS-induced oxidative injury. The effect of Qi seems to be related to the inhibition of oxidative injury on mitochondrial membranes caused by ROS. Therefore, Qi would have a beneficial effect on protecting mitochondria; thus, it would maintain efficient cellular metabolism and decrease the chance of unnecessary apoptosis.

'Qi-energy', which can be enhanced through the practice of Nishino Breathing Method (NBM), was reported to have beneficial health effects. It has been known for 20 years that the practitioners of Qi experienced beneficial health effects (Yumi, 2005). It was shown that the practice increased immune activity and decreased the stress level of the practitioners (Kimura *et al.*, 2005). From the collaboration with Master Nishino, Ohnishi *et al.* showed that 'Qi' is not a paranormal or parapsychological phenomenon, but a natural phenomenon. An interesting observation from the standpoint of CAM was that the Qi-energy, which inhibits cell division of cultured cancer cells (Ohnishi *et al.*, 2005) or protects isolated mitochondria from oxidative injury, was the same as that which could move other individuals in the Taiki-practice (Ohnishi and Ohnishi, 2006). This suggests that the training gained from the Taiki-practice may produce beneficial health effects. This is the reason why they are studying the mechanism behind the Taiki-practice.

Ohnishi *et al.* explain the philosophical and psychological background of Qi, emphasize that the unique aspects of Eastern philosophy are 'non-linearity' and 'holistic' approach and then present physics aspect of Qi. Their experiments demonstrated that a 'Qi-beam' carries 'entropy' (or information), which is different from 'energy' (Ohnishi and Ohnishi, 2009a). We believe that the human will uncover the secret of Qi in the near future with the rapid development of modern life science.

8. The significance of studying Qi

The difference between the cultures in the West and the East may be described by the difference between 'linear philosophy' and 'nonlinear philosophy'. Since Qi phenomena are essentially nonlinear, a straightforward application of linear philosophy may not be effective in its study. We hope that the study of Qi phenomena may help bridge some of the apparent difference between Western and Eastern culture. As Flowers mentioned, in the Christian West, God was the center of everything as opposed to Qi being the center of everything in the East. Qi may be another name of 'life'. As Flowers beautifully described, Qi may represent the entity of life itself (Flowers, 2006). Then, the understanding of Qi may shed light on other aspects of biological sciences. We hope that the study of Qi might help to unite more aspects of Eastern and Western philosophy.

Understanding of Qi will help bridge Western and Eastern viewpoints, According to Eastern thought, the universe has 'life' and the function of 'life' is represented by Qi. Qi flows and circulates throughout the universe and through each human being. Qi is a non-linear phenomenon, and therefore, it can function as an essential element of life and the universe (both of which are non-linear). If Western people could understand Qi more, they would incorporate holistic Eastern philosophy into their own philosophical system. Then, mind and body, as well as life and its environment, will be viewed as a unified entity, and the world would finally become a better place to live.

The concept of Qi would be of great value towards this direction, as it is understood as a kind of 'energy' of mind/body as a whole. If, therefore, there was some concrete method to enhance (strengthen) Qi, it would become one of the cornerstones of holistic medicine of the future. Thus, from the medical point of view, Qi can be seen as the totality of the body's healing systems or defense mechanisms which include the immune system as their essential part. Qi has both energy and entropy (information) aspects. The practice of breathing to enhance the Qi level may in-essence help to restore the original ability of human beings. Therefore, it may contribute to improve our health, wellness and life itself.

Qi phenomenon seems to be characteristic to the nonlinear nature of life. If so, the study of Qi may help deepen our understanding on our life and the universe itself. Since Qi is related to our life activity, the understanding of Qi would contribute to the elucidation of the beautiful nature of life itself. Further development and understanding of Qi may help round out our belief in technology-oriented modern science which lacks humanistic aspects. This may help to transform the 'Century of Death' to the 'Century of Life'. The 19th century was the age of the 'industrial revolution' which was symbolized by an invention of a steam engine. The 20th century is the age of 'nuclear energy'. Then, what would make the 21st century more humanistic so that history might regard it as a century of life? The pursuit of studies on Qi might be a positive step. In conclusion, Qi phenomenon is not paranormal. It is a normal and real phenomenon and can be the object of rigorous scientific study. If the question is posed, 'Why do you study Qi?' We will answer, as a famous mountain climber once said, 'Because it is there!' We believe that further analysis of Qi may open up a new horizon in life science.

9. The comparisons between Qi and bioenergy

Qi, an important category in the ancient Chinese philosophy, is a simple understanding of natural phenomena. According to ancient Chinese philosopher, Qi is the most basic material that constitute the world, the everything in the universe were produced by the motion of Qi, and it is roughly similar to the concept material of Western philosophy. The theory of Qi in ancient philosophy was introduced into the medical field, the basic theory of Qi in traditional Chinese medicine (TCM) was formed, i.e., the concept of Qi in TCM was established during the mutual penetration between the materialist philosophy and medicine in ancient China, it is a concept of material. In TCM, Qi is constantly in motion, is the subtle substance with a strong vitality which constitute the human body and maintain the activities of human life, is one of the most basic material, it is also known as the "essence Qi". When the concept Qi in TCM was used to discuss the human body, it often has the meaning of both life material and physiological functions. Therefore, Qi in TCM is one of the most important basic concepts. Bioenergetics research in life sciences have played an important role, Mitchell's chemiosmotic theory earned the 1978 Nobel Prize in Chemistry, as the coupling between electron transport in the respiratory chain and adenosine diphosphate (ADP) phosphorylation which is caused by electrochemical gradient of protons between internal and external mitochondrial membrane was expounded; Nobel Prize in Chemistry in 1997 was awarded academician PD Boyer in the U.S. Academy of Sciences for elucidating generation mechanism of adenosine triphosphate (ATP)—the most important energy molecules. The work was closely related to the energy production and consumption which is required for life activities, and the binding-changes and rotation-catalytic mechanism of ATP synthase was proposed. ATP synthase is the smallest molecular motor in the world. In this paper, the relationship between Qi and bioenergy was approached to.

9.1 The generation of Qi and ATP
9.1.1 The generation of Qi
Qi in TCM, constitute the body and maintain life activities, has the following three sources and is a combination of them. (i). Congenital essence: This essence, which is born before the body, is the basic material of life, is intrinsic from the parents. (ii). Acquired essence: is acquired from the diet to obtain nutrients from the transportation and transformation through the spleen and stomach, that is, the essence of water and food. (iii). The clear air in the nature: the fresh air inhaled through the breathing exercise of lungs.

From the generation process of Qi, Qi depends on the normal function of the organs and tissues of the body, but the physiological functions of the viscera kidney, spleen and stomach, lungs are closely related to it. The lung, being the dominator of Qi, operates the Qi of the whole body; spleen and stomach, being the acquired foundation, their function of transformation and transport is particularly important in the Qi generation process; kidney, being the source of Qi generation and the congenital foundation, store the essence of life which includes congenital and acquired essence. For example, Qi, blood and body fluid are formed in the following manner: ingested food is changed into food essence, and food essence is, in turn, transformed into Qi, blood or body fluid, and these can then be changed into any one of the others according to the physiological need of the body. The waste from the eaten food and the products produced in the course of metabolism are changed, separately, into feces, urine and sweat which are ready to be removed from the body.

The Qi in the human body is different in classification and formation. But, generally speaking, it has no more than two sources. One is the innate vital substance one inherits from one's parents before birth. The other is the food essence and fresh air one receives from air, water and food in the natural world. The materials obtained in the two ways above have to be processed and transformed by the viscera and bowels before becoming the Qi of the human body. The process for Qi to be formed is as follows: The innate vital substance acted on by the kidney comes out of the gate of life (the portion between the two kidneys) and goes up to the middle warmer. There it combines with the food essence coming from the spleen and continues upwards until it combines with the fresh air inhaled by the lung. The food essence transformed and transported by the Spleen must be sent up to the Lung to combine with fresh air to produce the nutrients necessary for man's life activities. Finally it turns into Qi. It is easy to see from the above that the Qi of the human body is formed through the joint work of the kidney, the spleen, the stomach and the lung in combining the innate vital substance taken from one's parents, the food essence received from water and food, and the fresh air obtained from nature.

9.1.2 The generation of ATP

The major function of mitochondria is the generation of ATP, the energy currency of the cell, by oxidative phosphorylation. Essential mechanisms of energy production, signaling, biosynthesis and apoptosis are contained within mitochondria, and their orchestration plays a determinant role in cell physiology (Benard et al., 2006; Bailey et al., 2005). Since mitochondria generate between 80% and 90% of all ATP produced in the cell, the rest of the energy was provided from anaerobic glycolysis and the conversion of creatine phosphate (PCr) by creatine kinase (CK) (Papa, 1996; Radda et al., 1995), it is understandable that in tissues like the cardiac muscle and liver (each hepatocyte contains 1000–2000 mitochondria) these organelles occupy 20–30% of the cell volume, having mitochondrial function, or dysfunction, a critical role in the performance of these tissues (Smith et al., 2008; Yang et al., 2010). An adult needs about 3000 kcal, or 400 mol ATP (about 200 kg) every day. Mitochondrial oxidative phosphorylation (OXPHOS) enzymes including 5 oligomeric protein complex, i.e. complex I (NADH dehydrogenase), complex II (succinate ubiquinone reductase), complex III (cytochrome c reductase), complex IV(cytochrome c oxidase, COX) and complex V(H^+-ATP synthase). Complex I and II capture electrons from the reduced coenzyme I (NADH) and succinate respectively, and transfer them to coenzyme Q (CoQ), CoQ is oxidized by complex III and IV. These complexes (except complex II) are coupled electron flow to proton pump and to ensure that the generated proton driving force was used by complex V to form ATP from ADP and phosphate (Pi) coupling reaction, each complex is composed by different subunits, and complex I, II, III and IV contain several redox active prosthetic groups (Papa, 1996).

Bio-energy materials - ATP generation process in modern medicine is as follows: ATP, the "Universal Currency" of bioenergy in the cell, is a direct provider of energy required for the body, provide efficient energy for any endergonic reactions. Therefore, life is basically dependent on the activities of ADP -ATP cycle. There are two types of ATP-generating mechanisms: substrate level phosphorylation in the original fermentation pathway and photophosphorylation and OXPHOS that use electron transport system in the evolutionary pathways. The efficiency for generating ATP of the latter is about 20 times compare to the former, the key reasons for high efficiency in photophosphorylation and OXPHOS system depend on the proton pumps and ATP synthase in biomembrane, for example, ATP synthase catalyze endergonic reaction by binding the protons that accumulated in one side of the membrane: ADP + Pi (phosphate) → ATP. Then, proton pump coupled with the electron transport system to generate energy.

Now, let's look at the overview of the mitochondrial ATP production. Mitochondria are intracellular organelles mainly devoted to energy production. From the point of the main generation process of bio-energy substance-ATP, at first, the three major nutrients carbohydrates, lipids and proteins are decomposed into the simple sugars, fatty acids and amino acids respectively by different enzymes in the body. Then pyruvate was generated from glucose by glycolysis, acetyl coenzyme A (CoA) was then formed from pyruvate through the pyruvate dehydrogenase complex, acetyl-CoA, can also be generated in mitochondria from fatty acids by β-oxidation, then enter the Krebs cycle, and the 20 kinds of standard amino acids that make up proteins can be decomposed in the body to generate acetyl-CoA, oxaloacetate, fumarate, succinyl-CoA and α-ketoglutaric acid and other substances to enter the citric acid cycle. The hydrogens stripped off in the Krebs cycle were accepted by nicotinamide adenine dinucleotide (NAD^+) or flavin adenine dinucleotide (FAD) to enter in the respiratory chain of inner mitochondrial membrane through a series of electron carriers (low potential to high potential), the electrons were finally transported to oxygen accompanied by the phosphorylation of ADP to generate ATP.

The following describes the basic processes occurring in a typical normal cell, using glucose as a major source of energy. The breakdown of glucose into water and CO_2 includes two steps, namely, glycolysis (the anaerobic phase) taking place in the cytoplasm, and OXPHOS (the aerobic phase) occurring in the mitochondria. Of the total yield of 38 ATP per mole of glucose, two are produced in the glycolysis process and 36 during the OXPHOS. It is important to note that oxygen availability in the mitochondrion is a critical factor for the normal ATP production in the cell. Glycolysis depends on the entrance of glucose from the capillary into the cell via the glucose transporter. The end product of glycolysis, pyruvate, is transported into the mitochondria by a specific carrier protein. The pyruvate is transformed, in the matrix of the mitochondria, into acetyl coenzyme A that activates the tricarboxylic acid (TCA) cycle. In the mitochondria, the TCA cycle generates NADH which enters the electron transport chain (ETC) leading to the OXPHOS that generates ATP (Mayevsky, 2009).

The mitochondrial respiratory chain consists of four enzyme complexes (complexes I–IV), and two mobile carriers (coenzyme Q and cytochrome c) along which the electrons liberated by the oxidation of NADH and $FADH_2$ are passed, and ultimately transferred to molecular oxygen. This respiratory process generates the electrochemical gradient of protons used by the F_1F_0 ATP synthase (i.e., complex V) to phosphorylate ADP and produce ATP. Briefly, nutrients such as glucose, amino acids and fatty acids are transformed by intermediary metabolism into their reduced equivalents (NADH, H^+ or $FADH_2$), which are further oxidized by the mitochondrion to generate ATP. Mitochondria of normal tissues typically oxidize combinations of these energy substrates (fatty acids, the glycolysis end product pyruvate and amino acids) to establish the electrochemical gradient of protons ($\Delta\mu H^+$) used by the F_1F_0-ATP synthase to produce ATP (Benard *et al.*, 2010). In this regard, mitochondria play a pivotal role by producing almost all the cellular energy (Freyre-Fonsecaa *et al.*, 2011).

It is quite evident that the generation of ATP requires both acquired essence — the essence of water and food (which can be regarded as decomposition products of the three major nutrients — monosaccharides, fatty acids and amino acids) and the clear Qi in the nature - the fresh air (mainly oxygen, around 90% oxygen inhaled by the body was consumed by the process of ATP production through mitochondrial electron transport), mitochondria are also needed. But modern biochemical research show that human mitochondria are maternally inherited, that is, mitochondria of everyone are from the mother genetically, and this can be called the congenital essence. Therefore, the Qi and ATP have common sources.

9.2 The functions of Qi and bioenergy

Generally speaking, Qi of the human body has five functions: promoting, warming, defending, consolidating and governing, promoting metabolism and transformation, these functions of Qi are consistent with those of energy metabolism. All cells in the body depend on a continuous supply of ATP in order to perform their different physiological and biochemical activities (Mayevsky, 2009). In modern medicine, all the physiological activities of the body are dependent on bio-energy source (ATP) generated by substance metabolism (including oxygen metabolism), various forms of physiological functions can be played by ATP through different effectors to maintain all life activities. Large amounts of ATP are used in muscle contraction, nerve impulse conduction, compound biosynthesis or other biological processes (Benard *et al.*, 2010).

Qi is a vigorous substance that flows fast in the human body. So it promotes the growth and development of the body, the movement, distribution and discharge of Blood and Body Fluids, and the physiological functional activities of viscera and bowels, channel, collateral, tissue and organ. Qi, as a Yang substance, heat source of the body, is rich in heat, which can warm viscera and bowels, channels, skin, and muscles and tendons, to maintain normal body temperature and the normal functional activities of these organs and tissues. This Qi function is of important to physiological significance of the human body. "Qi hua" is a specific term in the science of TCM. It refers, in general, to various kinds of changes taking place in the body under the action of Qi. Specifically, it refers to the metabolism of fundamental substances, Qi, blood and body fluid, and the transformations which can occur between them, it is actually material conversion and energy conversion process. Although the above mentioned five functions of Qi differ from each other, they enjoy close cooperation and mutual support. Qi is the foundation of all movement and growth in the body.

According to TCM, "if Qi gets together, it will result to the birth; if Qi is harmonious, then the human body is healthy; if Qi is disordered, the human will be sick; if Qi is depleted, the human will die." According to the modern life science, energy metabolism is the center for life activity, if the energy metabolism is normal, the body can carry out normal vital activities, If no bio-energy is supplied for the body, the life activities cease immediately. Therefore, Qi and bioenergy have identical functions.

10. The effects of QIHM and QRHM on energy metabolism—An experimental perspective

ABSTRACT Aims: TCM practitioners usually compose prescriptions made up of Qi-invigorating herbal medicines (QIHM) or Qi-flow regulating herbal medicines (QRHM) for Qi system diseases, and have accumulated abundant clinical experience for a long time. To approach to the nature of Qi in TCM from bioenergetics, the effects of QIHM (ginseng, astragalus root, pilose asiabell root, white atractylodes rhizome) and QRHM (immature bitter orange, magnolia bark, green tangerine and lindera root) on oxidative phosphorylation (OXPHOS), bioenergy level and creatine kinase activities were investigated.

Methods: QIHM and QRHM were administered by oral gavage daily for 10 days. Mice liver mitochondria were isolated by differential centrifugation. The effects of QIHM and QRHM on energy metabolism were studied from the production, regulation, and storage of bioenergy. Mitochondrial OXPHOS curve was determined by Clark oxygen electrode method. The levels of adenosine triphosphate (ATP), adenosine diphosphate (ADP) and adenosine monophosphate (AMP) in liver cells were determined by reversed-phase high performance liquid chromatography (RP-HPLC), adenylate energy charge (AEC), total adenylate pool (TAP) were calculated. The creatine kinase (CK) activities in mice skeletal muscle were determined by a commercial monitoring kit. The regularity of action of QIHM and QRHM were analyzed and concluded.

Results: Ginseng and astragalus root can decrease oxygen consuming rate and respiratory control ratio (RCR) of liver mitochondria obviously, we consider this is appearance of lowering standard metabolic rate and is a kind of protective adaptation. QRHM can increase P/O ratio and RCR. Both QIHM and QRHM can stimulate activity of CK significantly in the storage of energy, and QRHM is stronger than QIHM. But it is worth notice that all the four QIHM can increase levels of ATP, AEC and TAP; on the contrary, all the four QRHM can decrease levels of ATP, AEC and TAP in liver cells. In a word, QIHM and QRHM increase and decrease bioenergy level of liver cells respectively *in vivo*. Therefore, Qi is closely related to bioenergy.

Conclusion: Qi and bioenergy have common sources and identical functions. QIHM and QRHM are able to improve and decrease the energy state of the body respectively. Qi and bioenergy have general characteristics in many aspects. The experiments provide scientific evidence for Qi in TCM is bioenergy.

Key words: Qi; bioenergy; Adenosine triphosphate; qi-invigorating herbal medicine; qi-regulating herbal medicine.

According to TCM theory, Qi (vital energy) refers to a kind of refined nutritive substance within the body. Qi is one of the most basic, the most important, and the most complicated concept in TCM. We propose a hypothesis that Qi is closely related to bioenergy according to the ancient concept of Qi and modern bioenergetics. TCM practitioners usually compose prescriptions made up of Qi-invigorating herbal medicines (QIHM) or Qi-flow regulating herbal medicines (QRHM) for Qi system diseases, and have accumulated abundant clinical experience for a long time. QIHM is a kind of herbal medicines which can invigorate Qi and treat syndromes of Qi deficiency, they have the effects of invigorating Qi, promoting the production of body fluid and tonifying the spleen and lung etc. QRHM is a kind of herbal medicines which can induce the flow of Qi, regulate the Qi system diseases and treat the syndromes of stagnation of Qi or rebellious Qi etc. They can activate Qi to reduce pain, depress upward-reverse flow of Qi, break the stagnant Qi to remove masses etc. QIHM and QRHM have similar nature and atributive channels, but their flavours are different significantly. QIHM taste sweet while QRHM taste acrid-bitter, and their compositions are also different. Although Qi of TCM is similar to the concept of modern medical bioenergy in some aspects, the energy nature of Qi still lacks convincing evidence. Therefore, we take it as our basic point to approach the characteristics of QIHM and QRHM on energy metabolism. We have approached the rules of QIHM and QRHM from the production (oxidative phosphorylation), storage (creatine kinase activity) and regulation (adenylate energy charge) of bioenergy (ATP). Since there is no direct detection method on Qi, the widely used QIHM (ginseng, astragalus root, pilose asiabell root, white atractylodes rhizome) and QRHM (immature bitter orange, magnolia bark, green tangerine and lindera root) were selected to study the effect on energy metabolism to approach to the nature of Qi in TCM.

Sasang constitutional medicine (SCM) is a unique traditional Korean therapeutic alternative form of medicine. In both SCM and TCM theories, Qi is the most essential element, the 'driving force' that constitutes the body and maintains the activities of life, visceral functions and metabolism. In a generalized scope, the essence of Qi in SCM can be compared with that of energy in modern physiology. The metabolic process in physiology provides energy, kinetic and potential energies, whereas metabolism in SCM produces and regulates Qi. Since catabolism breaks own complex molecules into simple ones and releases kinetic energy, this pathway can be compared with the process of consuming Qi in SCM. Similarly, anabolism, which links together simple molecules to form more complex molecules and stores potential energy, is comparable with the process of producing and storing Qi in SCM. In terms of interior–exterior exchange, the process of taking up raw materials from the external environment to produce Qi in SCM (function of the spleen) corresponds to the process of digestion and absorption of food and water and inhaling air in physiology (Kim and Pham, 2009). To approach to the nature of Qi in TCM from bioenergetics, the effects of QIHM and QRHM on oxidative phosphorylation (OXPHOS), bioenergy level and creatine kinase (CK) activities were investigated.

Materials and methods

Animals and materials

Male Kunming mice (Grade II, Certificate No 2002-5), weighing 22±2.0 g each, were purchased from Experimental Animal Center, Dalian University. All mice were cared for according to the Guiding Principles in the Care and Use of Animals. The experiment was approved by Medical College Council on Animal Care Committee of Dalian University (China) in accordance with NIH guidelines (NIH, 2002). Rodent laboratory chow and tap water were available *ad libitum* during the period. Spherisorb C_{18} reversed-phase chromatographic column (4.6 mm×250 mm, 5 μm particle size) was produced by Dalian Institute of Chemistry and Physics, Chinese Academy of Sciences. Adenosine triphosphate (ATP), adenosine diphosphate (ADP), adenosine monophosphate (AMP), 2-Thiobarbituric acid (TBA), and 1,1,3,3-tetraethoxypropane (TEP) were from Sigma Chemical (St Louis, MO, USA). N-2-Hydroxyethylpiperazine-N'-2-ethane sulfonic acid (HEPES) was from Merck (Darmstadt, Germany). Coomassie Brilliant Blue G-250 (CBBG-250) was purchased from Fluka (Bushs SG, Switzerland). Bovine serum albumin (BSA) was from Boehringer Mannheim Corp. (Indianapolis, IN, USA). Tris(hydroxymethyl)aminomethane (Tris) was from Gibco BRL

(Grand Island, NY, USA). A commercial creatine kinase monitoring kit [N-acetyl-L-cysteine(NAC)-activated] was from Beijing Zhongsheng High-Tech Bioengineering Company (Beijing, China). All other chemicals and solvents used in the study were of analytical grade made in China. Ginseng, astragalus root, pilose asiabell root, white atractylodes rhizome, immature bitter orange, magnolia bark, green tangerine and lindera root, are *Panax ginseng* C.A. Mey (Tongrentang red ginseng), *Astragalus membranaceus* (Fisch.) Bge.var. mongholicus (Bge.) Hsiao, *Codonopsis pilosula* (Franch.) Nannf, *Atractylodes macrocephala* Koidz, *Citrus aurantium* L, *Magnolia officinalis* Rehd et Wils, *Citrus reticulate* Blanco and *Lindera aggregate* (Sims) Kosterm respectively, were purchased from Beijing Tongrentang Drugstore, and identified by professor Li Jiashi at Beijing University of Traditional Chinese Medicine.

Preparation of the aqueous extracts of QIHM and QRHM

Powdered dry ginseng, astragalus root, pilose asiabell root, white atractylodes rhizome, immature bitter orange, magnolia bark, green tangerine and lindera root were immersed in distilled water (the ratio of the drug and distilled water was 1:10) for 0.5 hour and extracted thrice with distilled water for 0.5 hour each in a boiling water bath. The filtrate was collected after filtration with gauze, mixed and condensed to 0.2 g crude drug/ml.

Animal groups

Mice in each QIHM and QRHM group (n=10) were administered respective aqueous extracts (4 g crude drug/kg/day) by oral gavage and mice in the control group received an equivalent volume of normal saline for 10 days, there are nine groups all together. All the mice were maintained with free access to food and drinking water.

Isolation of liver mitochondria

Mitochondria were isolated by differential centrifugation using a modified version of the protocol of Michele *et al.* (1992). Mice were dislocated and their livers were removed immediately and placed in an ice-cold isolation medium (containing 0.25 M sucrose, 0.5 mM EDTA and 3 mM HEPES, pH 7.4). Livers were homogenized with a motor-driven Teflon pestle in wet ice at 0°C. Following homogenization, samples were centrifuged at 1,000 g for 10 min. This, and all other centrifugation steps, used a Beckman JA-25.50 rotor and Beckman J$_2$-MC centrifuge at 4°C. Supernatants were removed and centrifuge at 12,000 g for 10 min. The pellets were washed twice in the isolation medium, and respun at 12,000 g. Following the final wash, mitochondria were resuspended in the same medium. Protein determinations were carried out using Bradford (1976) method.

Measurement of oxidative phosphorylation curve of liver mitochondria

Respiratory control ratio (RCR) of liver mitochondria was measured using the method described by Estabrook (1967). Oxygen consumption was measured at 30°C in a closed, stirred, and thermostatted glass vessel equipped with a Clark-type oxygen electrode in 2.0 ml respiration buffer. The respiration buffer (pH 7.4) consisted of sucrose 225 mM, EDTA 1 mM, MgCl$_2$ 5 mM, KCl 15 mM, KH$_2$PO$_4$ 15 mM, Tris 50 mM, L-glutamic acid 5 mM, DL-malate 10 mM, and mitochondrial protein 5 g/L. Respiratory state 3 (S$_3$) was the oxygen (O$_2$) consumption by mitochondria in the presence of substrate after the addition of 0.25 mM adenosine diphosphate (ADP, ADP is a potent stimulator of mitochondrial respiration). Respiratory state 4 (S$_4$) was the oxygen consumption when all the ADP has been phosphorylated. S$_3$ and S$_4$ can be calculated according to the oxidative phosphorylation

(OXPHOS) curve. Respiration rates were expressed in nanomoles atom O per minute per milligram of protein. RCR was the ratio of S_3 to S_4 respiration. P/O ratio is the number of ADP molecules phosphorylated per oxygen atom reduced.

Determination of creatine kinase activity

Mice were killed via dislocation, and skeletal muscle from the hind leg was rapidly removed, weighed and made into 1% homogenates with normal saline at 0°C. 2.0 ml homogenate was centrifuged at 2,000 g for 5 min, 100 μl supernatant was added to 900 μl normal saline and mixed, 10 μl of which was used for determination of creatine kinase (CK) activity. CK activity was measured by using a commercial CK monitoring kit [N-acetyl-L-cysteine(NAC)-activated], following the manufacturer's protocol.

Measurement of ATP, ADP, and AMP in liver cells by HPLC

Mice were killed via dislocation, and livers were rapidly removed, weighed and made into 10% homogenates with normal saline at 0°C, 1 ml of ice-cold 0.3 M perchloric acid was added to 1 ml of 10% liver homogenates that were kept on ice for an additional 5 min. Harvested materials were centrifuged at 15,000 g at 4°C for 10 min. The supernatant was neutralized with 80 μl of 3 M KOH, and tubes were kept on ice for an additional 30 min. The resulting precipitate was removed by centrifugation, and the supernatant was stored at -80°C until it was analyzed. 10 μl of neutralized cell extract was used for determination of ATP, ADP, and AMP in liver cells, which was carried out by gradient RP-HPLC (reversed-phase high performance liquid chromatography) with ultraviolet detector at room temperature and with mobile phase at a rate of 0.8 ml/min. Mobile phases used for the gradient system were buffer A (0.05 M KH_2PO_4-K_2HPO_4, pH 6.0) and buffer B, consisting of buffer A plus 10% methanol (v/v). All buffers and solutions used for HPLC analysis were filtered and degassed through a 0.45 μm filter. Gradient elution procedure: buffer A was used as mobile phase between 0 and 3 min, buffer A was changed from 100% to 0% and buffer B from 0% to 100% between 3 and 6 min, buffer B was mobile phase between 6 and 9 min, buffer A was the mobile phase after 9 min, all the running time was 12 min, the detection wavelength was set at 254 nm. ATP, ADP and AMP quantitation in liver cells was calculated by computing the peak area of them, identification and quantitative measurements of nucleotides were carried out by the injection of standard solutions of nucleotides with known concentrations. Standard curves were plotted for individual compounds and were used to determine the contents of ATP, ADP, and AMP in each sample. Total adenylate pool (TAP) and adenylate energy charge (AEC) were calculated by the following formulas respectively: TAP = [ATP] + [ADP] + [AMP], AEC = ([ATP] + 0.5[ADP])/TAP. AEC represents a linear measure of the metabolic energy stored in the adenine nucleotide system.

Statistical analysis

Data were expressed as means±SD and statistical differences between groups were analyzed by Student's t test which was performed using SPSS 16.0 statistical software (SPSS Inc., Chicago, Illinois, USA). The probability (P) values <0.05 were considered to be statistically significant.

Results

The effects of QIHM and QRHM on OXPHOS of liver mitochondria

The liver is known to be the hub of the metabolism; it plays a major role in controlling glucose storage and flux. It is also known that, during heat stress, both lipids and carbohydrate stores can be mobilized for energy generation to attenuate the stress response (Manoli et al., 2007). In addition, many biochemical studies have been performed using mitochondria from liver cells. The rate of ATP synthesis and oxygen consumption (respiratory state 3) driven by complex I substrates, the respiratory control ratio (RCR) and P/O ratio were reduced in liver mitochondria by ginseng and astragalus root, but there were no significant effect on state 4 ($P > 0.05$) (Table 1). It showed that the efficiency of ATP production via ADP phosphorylation was decreased. In perfectly coupled mitochondria, there would be no proton leak across the inner mitochondrial membrane, and the entire gradient generated by the respiratory chain would be used to generate ATP (Boudina and Dale Abel, 2006). Control of oxidative phosphorylation (OXPHOS) allows a cell to produce only the precise amount of ATP required to sustain its activities. Recall that under normal circumstances, electron transport and ATP synthesis are tightly coupled. The value of P/O ratio (the number of molecules of Pi consumed for each oxygen atom reduced to H_2O) reflects the degree of coupling observed between electron transport and ATP synthesis (Mckee and Mckee, 1999). Oxygen consumption increase dramatically when ADP is supplied. The control of aerobic respiration by ADP is referred to as respiratory control. Substrate oxidation accelerates only when an increase in the concentration of ADP signals that the ATP pool needs to be replenished. This regulation matches the rates of phosphorylation of ADP and of cellular oxidations via glycolysis, the citric acid cycle, and the electron-transport chain to the requirement for ATP (Horton, et al., 2002).

Ginseng and astragalus root can decrease oxygen consuming rate and RCR of liver mitochondria obviously, I consider this is appearance of lowering standard metabolic rate and is a kind of protective adaptation. Qi deficiency patients need nutritional supplements, adequate rest, and should reduce energy consumption, ginseng and astragalus root can just achieve this goal, while the effect of other QIHM is not obvious. All the four QRHM can increase RCR and P/O ratio (Table 1).

The effects of QIHM and QRHM on creatine kinase activities

Although ATP is the instantaneous donor of bio-energy in the body, it can not be stored, but phosphocreatine (PCr) can. Among the energy metabolism enzymes in the muscle cells, creatine kinase (CK, EC 2.7.3.2) plays a significant role in energy homeostasis. CK is distributed in skeletal muscle, heart, brain and other tissues and catalyzes the reversible conversion from ATP and creatine (Cr) to ADP and phosphocreatine (PCr, high energy phosphate able to supply ATP on demand) (Zhao et al., 2007; Brancaccio et al., 2007). CK performs a pivotal physiological role in high energy consuming tissues, by acting as an energy buffering and transport system between the sites of ATP production and consumption by ATPases (Bessman and Geiger, 1981). Creatine kinase rapidly provides ATP to highly energy-demanding processes, the rate of transfer of the phosphoryl group from PCr to ADP by CK is greater than the maximum rate of ATP generation by OXPHOS, and this ensures rapid resynthesis of ATP (Wallimann et al., 1998). High tissue CK activity, whether constitutive, induced, or both, may rather directly enhance contractile responses by enhancing cellular energy and contractile reserve (Brewster et al., 2007). Greater CK activity could bind more ADP and increase the rate of the conversion of ADP to ATP, which could reduce the relative levels of local ADP at the contractile proteins (Clark, 1994). CK enhances ATP buffer capacity. We believe that high CK activity may be quite beneficial for rapid and dynamic energy demand. Thus, increased CK activity in muscle tissue might lead to hyperdynamic activity. Both QIHM and QRHM can stimulate activity of CK significantly in the storage of energy, and QRHM is stronger than QIHM (Table 1).

Group	State 3 (nmol /min/mg)[d]	State 4 (nmol /min/mg)[d]	RCR	P/O	CK (U/μg)[e]
Control	83±11	19.4±2.6	4.2±0.6	2.61±0.28	2.25±0.28
Panax ginseng	66±11[b]	18.3±1.9	3.6±0.4[a]	2.21±0.30[b]	2.58±0.26[a]
Astragalus membranaceus	68±13[a]	18.0±2.5	3.7±0.4[a]	2.32±0.24[a]	2.60±0.29[a]
Codonopsis pilosula	80±15	18.3±2.2	4.3±0.6	2.66±0.26	2.59±0.29[a]
Atractylodes macrocephala	81±14	19.1±1.8	4.2±0.7	2.60±0.28	2.63±0.32[a]
Citrus aurantium	91±10	18.5±2.9	4.9±0.4[b]	2.89±0.27[a]	3.32±0.27[b]
Magnolia officinalis	99±13[b]	19.0±2.1	5.1±0.5[b]	2.92±0.34[a]	3.20±0.44[b]
Citrus reticulate	96±12[a]	19.3±2.2	4.9±0.6[a]	2.88±0.22[a]	3.09±0.49[b]
Lindera aggregate	86±16	16.6±2.3[a]	5.2±0.7[b]	2.93±0.31[a]	3.23±0.35[b]

[d] nanomole O_2 per minute per milligram protein (nmol O_2 min^{-1} mg protein^{-1}). [e] Unit of CK activity per microgram protein (U μg protein^{-1}). [a] P <0.05 vs Control. [b] P <0.01 vs Control.

Table 1. Effects of QIHM and QRHM on respiratory function of liver mitochondria and CK activities in vivo (n=10, mean ± standard deviation).

The effects of QIHM and QRHM on energy state of mice hepatocyte in vivo

Adenylate energy charge (AEC) is a sign parameter of cellular energy state (the higher [ATP], the larger the AEC, the higher [AMP], the smaller the AEC), when the tissue's ATP level increased, the pathway for generating ATP would be inhibited; When ATP levels drop due to over consumption of energy by the body, the pathway for generating ATP would be stimulated. AEC represents a linear measure of the metabolic energy stored in the adenine nucleotide system. AEC remained at a fairly narrow range of changes, just like pH value in the cells, energy charge also has a buffering effect, AEC of the most cells fluctuate in the 0.8-0.95 range. Ginseng is commonly known as a high-level herb for tonifying Qi, according to our former study, *Panax ginseng* polysaccharide could increase levels of ATP, TAP and AEC in liver cells under chronic hypoxia condition, therefore, improving energy status, protect mitochondria by inhibiting mitochondrial swelling (Li et al., 2009). It is worth notice that all the four QIHM can increase levels of ATP, AEC and TAP, the effect of ginseng is the most potent; on the contrary, all the four QRHM can decrease levels of ATP, AEC and TAP in liver cells. All the four QIHM can't affect the levels of ADP and AMP; while all the four QRHM can decrease levels of ADP, and increase levels of AMP in liver cells. In a word, QIHM and QRHM increase and decrease bioenergy level of liver cells respectively in vivo. Therefore, Qi is closely related to bioenergy. This result shows that the decreased energy state of the body can be improved by taking QIHM and the effect of QRHM is contrary to that of QIHM. Therefore, the effects on energy regulation of two types of Qi system drugs are different (Table 2).

The similarities and differences in natures, tastes, channel tropism and compositions

Qi is an important concept in physiology and pathology of TCM, directed towards the two main therapeutic principles of Qi—qi-invigoration and qi-flow regulation are self-evidently extreme important. The two therapeutic principles are closely related, complementary and two-way adjustable, and difficult to substitute by others. If they are used properly, they will play an important clinical role in overcoming various difficult diseases. Since there is no direct detection method on Qi, the widely used QIHM (ginseng, astragalus root, pilose asiabell root, white atractylodes rhizome) and QRHM (immature bitter orange, magnolia bark, green tangerine and lindera root) were selected to study the effect on energy metabolism to approach to the nature of Qi in TCM, Comparison of the regulatory role of QIHM and QRHM are summarized as follows.

Group	ATP/ (mmol·L⁻¹)	ADP/ (mmol·L⁻¹)	AMP/ (mmol·L⁻¹)	TAP/ (mmol·L⁻¹)	AEC
Control	1.02±0.28	0.78±0.20	0.09±0.07	1.89±0.33	0.745±0.021
Panax ginseng	1.41±0.36[a]	0.86±0.24	0.07±0.05	2.34±0.46[a]	0.786±0.031[b]
Astragalus membranaceus	1.36±0.31[a]	0.84±0.23	0.11±0.05	2.31±0.38[a]	0.770±0.026[a]
Codonopsis pilosula	1.33±0.22[a]	0.85±0.25	0.12±0.08	2.30±0.32[a]	0.763±0.015[a]
Atractylodes macrocephala	1.25±0.19[a]	0.81±0.26	0.10±0.06	2.16±0.28	0.764±0.016[a]
Citrus aurantium	0.70±0.26[a]	0.53±0.14[b]	0.25±0.12[b]	1.48±0.27[b]	0.651±0.024[b]
Magnolia officinalis	0.71±0.23[a]	0.61±0.13[a]	0.19±0.09[a]	1.51±0.23[b]	0.673±0.033[b]
Citrus reticulate	0.75±0.25[a]	0.49±0.14[b]	0.27±0.12[b]	1.51±0.26[a]	0.660±0.028[b]
Lindera aggregate	0.61±0.22[b]	0.47±0.16[b]	0.29±0.13[b]	1.37±0.21[b]	0.618±0.027[b]

All values are mean±SD (n=10). [a]P <0.05, [b]P <0.01 versus Control group. Each value expressed in mmol·L⁻¹ (ATP, ADP, AMP, TAP) or as a ratio (AEC). ATP: adenosine triphosphate; ADP: adenosine diphosphate; AMP: adenosine monophosphate; TAP: total adenylate pool; AEC: adenylate energy charge

Table 2. The effects of QIHM and QRHM on energy status of mice hepatocytes *in vivo* (n=10, mean ± standard deviation).

The channel tropism of QIHM and QRHM are all the spleen, lung and stomach channel, this shows that they have common target sites in the body. The natures of QIHM are mild or warm, and QRHM are warm, the properties of the two kinds of medicines are similar. QIHM are sweet taste, medicines with sweet taste have the effects of invigoration, normalizing the function of the stomach and spleen, and buffering emergency, etc. they are usually used for tonifying deficiency, easing the pain, and harmonizing the property of different drugs, they are mostly moist and good at nourishing and moistening dryness evil. QRHM are bitter and/or hot tastes, medicines with bitter taste have the effects of purgation and drying the wetness evil etc. medicines with hot taste have the effects of dispersing, promoting the circulation of qi and blood. Therefore, QIHM and QRHM have obviously different effects due to the different tastes. All the QIHM contain more water-soluble carbohydrate due to the sweet taste, and almost all QRHM don't contain or contain less water-soluble carbohydrate composition, most of them contain volatile components (Zheng et al., 1998). Therefore, QIHM and QRHM have obviously different components due to the different tastes (Table 3).

Effects	Items	QIHM	QRHM
Same or similarities	1. channel tropism	spleen, lung and stomach	spleen, lung and stomach
	2. natures	mild or warm	warm
	3.CK activity	increase	increase
Cross effects	1. RCR	decrease or no effect	no effect or increase
	2. oxygen consumption rate	decrease or no effect	no effect or increase
Differences	1. tastes	sweet	bitter and/or hot
	2. compositions	more carbohydrate	volatile components
	3. bioenergy level	increase	decrease

Table 3. Comparisons of the regularity between QIHM and QRHM

11. Conclusion

Qi, is the most basic, the most important and the most nebulous concept, and can be called the biggest enigma in TCM. Research on the nature of Qi in TCM has important theoretical and clinical significance. By analyzing and concluding generation process and function of Qi and bio-energy (ATP), and the effects of Qi-invigorating herbal medicines (QIHM) and Qi-regulating herbal medicines (QRHM) on energy metabolism, the following conclusions can be drawn: Qi and bioenergy have common source and identical functions. Regulation on energy metabolism by QIHM and QRHM showed significant differences due to the different chemical compositions and flavors, QIHM and QRHM are able to improve and decrease the energy state of the body respectively. QIHM invigorate "Qi" through increased intracellular ATP level; and QRHM regulate "Qi" by reducing intracellular ATP levels. Thus, there are many common natures between Qi and bio-energy. Studies on the nature of Qi in TCM should be carried out in other areas of life science due to the wide implications for Qi. With the rapid development of modern life science, we believe that mankind will reveal the truth of the enigma in the near future, it would be better for clinical services.

Without having a scientific model, we cannot advance the research. A future step in Qi research would be to set up effective model to assess Qi effect and identify the effect of Qi on energy metabolism which plays the central role in life activities. If such a model is found, then, the next task might be to find the mechanism of how Qi act. We have a long way to go, but at least, we now have a model which is based upon biochemical pharmacology. With this, we can advance our search to understand the mechanisms of Qi-related phenomena and Qi-healing processes, which have been known for 4000 years.

12. References

Abbott RB, Hui K-K, Hays RD, Li M-D, Pan T. A randomized controlled trial of tai chi for tension headaches. Evid Based Complement Alternat Med 2007; 4: 107 - 113.

Bailey SM, Landar A, Darley-Usmar V. Mitochondrial proteomics in free radical research. Free Radic Biol Med 2005; 38: 175–188.

Benard G, Bellance N, Jose C, Melser S, Nouette-Gaulain K, Rossignol R. Multi-site control and regulation of mitochondrial energy production. Biochim Biophys Acta 2010; 1797: 698–709.

Benard G, Faustin B, Passerieux E, Galinier A, Rocher C, Bellance N et al. Physiological diversity of mitochondrial oxidative phosphorylation, Am J Physiol Cell Physiol 2006; 291: C1172–C1182.

Bessman SP, Geiger PJ. Transport of energy in muscle: the phosphorylcreatine shuttle. Science 1981; 211: 448–452.

Boudina S, Dale Abel E. Mitochondrial uncoupling: A key contributor to reduced cardiac efficiency in diabetes. Physiology 2006; 21:250-258.

Boveris A, Cadenas E. Mitochondrial production of superoxide anions and its relationship to the antimycin-insensitive respiration. FEBS Lett 1975; 54:311-314.

Bradford MM. A rapid and sensitive method for the quantation of microgram quantities of protein utilizing the principle of protein-dye binding. Anal Biochem 1976; 72:248-254.

Brancaccio P, Maffulli N, Limongelli FM. Creatine kinase monitoring in sport medicine. Br Med Bull 2007; 81-82: 209-230.

Brewster LM, Clark JF, van Montfrans GA. Is greater tissue activity of creatine kinase the genetic factor increasing hypertension risk in black people of sub-Saharan African descent? J Hypertens 2007; 18: 1537-1544.

Chai C, Kou J, Zhu D, Yan Y, Yu B. Mice exposed to chronic intermittent hypoxia simulate clinical features of deficiency of both Qi and Yin syndrome in traditional Chinese medicine. Evid Based Complement Alternat Med 2009; doi:10.1093/ecam/nep226

Chance B, Williams GR. Respiratory enzymes in oxidative phosphorylation. I. Kinetics of oxygen utilization. J Biol Chem 1955; 217:383-393.

Chang SO. The nature of touch therapy related to Ki: practitioners' perspective. Nurs Health Sci 2003; 5: 103 – 114.

Chen K. An analytic review of studies on measuring effects of external QI in China. Altern Ther Health Med 2004;10:38 – 50.

Chien CH, Tsuei JJ, Lee SC, Huang YC , Wei YH. Effect of emitted bioenergy on biochemical functions of cells. Am J Chin Med 1991; 19: 285–292.

Clark JF. The creatine kinase system in smooth muscle. Mol Cell Biochem 1994; 133–134:221–232.

Estabrook RW. Mitochondrial respiratory control and the polarographic measurement of ADP:O ratios. Methods Enzymol 1967; 10: 41-47.

Flowers J. What is Qi? Evid-based Complement Altern Med 2006; 3:551-552.

Freyre-Fonsecaa V, Delgado-Buenrostroa NL, Gutiérrez-Cirlosb EB, Calderón-Torresa CM, Cabellos-Avelarb T, Sánchez-Pérezc Y et al. Titanium dioxide nanoparticles impair lung mitochondrial function. Toxicology Letters 2011; 202: 111–119.

Fukushima M, Kataoka T, Hamada C, Matsumoto M. Evidence of Qigong energy and its biological effect on the enhancement of the phagocytic activity of human polymorphonuclear leukocytes. Am J Chin Med 2001; 29: 1–16.

Green DR, Reed JC. Mitochondria and apoptosis. Science 1998; 281: 1309–1312.

Hankey A, McCrum S. Qigong: life energy and a new science of life. J Altern Complement Med 2006; 12:841 – 842.

Horton HR, Moran LA, Ochs RS, Rawn JD, Scrimgeour KG. Principles of Biochemistry (third edition), New Jersey: Science Press and Pearson Education North Asia Limited, 2002.

Ikeda S, Kaneko M, Kumazawa Y, Nishimura C. Protective activities of a Chinese medicine, Hochu-ekki-to, to impairment of hematopoietic organs and to microbial infection. Yakugaku Zasshi 1990; 110: 682-687.

Ishikawa H, Manabe F, Zhongtao H, Yoshii S, Koiso K. The hormonal response to HCG stimulation on patients with male infertility before and after treatment with hochuekkito. Am J Chin Med 1992; 20: 157–165.

Ito H, Shimura K. Studies on the antitumor activity of traditional Chinese medicine. Gan-To-Kagaku-Ryoho 1985; 12: 2145–2148.

Jacobson MD, Weil M, Raff MC. Programmed cell death in animal development. Cell 1997; 88: 347–354.

Kawakita T, Nomoto K. Immunopharmacological effects of Hochu-ekkito and its clinical application. Prog Med 1998; 18: 801–807.

Kiang T. Chinese 'Nature Magazine': Chinese style. Nature 1978; 275: 697.

Kim JY, Pham DD. Sasang constitutional medicine as a holistic tailored medicine. Evid-based Complement Altern Med 2009; 6(S1):11–19.

Kimura H, Nagao F, Tanaka Y, Sakai S, Ohnishi ST, Okumura K. Beneficial effects of the Nishino Breathing Method on the immune activity and stress level. J Altern Complement Med 2005;11:285 – 291.

Kobayashi H, Ishii M. Mind–body, Ki (Qi) and the skin: Commentary on Irwin's 'Shingles immunity and health functioning in the elderly: Tai Chi Chih as a behavioral treatment'. Evid-based Complement Altern Med 2005; 2(1):113–116.

Koshikawa N, Imai T, Takahashi I, Yamauchi M, Sawada S, Kansaku A. Effect of Hochuekki-to, Yoku-kan-san and Saiko-ka-ryukotsu-borei-to on behavioral despair and acetic acid-induced writhing in mice. Meth Findings Exp Clin Pharmacol 1998; 20: 47–51.

Lee M. Effects on *in vitro* and *in vivo* qi-therapy on neutrophil superoxide generation in healthy male subjects. Am J Chin Med 2003; 31:623 – 628.

Lee MS, Huh HJ, Jang HS, Jeong SM, Ryu H, Chung HT. Effects of Qi-therapy on *in vitro* natural killer cell cytotoxic activity. Am J Chin Med 2001a; 29: 17–22.

Lee MS, Huh HJ, Jang HS, Ryu H, Chung HT. Psychoneuroimmunological effects of Qi-therapy: preliminary study on the level of anxiety, mood, cortisol and melatonin, and cellular function of neutrophil and natural killer cell. Stress and Health 2001b; 17: 17–24.

Lee MS, Yang KH, Huh HJ, Kim HW, Ryu H, Lee HS *et al.* Qi-therapy as an intervention to reduce chronic pain and to enhance mood in elderly subjects: a pilot study. Am J Chin Med 2001c; 29: 237–245.

Li XT, Chen R, Jin LM, Chen HY. Regulation on energy metabolism and protection on mitochondria of Panax ginseng polysaccharide. Am J Chin Med 2009; 37(6): 1139-1152.

Li XY, Takimoto H, Miura S,Yoshikai Y, Matsuzaki G, Nomoto K. Effect of a traditional Chinese medicine, Bu-zhong-yi-qi-tang (Japanese name: Hochu-ekki-to) on the protection against Listeria monocytogenes infection in mice. Immunopharmacol Immunotoxicol 1992; 14: 383–402.

Lorenzo HK, Susin SA, Penninger J, Kroemer G. Apoptosis inducing factor (AIF): a phylogenetically old, caspase-independent effector of cell death. Cell Death Differ 1999; 6:516–524.

Machi Y. The Science of Ki. Tokyo: Tokyo Denki University Press, 1993 (in Japanese).

Manoli I, Alesci S, Blackman MR, Su YA, Rennert OM, Chrousos GP. Mitochondria as key components of the stress response. Trends Endocrinol Metab 2007; 18: 190–198.

Mayevsky A. Mitochondrial function and energy metabolism in cancer cells: Past overview and future perspectives. Mitochondrion 2009; 9: 165–179.

Mckee T, Mckee JR. Biochemistry: An Introduction (second edition). New York: McGraw-Hill Companies, Inc. 1999.

Michele AS, Jhon Z, Alain YF, Lee CP. Ischemic injury to rat forebrain mitochondria and cellular calcium homeostasis. Biochim Biophys Acta 1992; 1134:223–232.

Mike Craske NJ, Turner W, Zammit-Maempe J, Lee MS. Qigong ameliorates symptoms of chronic fatigue: A pilot uncontrolled study. Evid-based Complement Altern Med 2009; 6: 265 – 270.

Murakami, Y. Clinical effect of hotyuekkito (bu-zhong-yi-qi-tang) on symptoms due to renal ptosis and stress incontinence. Hinyokika Kiyo 1988; 34: 1841–1843.

Narita M, Shimizu S, Ito T, Chittenden T, Lutz RJ, Matsuda H *et al.* Bax interacts with the permeability transition pore to induce permeability transition and cytochrome c release in isolated mitochondria. Proc Natl Acad Sci USA 1998; 95:14681–14686.

Nishino K. The Breath of Life: Using the Power of Ki for Maximum Vitality. Tokyo, New York, London: Kodansha International, 1997.

Nishino K. Nishino Breathing Method: Activation of Life Energy. Tokyo: Kodansha, 2004 (in Japanese).

Nishino K. The Nishino Breathing Method (in Japanese). In: Arita H, (ed). The Dictionary of Respiration. Tokyo: Asakura Book Publishing Co., 2006; 678 – 697.

Ohnishi ST. Ki: A key to transform the century of death to the century of life. Evid-based Complement Altern Med 2007; 4: 287–292.

Ohnishi ST, Nishino K, Uchiyama K, Ohnishi T, Yamaguchi M. Ki-energy (life-energy) stimulates osteoblastic cells and inhibits the formation of osteoclast-like cells in bone cell cultured models. Evid-based Complement Altern Med 2007; 4: 225–232.

Ohnishi ST, Ohnishi T. The Nishino breathing method and Ki-energy (Life-energy): A challenge to traditional scientific thinking. Evid-based Complement Altern Med 2006; 3: 191–200.

Ohnishi ST, Ohnishi T. Philosophy, psychology, physics and practice of Ki. Evid-based Complement Altern Med 2009a; 6(2): 175–183.

Ohnishi ST, Ohnishi T. How far can Ki-energy reach? – A hypothetical mechanism for the generation and transmission of Ki-energy. Evid-based Complement Altern Med 2009b; 6(3): 379–391.

Ohnishi ST, Ohnishi T, Nishino K. Ki- Energy (Life-Energy) protects isolated mitochondria from oxidative injury. Evid-based Complement Altern Med 2006; 3: 475–482.

Ohnishi ST, Ohnishi T, Nishino K, Tsurusaki Y, Yamaguchi M. Growth inhibition of cultured human carcinoma cells by Ki-energy (Life Energy): Scientific study of Ki-effect on cancer cells. Evid-based Complement Altern Med 2005; 2: 387–393.

Olalde JA. The systemic theory of living systems and relevance to CAM. Part I: The theory. Evid Based Complement Alternat Med 2005; 2: 13 – 18.

Papa S. Mitochondrial oxidative phosphorylation changes in the life span. Molecular aspects and physiopathological implications. Biochim Biophys Acta 1996; 1276:87–105.

Radda GK, Odoom J, Kemp G, Taylor DJ, Thompson C, Styles P. Assessment of mitochondrial function and control in normal and diseased states. Biochim Biophys Acta 1995; 1271:15-19.

Shah S, Ogden AT, Pettker CM, Raffo A, Itescu S, Oz MC. A study of the effect of energy healing on *in vitro* tumor cell proliferation. J Altern Complement Med 1999; 5: 359–365.

Shih HC, Chang KH, Chen FL, Chen CM, Chen SC, Lin YT *et al.* Anti-aging effects of the traditional Chinese medicine Bu-Zhong-Yi-Qi-Tang in mice. Am J Chin Med 2000; 28: 77-86.

Shimizu S, Narita M, Tsujimoto Y. Bcl-2 family proteins regulate the release of apoptogenic cytochrome c by the mitochondrial channel VDAC. Nature 1999; 399: 483-487.

Shin MS. Brief view of chi and alternative therapy. Orient Pharm Exp Med 2002; 2: 1 - 16.

Shinagawa Y. The Science of Qigong (in Japanese). Tokyo: Kobunsha, 1990.

Shinnick P. Qigong: where did it come from? Where does it fit in science? What are the advances? J Altern Complement Med 2006; 12: 351 - 353.

Smith JR, Matus IR, Beard DA, Greene AS. Differential expression of cardiac mitochondrial proteins. Proteomics 2008; 8: 446-462.

Susin SA, Lorenzo HK, Zamzami N, Marzo I, Brothers G, Snow B *et al.* Molecular characterization of mitochondrial apoptosis-inducing factor. Nature 1999; 397: 441-446.

Terasawa K. Evidence-based reconstruction of Kampo medicine: part II—the concept of Sho. Evid Based Complement Alternat Med 2004; 1: 119-123.

Thompson CB. Apoptosis in the pathogenesis and treatment of disease. Science 1995; 167: 1456-1462.

Wallimann T, Dolder M, Schlattner U, Eder M, Hornemann T, O'Gorman E *et al.* Some new aspects of creatine kinase (CK): compartmentation, structure, function and regulation for cellular and mitochondrial bioenergetics and physiology. Biofactors 1998; 8 :229-234.

Weze C, Leathard HL, Grange J, Tiplady P, Stevens G. Healing by gentle touch ameliorates stress and other symptoms in people suffering with mental health disorders or psychological stress. Evid Based Complement Alternat Med 2007; 4: 115 - 123.

Xing C. Chinese Acupuncture and Moxibustion. Beijing, China: Foreign Languages Press, 1987.

Yang L, Tan GY, Fu YQ, Feng JH, Zhang MH. Effects of acute heat stress and subsequent stress removal on function of hepatic mitochondrial respiration, ROS production and lipid peroxidation in broiler chickens. Comparative Biochemistry and Physiology, Part C, 2010; 151: 204-208

Yuasa Y. The Body, Self-Cultivation and Ki-energy (translated by S. Nagatomo and M.S. Hull). Albany, NY: State University of New York Press, 1993.

Yumi K. The Ultimate Example of Nishino Breating. In: Nishino K. (ed). Method: Everyday of Yumi Kaoru with Slim and Bouncing Body. Tokyo: TAKE Shobo Pub. Co., 2005 (in Japanese).

Zhao TJ, Yan YB, Liu Y, Zhou HM. The generation of the oxidized form of creatine kinase is a negative regulation on muscle creatine kinase. J Biol Chem 2007; 282: 12022-12029.

Zheng HZ, Dong ZH, Yu J. Modern Studies and Application of Tradional Chinese Herbal Medicine. Beijing: Xueyuan Press, 1998 (in Chinese).

Part 2

Clinical Practice

5

Hyperspectral Imaging
Technology Used in Tongue Diagnosis

Qingli Li
Key Laboratory of Polor Materials and Devices, East China Normal University
China

1. Introduction

Traditional Chinese Medicine (TCM) is a range of medical practices used in China for more than four millenniums, a treasure of Chinese people (Lukman, He, & Hui, 2007). The important role of TCM and its profound influence on the health care system in China is well recognized. The West also has drawn the attention towards various aspects of TCM in the past few years (Chan, 1995). TCM consists of a systematized methodology of medical treatment and diagnosis (Watsuji, Arita, Shinohara, & Kitade, 1999). According to the basic concept of TCM, the different body-parts, zang-viscera and fu-viscera, the meridians of the body are linked as an inseparable whole. The inner abnormality can present on outer parts, while the outer disease can turn into the inner parts (Bakshi & Pal, 2010). Therefore, some diseases can be diagnosed from the appearance of the outer body. As the significant component part of TCM theory, TCM diagnostics includes two parts: TCM Sizhen (the four diagnosis methods) and differentiation of syndromes. The TCM physician experience the gravity of health condition of a sick person by means of the four diagnosis methods depending on the doctor's body "sensors" such as fingers, eyes, noses etc. Generally, TCM Sizhen consists of the following four diagnostic processes: inspection, auscultation and olfaction, inquiry, and pulse feeling and palpation (Nenggan & Zhaohui, 2004).

In the inspection diagnostic process, TCM practitioners observe abnormal changes in the patient's vitality, colour, appearance, secretions and excretions. The vital signs encompass eyes, tongue, facial expressions, general and body surface appearance. The inter-relationship between the external part of the body such as face and tongue and the internal organ(s) is used to assist TCM doctors to predict the pathological changes of internal organs. In the auscultation and olfaction process, the doctor listen the patient's voice, breathing, and coughing used to judge the pathological changes in the interior of the patient's body. Inquiry diagnosis method is refer to query patient's family history, feelings in various aspects, such as chills and fever, perspiration, appetite and thirst, as well as pain in terms of its nature and locality. Palpation approach involves pulse diagnosis (Siu Cheung, Yulan, & Doan Thi Cam, 2007). The palpation diagnosis has been accepted as one of the most powerful method to give information for making diagnosis from ancient time till now. The pulse waves are measured at six points near the wrists of both hands. The waves are different each other and give us information about different organs (Hsing-Lin, Suzuki, Adachi, & Umeno, 1993). Tongue diagnosis is another inspection diagnostic method which observes the abnormal changes in the tongue proper and the tongue coating to diagnose diseases. This method offers many advantages, such as non-invasive, simple and inexpensive. Tongue diagnosis is one of the most precious and widely used diagnostic methods in TCM, as well as it is great valuable in both clinic applications and self-diagnosis (Bo Pang, Wang, Zhang, & Zhang, 2002). Human tongue is one of the important organs of the body, which carries abound of information of the health status. The information often include tongue colour, tongue fissures or cracks, sublingual veins, tongue coating, etc. There are close relations between these information and our health conditions (Siu Cheung et al., 2007). Whenever there is a complex disorder full of contradictions, examination of the tongue can often quickly clarify the main pathological processes. The tongue's appearance is also a useful gauge for monitoring the improvement or deterioration of a patient's condition (B Pang, Zhang, & Wang, 2005). Therefore, tongue diagnosis is one of the few diagnostic techniques that accord with the most promising direction in the 21st century: no pain and no injury (B. Pang, Zhang, & Li, 2004).

As a convenient and non-invasive method, there are some significances of tongue diagnosis such as judge the exuberance or decline of the genuine Qi, distinguish the nature of disease, detect the location of disease, and infer the tendency of disease (Bakshi & Pal, 2010). However, traditional tongue diagnosis method has inevitable limitations that impede its medical applications. First, the clinical competence of tongue diagnosis is determined by the experience and knowledge of the TCM doctors which has the problem of objectification and standardization. Second, tongue diagnosis is usually based on the detailed visual discrimination, which depends on the subjective analysis of the examiners, makes the diagnostic results unreliable and inconsistent. Thirdly, traditional tongue diagnosis is intimately related to the identification of syndromes, and it is not very well understood in Western medicine and modern biomedicine (B. Pang et al., 2004). Finally, the change of the inspection circumstance like a light source affects the diagnosis result a lot (Kim, Do, Ryu, & Kim, 2008). Therefore, it is necessary to develop some quantitative and objective diagnostic standard for tongue diagnosis.

Nowadays, the rapid progress of information science and technology promotes the automatization of tongue diagnosis based on modern image processing and pattern recognition approaches (B. Pang, David, & Wang, 2005). There has been some work on computerized tongue diagnosis, and many issues of standardization and quantification have been resolved. In recent years, some computer-aided tongue diagnosis systems based on the texture, colour and other proper of tongue image have been developed (Wenshu, Shenning, Shuai, & Su, 2009). These systems include the Computerized Tongue Diagnosis System in TCM (Jiang, Chen, & Zhang, 2000), Automatic Recognition System of TCM Tongue Diagnosis, TID-2000 TCM Tongue Diagnosis Expert System (X. Yu et al., 1994), Tongue Imaging Analysis Instrument (Shen et al., 2003), Automatic Tongue Diagnosis System (Lun-chien, Hou, Ying-ling, Chiang, & Cheng-chun, 2009), computer aided tongue diagnosis system (CATDS) (Zhang, Wang, Zhang, Pang, & Huang, 2005), a prototype of tongue diagnosis support system (Ikeda, Fujiwara, & Yoshida, 2006), and Imaging System for Tongue Inspection (Yang, 2002), etc. In addition, Hong Kong Institute of Technology and Harbin Institute of Technology had made progresses in TCM automatic analysis of tongue image and had built a database with more than 5000 instances of tongue images (X. Yu et al., 1994). Some image processing and pattern recognition algorithms based on these tongue images have also been presented. On automated tongue body segmentation, Li, et al. proposed an improved snake algorithm (W. Li, Zhou, & Zhang, 2004). David Zhang, et al.

have presented a series of tongue body segmentation algorithms such as the Bi-elliptical deformable contour (REDC) algorithm (Bo Pang et al., 2002; B Pang et al., 2005), the combination of polar edge detection and active contour model (Zuo, Wang, Zhang, & Zhang, 2004), etc. Yang, et al. presented the colour active contour models to segment the tongue body (S. Yu, Yang, Wang, & Zhang, 2007). Some other algorithms also have been presented to analyze the tongue color (C. H. Li & Yuen, 2002; Y. G. Wang, Yang, & Zhou, 2007; Zhang, Wang, & Jin, 2005), tongue shape (Z. Liu, Jing-Qi, Tao, & Qun-Lin, 2006; Xu, Tu, Ren, & Zhang, 2008), sublingual veins (Chiu, Lan, & Chang, 2002; Yan, Wang, & Li, 2009; Yan, Yu, Wang, & Li, 2008), tongue fissures and cracks (L. L. Liu & Zhang, 2007; L. L. Liu, Zhang, Kumar, & Wu, 2008; Yue Zhou, Li Shen, & Jie Yang, 2002), tongue coating (Kim et al., 2008; Wu, Zhang, Li, Wang, & Yang, 2008), etc. These studies prove that the accurate segmentation of tongue body and extraction of tongue features is important for computerized tongue diagnosis. Although many issues of standardization and quantification problems have been resolved by these methods, there are still some difficulties because of the limitations of images captured by traditional CCD cameras. For example, the principal difficulties are that when these images are used it is difficult to distinguish in RGB colour space between the tongue and neighbouring tissues that have a similar colour. It is difficult to distinguish between tongue coating and tongue substance and to discrimination the colour automatically and quantificationally. The thickness and transparence of the sublingual mucosa covering the sublingual veins may change due to the different degrees of varicosity. For these reasons, current methods of tongue feature extraction or diagnosis perform well only on tongue images acquired under some special conditions and often fail when the quality of image is less than ideal. Therefore, automatic tongue diagnosis becomes difficult due to the limited information of common digital images, the variation of the illumination, etc. This will undoubtedly limit the applications of these approaches in clinical medicine.

Hyperspectral imaging technology, which comes from the remote sensing field (Chiou, 1984; Harsanyi & Chang, 1994), may offer a solution for these constraints. Hyperspectral remote sensing exploits the fact that all materials reflect, absorb, and emit electromagnetic energy, at specific wavelengths, in distinctive patterns related to their molecular composition (Manolakis & Shaw, 2002). If we introduce this technology to the biomedical diagnosis field, some pathological changes of organism or tissues can be detected and quantificationally analysed in a new way. Actually, hyperspectral imaging of human tissue have been used for many years for characterization and monitoring of applications in biomedicine (Chaudhari et al., 2005; Demos & Ramsamooj, 2003; Timlin J A, 2004). In our previous work, we have developed a microscopic pushbroom hyperspectral imaging system (MPHI) and apply it to analyse the rat retinal sections (Qingli Li, Wang, Zhang, Xu, & Xue, 2010; Qing Li Li, Xue, Xiao, & Zhang, 2007), human blood cells(Qingli Li, Dai, Liu, & Liu, 2009), etc. All these studies show that the hyperspectral imaging technology has significantly advanced in the area of biomedical imaging and early diagnosis. According to the electromagnetic theory, pathological changes of the object surface have a close relationship with its spectrum (Irigoyen & Herraez, 2003; Somosy, Bognar, Thuroczy, & Koteles, 2002). If hyperspectral imaging technology is introduced to computerized tongue diagnosis, both spatial and spectral data, which contain the pathological information of the tongue surface, can be obtained. Therefore, new algorithms should be developed to take advantage of the rich hyperspectral data not found in traditional CCD-based images. In this chapter, an acousto-optic tunable filter (AOTF) based hyperspectral tongue imaging system as well as its applications in computerized tongue diagnosis are presented. The remainder of the chapter is organized as follows. In Section 2 we describe the setup of the hyperspectral tongue imaging system (HTIS). Section 3 proposes the hyperspectral tongue images and the data preprocessing method. Section 4 briefly introduces the tongue body segmentation method based on hyperspectral tongue images. In Section 5, we describe the tongue colour analysis algorithm based on HTIS. In Section 6, tongue cracks extraction algorithm is presented. In Section 7, sublingual veins extraction algorithm based on the new system is proposed. Our conclusions are presented in Section 8.

2. Hyperspectral tongue imaging system

Most contemporary research on computerized tongue analysis focuses on operations in the gray-scale or colour [red-green-blue (RGB)] images (K. Q. Wang, Zhang, & Li, 2001). These images are captured by traditional charge coupled device (CCD) cameras which can only provide the spatial and colour information of tongue surface. The information contained in the CCD based images may not sufficient for computerized tongue diagnosis. Different from the traditional CCD cameras, hyperspectral imaging sensors in the reflective region of the spectrum (sometimes referred to as imaging spectrometers) can acquire digital images in many contiguous and very narrow spectral bands that typically span the visible, near-infrared, and even mid-infrared portions of the spectrum. This enables the construction of an essentially continuous radiance spectrum for every pixel in the scene. Thus, hyperspectral data exploitation makes possible the automatization and quantification of tongue diagnosis based on their spatial and spectral signatures.

In the past few years, we have developed the pushbroom hyperspectral tongue imaging (PHTI) system and found some useful applications in tongue diagnosis (Qingli Li, Liu, Xiao, & Xue, 2008; Q L Li, Xue, & Liu, 2008; Q. L. Li, Xue, Wang, & Yue, 2006). This PHTI system can capture tongue images from 400 nm to 800 nm with spectral resolution at 5 nm. The number of the efficient pixel is 652*620 for each single band image. However, this system needs pushbroom in one of the spatial dimensions to get the hyperspectral image of the whole scene, which makes the process time-consuming. To overcome this problem, we developed an acousto-optic tunable filter (AOTF) based hyperspectral tongue imaging system recently. AOTF is a rapid wavelength-scanning solid-state device that operates as a tunable optical band pass filter. The acoustic wave is generated by radio-frequency signals, which are applied to the crystal via an attached piezoelectric transducer (Inoue & Penuelas, 2001). When such a filter is placed in the optical train of a camera, different wavelengths can pass through it as a function of time. Unlike in a grating based instrument, no motion of the imager or object is required to obtain a complete image cube (Gupta, 2003). This new system offers the advantage of having no moving parts, having simple and compact structure, and can be scanned at very high rate which is more suitable for tongue imaging than the pushbroom one.

The instrument hardware of the AOTF based HTIS is shown in figure 1. The system consists of a camera lens (Nikon AF-S DX 18-200 mm VR II lens), an AOTF (Brimrose, CVA-200), an AOTF controller (radio-frequency drive unit), a CCD camera (Beijing JionHope Technology Ltd., AM1530), a data collection board, and a computer. From the figure we can see that the instrument has similar configuration compared with the standard CCD cameras commonly used by most contemporary research except that an AOTF adapter was coupled between camera lens and CCD in the new system. The dimension of the AOTF based HTIS is 408 mm

(L) × 77 mm (H) × 77 mm (W) as the size of Nikon AF-S DX 18-200 mm VR II lens is 96 mm (L) × 77 mm (Φ), AOTF adapter is 254 mm (L) × 60 mm (H) × 67 mm (W), and CCD is 58 mm (L) × 58 mm (H) × 58 mm (W). The AOTF adapter with Brimrose synthesizer electronics can provide narrow bandwidth, rapid wavelength selection, and intensity control. The high spatial resolution of the AOTF camera is ≥ 100 line pair/mm @ 532 nm. The designed wavelength ranges is 400 - 1000 nm and the spectral resolution is 2 - 6 nm (2 nm @ 543 nm; 5 nm @ 792 nm). The minimum wavelength selection sweep interval of the AOTF is 20 ns, which can meet the imaging speed demand of tongue. The block diagram of the computer controlled experimental setup for the AOTF-based HTIS is shown in figure 2. The tongue surface is illuminated by the light sources under the control of computer. The reflected light by tongue surface are firstly collected via the camera lens, then diffracted by the AOTF adapter, and imaged on the CCD detector at last. The new system can capture image scenes in contiguous but narrow spectral bands under the control of the AOTF controller. The hyperspectral tongue images provided by the instrument can be visualized as a 3D cube (Figure 3) because of its intrinsic structure, where the cube face is a function of the spatial coordinates and the depth is a function of wavelength. In this case, each spatial point on the face is characterized by its own spectrum (often called spectral signature). This spectrum is directly corresponds to the amount of energy that the tongue represented, as hyperspectral sensors commonly utilize the simple fact that a tongue can emits light in certain frequency bands. Consequently, the hyperspectral tongue image data provides a wealth of information about an image scene which is potentially very helpful to tongue diagnosis.

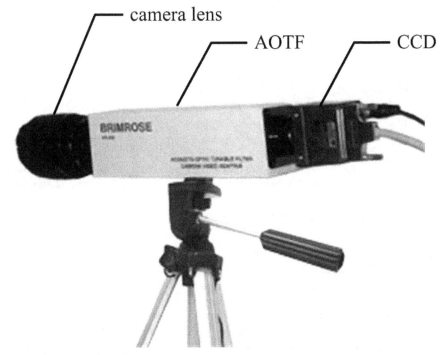

Fig. 1. Actual picture of HTIS

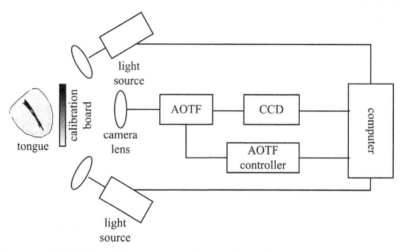

Fig. 2. Diagram of AOTF-based hyperspectral tongue imaging system

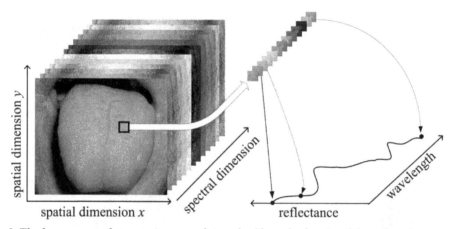

Fig. 3. The hyperspectral tongue imagery data cube (the cube face is a false colour image with the 758 nm, 634 nm, and 430 nm single-band images as the R, G, and B channels)

3. Hyperspectral tongue images and pre-processing

3.1 Hyperspectral tongue images

As one of the most important diagnostic methods in traditional Chinese medicine (TCM), tongue diagnosis inspects tongue to examine the physiological function and pathological changes of human body (Yan et al., 2009). Therefore, it is very important to capture the whole information of tongue surface for computerized tongue diagnosis. Most existing computerized tongue diagnosis methods are using tongue images captured by traditional CCD cameras (colour-based imaging methods). These colour-based images are commonly captured and displayed as a set of three black and white images collected with red (R), green (G), and blue (B) light, i.e., at wavelengths of approximately 630 nm, 545 nm, and 435 nm, respectively (Ballard & Brown, 1982). These wavelengths are chosen to match the spectral response of the human eye (Irigoyen & Herraez, 2003; Ornberg, Woerner, & Edwards, 1999). The relationship between the hyperspectral tongue images and the colour-based RGB images can be presented by figure 4. From the figure it can be seen that the hyperspectral tongue images not only contain the whole information that RGB images contained, but also can provide some information that the RGB images not contained. Although the colour-based tongue image processing is not a very difficult task, it may be neglect some details that dose not exist in the original RGB image in some cases. When the hyperspectral tongue images are used in tongue diagnosis, all bands which cover the wavelength range from 400 nm to 1000 nm will participate in the process. So the hyperspectral-based method can get more information than the colour-based imaging methods. In addition, this is not the only reason that we introduce hyperspectral imaging technology to computerized tongue diagnosis. The technology may also have some other good applications in this field, such as tongue body segmentation, tongue colour discrimination, tongue coating analysis, tongue sublingual veins recognition, etc. Therefore, hyperspectral imaging technology is more useful than traditional CCD cameras in modernization of TCM. Figure 5 illustrate a representative subtotal of hyperspectral images captured at various wavelengths of tongue surface and sublingual veins using the AOTF-based HTIS, respectively. From the figures it can be seen that there are different tongue features in different single band images.

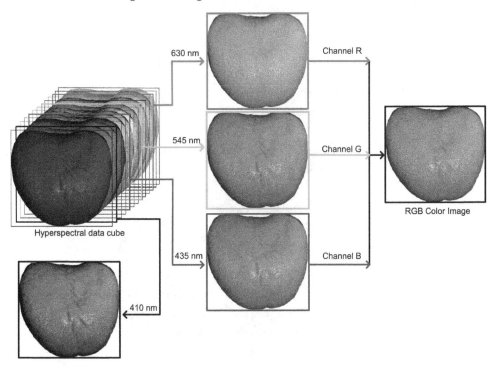

Fig. 4. Relationship between hyperspectral images and colour-based RGB images

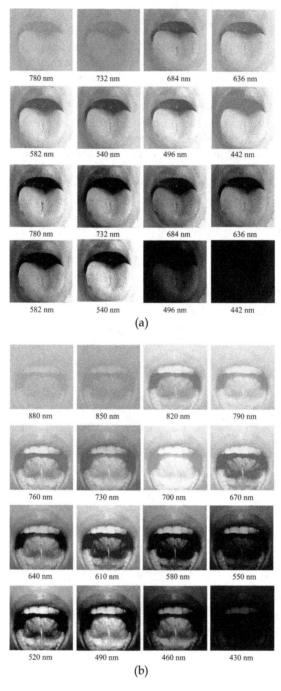

Fig. 5. Single band images of (a) tongue surface and (b) sublingual veins

3.2 Spectral response calibration

One of the big advantages of the HTIS over conventional imaging techniques is the fact that it is capable of acquiring both spatial and spectral information of tongue surface. The spectral response range of the hyperspectral tongue images covering the whole visible wavelength, it can provide more information than the RGB images captured by the traditional CCD. Therefore, it is possible to identify tongue features automatically based on spectral signatures extracted from the hyperspectral tongue images. As the spectral response of the HTIS is inhomogeneous, some data pre-processing procedure should be performed before the spectra extraction. To calibrate the spectral response of the HTIS, a white plane made of Teflon is selected to be the reference plane. Before tongue image collection, a scene of hyperspectral images of the reference plane is captured. Figure 6 shows a typical intensity curve of a pixel extracted from the hyperspectral data of the reference white plane. This curve can be used to represent the spectral response of the HTIS to some extent according to its optical model and sensor model. We define the gray correction coefficient to calibrate the spectral response of the system. The gray correction coefficient k $(i, j; \lambda)$ of each pixel can be calculated by the following formula:

$$k(i,j;\lambda) = \frac{DN(i,j)}{DN(i,j;\lambda)} \tag{1}$$

where k $(i, j; \lambda)$ is the gray correction coefficient of pixel (i, j) in band λ; $DN(i, j; \lambda)$ is the gray value of pixel (i, j) in band λ of the reference hyperspectral data; $DN(i, j)$ is the average gray value of pixel (i, j) in all bands, it can be calculated according to the following formula:

$$DN(i,j) = \left(\sum_{\lambda=1}^{N} DN(i,j;\lambda) \right) / N \tag{2}$$

where N is the total band number of the hyperspectral data. Then, the hyperspectral data of tongue can be calibrated with the gray correction coefficient and the true intensity curve can be extracted. The calibration formula is as follows:

$$DN'(i,j;\lambda) = DN(i,j;\lambda) \cdot k(i,j;\lambda) \tag{3}$$

where DN' $(i, j; \lambda)$ is the gray value of pixel (i, j) at wavelength λ after calibration. In order to assess the efficiency of the calibration method, another white plane is selected as the sample and the hyperspectral data is collected under the same working conditions with the reference plane. Figure 7 shows an intensity curve of the same pixel extracted from the hyperspectral data of the sample white plane before and after calibration respectively. From the figure it can be seen that the intensity curve of the sample white plane is close to the theoretical value after calibration. Then we can get the real tongue intensity curve from the hyperspectral tongue images with the spectral response calibration method.

4. Tongue body segmentation

Currently there are two main issues in computerized tongue analysis. One is the objective representation of tongue's colour, texture and coating with the help of image analysis technology (Zheng, Yang, Zhou, & Wang, 2006). The other is automatic tongue body segmentation. Tongue body segmentation is the primitive work of tongue image analysis. Recently, the main segmentation algorithms are threshold segmentation algorithm, region grow method, watershed algorithm, BEDC algorithm (B Pang et al., 2005), active contour model (for example the snake method (W. Li et al., 2004)), etc. However, these methods can not give satisfied results in the tongue segmentation application. The reason is that the automatic segmentation of anatomical structures in traditional monochromatic images is often performed using model-based nonrigid registration methods. That is to say, an automatic segmentation of a certain structure can be obtained by registering a labelled model, typically generated in a manual segmentation process, to another data set containing the structure of interest. This registration is difficult and laborious (Crum, Hartkens, & Hill, 2004). This is a problem that might be solved if the variability in the spectra of different tissue types could be used to distinguish between the human tongue and the nontongue biological substances in hyperspectral image space (Z. Liu, Yan, Zhang, & Li, 2007).

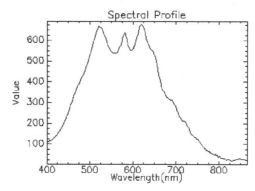

Fig. 6. An intensity curve extracted from the hyperspectral data of the white plane.

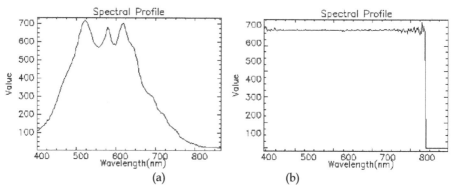

(a)   (b)

Fig. 7. Spectral response calibration result (a) before calibration and (b) after calibration.

After capture the hyperspectral tongue images, an algorithm which can simultaneously utilizes both the spatial and spectral information of the hyperspectral tongue imagery data can be used to segment the tongue body. To evaluate the effectiveness of the hyperspectral based method, we use a spectral angle mapper (SAM) based automatic tongue segmentation algorithm to segment tongue body. The SAM is an automated method for directly comparing image spectra to known spectra (usually determined in a lab with a spectrometer) (Kruse, Lefkoff, & Boardman, 1992). This method treats both spectra (the questioned and known) as vectors and calculates the spectral angle between them. This method is insensitive to illumination since the SAM algorithm uses only the vector direction and not the vector length. Figure 8 show the core of the SAM based automatic tongue segmentation algorithm. First, a transformed image cube (the SAM cube) is constructed by applying the SAM algorithm with each pixel in the original $N*N$ cube with each and every other pixel in the original hyperspectral tongue imagery data cube. In other words, band 1 of the transformed SAM cube contains the spectral angle of the spectrum in pixel location (sample 1, line 1) with every other spectrum in the cube. Band 2 of the SAM cube contains the spectral angle of the spectrum in pixel location (1, 2) with every other spectrum in the original cube, etc. Thus, a 'spectrum' from the SAM cube contains information about tongue edge. The spectra of the SAM cube are then analyzed, each in turn, for edge detection. In other words, a one-dimensional edge detection technique is applied to the one-dimensional data of each SAM cube spectrum. The SAM cube spectrum band number corresponds to pixel address in the original hyperspectral tongue imagery data cube. Thus, when an edge is detected in the analysis of an SAM cube spectrum, the 'band number' of the edge is converted to the (sample, line) address of the original hypspectral tongue imagery data cube and a point is plotted on a separate output plane indicating the presence of the edge (Resmini, 2004). So the SAM based automatic tongue segmentation algorithm converts a two-dimensional kernel-based edge detection problem into a series of one-dimensional edge detection problems.

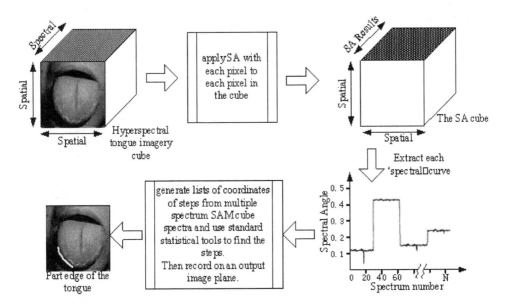

Fig. 8. The core of the SAM based automatic tongue segmentation algorithm

To evaluate the new automatic tongue body segmentation method, several hyperspectral tongue images were captured by the AOTF based system. After the pre-processing and calibration of the hyperspectral data, we can extract the transmittance spectra of each pixel in the whole scene. Then the SAM based automatic tongue segmentation algorithm was used to segment tongue body from the hyperspectral images. Figure 9 shows the segment results by the new algorithm. The results demonstrate the efficiency of this approach.

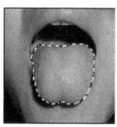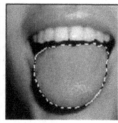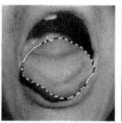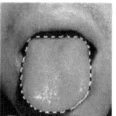

Fig. 9. Tongue body segmentation results

5. Tongue colour analysis and discrimination

In the area of computer-assisted medical diagnosis, colour image analysis can be a useful aid in standardization and automation. Colour image analysis has been applied to assess the power of new drugs on the spreading of skin erythema (Nischik & Forster, 1997), to the identification of skin tumour border (Hance, Umbaugh, & Moss, 1996), assessment and tracking of wound severity (Hansen, Sparrow, & Kokate, 1997), and matching tongue colour images for tongue diseases diagnosis (C. H. Li & Yuen, 2002), etc. These researches show that different colours of organism have some relationship with its physiological functions and changes. So the colour retrieval from images automatically and quantitatively is very important for the purpose of disease diagnosis and prognosis assessment.

Tongue colour is one of the most important pathological features for computer aided tongue diagnosis system. By the use of digital imaging and processing technology, some physiological information of human body condition can be retrieved by analyzing colour features and colour differences extracted from tongue images (X. Wang & Zhang, 2010). For the CCD based RGB colour tongue images, colour image matching can be performed using colour coordinates or based on colour histograms of images in different colour spaces. Therefore, in order to get consistent and standard colour perception of tongue images for tongue analysis, further colour correction to determine the mapping algorithm between its unknown device-dependent RGB colour spaces and a particular known device-independent colour space is necessarily needed. In the past few years, some algorithms in colour correction of tongue images have been developed, such as polynomial-regression-based algorithm and support-vector regression (SVR)-based algorithm (Zhang, Wang, & Jin, 2005), the optimized tongue colour correction scheme (X. Wang & Zhang, 2010), etc. Although these methods can extract some tongue colour features, there are still some difficulties because of the limitations of RGB images captured by the traditional CCD cameras. The principal difficulties are first that when these images are used it is difficult to distinguish in RGB colour space between the tongue and neighbouring tissues that have a similar colour, second it is difficult to distinguish between tongue coating and tongue substance, and third it is also difficult to discrimination the colour automatically and quantificationally. Finally, colour distortion of tongue image, which is often caused by the inconstancy of lighting conditions, can seriously affect the validity of diagnosis results and furthermore, impair the interchange ability among tongue images captured by different devices. For these reasons, current methods of tongue colour calibration or recognition perform well only on tongue images acquired under some special conditions and often fail when the quality of image is less than ideal (Y. G. Wang et al., 2007). So tongue colour analysis becomes difficult due to the limited information of common digital images, the variation of the illumination, etc. According to the principle of physics, colours of an object surface have close relationship with its spectrum (Irigoyen & Herraez, 2003). As spectra of an organism in the range of wavelengths of the visible light (among 400 nm–750 nm approximately) completely includes the RGB colour space, spectra can be used to retrieve tongue colours more accurately. When the HTIS is used in tongue diagnosis, new automatic tongue colour calibration and discrimination method based on hyperspectral images can be used to recognize and classify tongue colours according to the spectral signatures rather than the colour values in RGB colour space. As different tongue colours have different reflectance spectral signatures, we use the SAM algorithm to classify tongue colours. This method is insensitive to illumination since the SAM algorithm uses only the vector direction and not the vector length. The result of the SAM tongue colour classification is an image showing the best match at each pixel. Then different tongue colours can be classified accurately by the SAM algorithm.

In the experiment, 230 scenes hyperspectral tongue images are selected for colour recognition test. The colours of tongue substances are quantized into six classes: light white, pale red, red, maroon, purple and reddish purple, while the colours of tongue coatings include four categories: white, light yellow, yellow and gloom. To evaluate the performance of the tongue colour classification method, four experienced doctors have been asked to label the reference samples, classify all of the 230 tongues using naked eyes, and evaluate the experimental results. Due to the discrepancy between inspection results of different doctors, we treated the consensus as the ground truth. The numbers of tongues corresponding to each category of substances and coatings were given in Tables 1

	color	light white	pale red	red	maroon	purple	reddish purple	Overall
recognize results	light white	25	1				1	
	pale red	2	53	3	1			
	red	1	4	30	3	1	1	
	maroon		2	1	45	1		
	purple		1	1	2	23	2	
	reddish purple		1			3	22	
Number of tongues		28	62	35	51	28	26	230
Rate of correctness (%)		89	85	86	88	82	85	86

Table 1. Colour recognition results and rates of correctness for different categories of substances

and Tables 2. The rate of correctness for each category of substances or coatings was defined as the percentage of the number of tongues classified correctly by the proposed method to the number of tongues in this category (Qingli Li & Liu, 2009). From Tables 1 and Tables 2 it can be seen that the proposed method has good performance in terms of the rates of correctness for colour recognition of coatings and substances. Therefore, hyperspectral tongue images can be used to tongue colour analysis and discrimination. This method is effective to reduce the colour difference between images captured using different cameras or under different lighting conditions, as the method recognize and classify tongue colours using their spectral signatures rather than their colour values in RGB colour space.

	color	white	light yellow	yellow	gloom	Overall
recognize results	white	35	3			
	light yellow	3	108	3		
	yellow	2	9	45	2	
	gloom		2	2	16	
Number of tongues		40	122	50	18	230
Rate of correctness (%)		88	89	90	89	89

Table 2. Color recognition results and rates of correctness for different categories of coatings

6. Tongue cracks extraction and classification

According to the TCM theory, human tongue carries abundant information about the health status of a person. Among the information that collected from tongue surface, the appearance of cracks has been known to have the greatest clinical importance. A crack tongue, also known as a scrotal tongue, is a benign condition characterized by deep grooves (fissures) in the dorsum of the tongue. Tongue cracks refer to the surface of the tongue covered with all kinds of cracks or lines in deep or shallow shape, which are induced by the fusion or separation of the ligular papillae. Normally, the tongue surface should be smooth and soft and show no cracks. When obvious cracks appear on the tongue surface, it suggests the deficiency of *Qi*-blood and the consumption of *Yin* by excessive heat and, sometimes, the blood stasis. For instance, a deep crack in the center reaching to the tip reflects hyperactivity of Heart fire (L. L. Liu & Zhang, 2007). In the past few years, many studies have been conducted on tongue cracks extraction and classification methods based on gray or colour images. Pham and Cai (Pham & Cai, 2004) constructed an algorithms to calculate six features on a tongue in order to analyze different types of tongue disease. These features include roughness, amount of fissures, a* and b* (chromatic dimensions of L* a* b* colour space), energy, and entropy functions computed from the gray level cooccurrence matrix. Liu and Zhang et al. (L. L. Liu & Zhang, 2007; L. L. Liu et al., 2008) presented a tongue crack detection scheme based on the wide line detector (WLD) algorithm. There are also other tongue cracks extraction algorithms, such as the multiscale edge detection algorithm (Shen et al., 2003), the 2D Gabor wavelet transform coefficient energy (GWTE) algorithm (Y Zhou, L Shen, & J Yang, 2002), and the tongue texture analysis method based on the gray covariance matrix model (B. Pang et al., 2004). Although these methods can extract tongue texture or cracks correctly from tongue images, some difficulties still exist in analyzing these features in detail because of the limitations of images captured by traditional CCD cameras.

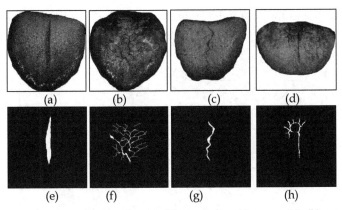

Fig. 10. Tongue cracks extraction results: (a)–(d) single band images, (e)–(h) extraction results by the hyperspectral-based method

In TCM, the appearance of obvious cracks on the tongue surface suggests the development of some pathological changes. According to electromagnetic theory, pathological changes of the object surface have a close relationship with its spectrum (Somosy et al., 2002). If hyperspectral imaging technology is introduced to computerized tongue diagnosis, both spatial and spectral data, which contain the pathological information of the tongue surface, can be obtained. Therefore, tongue cracks can be extracted by some new algorithms which can take advantage of the rich hyperspectral data not found in traditional CCD images (Q. L. Li, Wang, Liu, Sun, & Liu, 2010). Generally, there are three steps in a typical tongue cracks extraction procedure, which is finding, tracking, and linking (L. L. Liu & Zhang, 2007). For hyperspectral tongue images, the spectral signatures should be added to the three stages to improve the extraction accurate. In the cracks finding stage, a target-constrained interference-minimized filter (Ren & Chang, 2000) is used to perform the extraction. The filter casts the detection of a foreground signature mixed with background signatures, as a linearly constrained adaptive beam-forming problem. This technique can be used to determine a vector operator that suppresses the undesired background signatures while enhancing that of the known target signature. After perform the cracks finding procedure, we can get a gradient image with tongue cracks seed images and some noisy pixels. Although the gradient image displays most connected cracks, some isolated spots and misidentified areas still exist in the image. So the tracking and linking process is performed to track the cracks candidates obtained in the first step. As tongue cracks commonly refer to the surface of the tongue covered with all kinds of connected cracks or lines in deep or shallow shape, a roving window of the Hueckel's operator (Ballard & Brown, 1982) is used to prolong or link the bright pixels on the histogram-sliced image. Then postprocessing is performed to reduce the misclassified pixels. Two morphological characteristics of tongue cracks are selected in this algorithm: length and area. The threshold values of them are set to 10 pixels and 100 pixels according to the evaluation standard commonly used by TCM doctors. Then the extracted cracks will be discarded if its length is very short or its area is too small. The final result shows a binary image to represent the extracted tongue cracks which can be classified easily. In the tongue cracks extraction experiment, four scenes of hyperspectral tongue images with different kind of cracks were selected and processed.

Figure 10 shows the extraction results by the proposed method. From the figure it can be seen that the hyperspectral-based tongue cracks extraction method is effective.

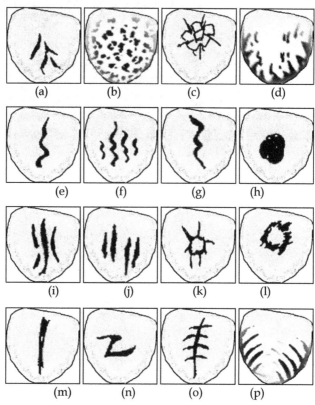

Fig. 11. Typical tongue crack categories

After tongue cracks extraction, they should be classified into several categories to help doctors to diagnose disease. According to the TCM theory, there are 16 kinds of typical tongue cracks as shown in figure 11 (named as Ba zi, Duo dian, Gui, Ju chi, Lai she, Qu chong, Qu she, Shi xin, Shui zi, Si zhi, Tai Yang, Xuan zhen, Yi zi, Yu gu, and Zuoyou pie cracks, respectively). These typical tongue cracks can be regarded as objects with different shapes which commonly observed in the clinical tongue diagnosis in TCM. We can classify these cracks by a shape classifier which comprises a feature extraction stage and a shape matching stage. Shape classification is a basic problem in computer vision. Its application has been found in various areas such as industrial part identification, target identification, character recognition, and medical diagnosis (He & Kundu, 1991). Shape can be represented either by its contour or by its region. Contour-based descriptors such as curvature, chain codes, Fourier descriptors, etc. have been widely used as they can preserve the local information that is important in classification of complex shapes (Thakoor, Gao, & Jung, 2007). Tongue cracks can be assumed to be formed by various segments, each of which has a constant curvature. Therefore, curvature can be chosen as the feature of contour-based shape descriptors and the hidden Markov model (HMM) (Thakoor et al., 2007) can be used as the framework of tongue cracks modelling and classification. Then the generalized probabilistic descent (GPD) method (Katagiri, Juang, & Lee, 1998) was used as a training algorithm for the tongue cracks classifier. At last, tongue cracks can be classified into different typical categories. To evaluate the hyperspectral based tongue cracks classify method, 480 scenes of hyperspectral tongue images were captured by the HTIS from in-patients in hospital. These tongue cracks can be divided into 16 typical classes named Class 1 ~ Class 16 which corresponding to figure 1 (a) ~ (p), respectively. The 16 typical tongue cracks are chosen according to the diagnostic criteria commonly used by TCM doctors (S. Wang, Wang, & Wang, 2001). The numbers of tongue cracks corresponding to each category classified by the proposed algorithm was given in Table 3 (the confusion matrix of classification). The rate of correctness for each category of cracks is defined as the percentage of the number of tongues classified correctly by the proposed method to the number of tongues in this category. From the table it can be seen that the proposed method has good performance in terms of the rates of correctness for tongue cracks classification. As a preliminary research, we just use the most simple classify method here. To classify tongue cracks more accurately, some other

Cracks type	C 1	C 2	C 3	C 4	C 5	C 6	C 7	C 8	C 9	C 10	C 11	C 12	C 13	C 14	C 15	C 16	Overall
Classification results																	
C 1	23			1													
C 2		12			2										1		
C 3	1		22				1				1						
C 4				50		1					2				1		
C 5				1	30									1			
C 6						38			2	1				1			
C 7							33							1			
C 8			1					25	4			4					
C 9		1			2			3	43			1			1		
C 10				2						17	1			1			
C 11	1		1								13						
C 12			1				1					29			2		
C 13			1									1	27				
C 14					3	1					1			16	1		
C 15		1			1			1							12		
C 16			2													32	
Number of tongues	25	14	25	54	33	44	37	29	49	19	16	33	32	18	15	37	480
Rate of correctness (%)	92	86	88	93	91	86	89	86	88	89	81	88	84	89	80	86	88

Table 3. Tongue cracks classification results and rate of correctness for each category

classification method such as support vector machines (SVM) should be used in the future as SVM is a more accurate classifier than the maximum likelihood method and can efficiently analyze hyperspectral data directly in the hyperdimensional feature space without the need for any feature-reduction procedure (Melgani & Bruzzone, 2002).

7. Sublingual veins analysis

According to TCM diagnostics theory, sublingual veins collateral stem from the base of tongue and connect directly with visceras, especially the heart, spleen, liver and kidney. Under normal conditions, they are bluish purple in colour and moist. These veins travel naturally without meandering, distending or exhibiting any varicosity. The sublingual veins are sensitive indicators of the blood stasis and show the activity of the blood circulation (Chiu et al., 2002). Inspection of sublingual veins can provide valuable insights into the healthy status of human body (Yan et al., 2009). However, the subjective characteristics of the traditional method impede this objective because sublingual vein diagnoses are usually based on detailed visual discrimination, which mainly depends on the subjective analysis of the examiners. Therefore, a quantitative analysis should produce the possibility of evaluating and classifying the severity of blood stasis in a less subjective way and deriving an automatic diagnostic procedure.

In recent years, some studies have shown that the accurate extraction of tongue features is important for computerized tongue diagnosis (Bakshi & Pal, 2010; Qingli Li & Liu, 2009; B. Pang et al., 2005; B. Pang et al., 2004). The automatic extraction of sublingual veins from complex scenes should also be foremost solved due to the qualities of segmentation directly influencing the subsequent feature extraction and recognition. Some experiments have been conducted on sublingual images acquired by an ordinary camera under a visible light source or an infrared light source for the extraction of sublingual veins. Takeichi and Sato (Takeichi & Sato, 1997) performed computer-assisted image analyses on the colour of the tongues of 95 medical students to enhance the accuracy and objectivity of sublingual veins inspections for determining blood stasis. This is a prior research on colour of sublingual veins. Then, Chiu et al. (Chiu et al., 2002) developed a computerized inspection system and presented a method to extract the chromatic and geometrical properties of sublingual veins quantitatively. Their system is also a colour based method that can extract the length, width, area, and colour information from the sublingual veins. Afterwards, Yan et al. (Yan et al., 2008) used monochrome industrial CCD with enhanced near infrared sensitivity to capture sublingual vein images. More recent studies by them (Yan et al., 2009) have focused on the pixel-based sublingual vein segmentation algorithm and adaptive sublingual vein segmentation algorithm for colour sublingual images with visible and low contrasts. Although many issues on the standardization and quantification of sublingual veins have been resolved, there are still some difficulties because of the limitations of these kinds of images (Q. Li, Wang, Liu, Guan, & Xu, 2011). For example, the thickness and transparence of the sublingual mucosa covering the sublingual veins may change due to the different degrees of varicosity. This change may lead to the sublingual veins being clear in some sublingual images but blurry in others, the contours of the sublingual veins are difficult to extract.

If the HTIS were used to capture the sublingual vein images, it can provide both the spectral and spatial information of the sublingual veins. The spectra extracted from the hyperspectral sublingual images can be represented as a non-stationary sequence of feature vectors, and the spectral correlation and band-to-band variability can be characterized using some models. For example, the SAM or the hidden Markov model (HMM) can be used to extract the sublingual veins from hyperspectral images. Unlike existing approaches, the new method can recognize sublingual veins using their spectral signatures rather than their gray values. To evaluate the effectiveness of the HTIS on sublingual veins analysis, some scenes of hyperspectral sublingual images were captured. Figure 5 (b) shows some single band images of sublingual veins. Here we use the improved spectral angle mapper algorithm to segment the sublingual veins. Spectral angle mapper (SAM) algorithm is a tool that permits rapid mapping of spectral similarity of one image spectrum to another spectrum (Kruse et al., 1992; Park, Windhama, Lawrencea, & Smitha, 2007). The algorithm determines the spectral similarity between two spectra by calculating the 'angle' between them. The angle between the endmember spectra vector and each pixel vector in N-dimensional space is compared. Smaller angles represent closer matches to the reference spectra. This algorithm can extract the target from hyperspectral images effectively by mapping the spectral similarity. However, the wavelengths often shift several bands with the influence of noise in the real HTIS which lead to some extraction errors. To overcome this disadvantage, an improved spectral angle mapper (ISAM) algorithm is used to extract the sublingual veins. The ISAM algorithm calculate the spectral angle (SA) not only between the reference spectral vector and the testing spectral vector, but also between the reference spectral vector and the testing spectral vector with shift 2 bands both forward and backward, respectively. Then the maximum was selected as the real SA value between the two vectors as the following formula

$$SA = Max\left(\alpha\left(\vec{T}_j, \vec{R}\right)\right) = Max\left(\cos\left(\sum_{i=1}^{N} t_{i+j} r_i \middle/ \sqrt{\sum_{i=1}^{N} t_{i+j}^2 \sum_{i=1}^{N} r_i^2}\right)\right) \tag{4}$$

where $j = -2, -1, 0, 1, 2$.

This method is insensitive to illumination since the ISAM algorithm uses only the vector direction and not the vector length. It also can reduce the wavelengths shift errors effectively. Figure 12 shows the extraction results by the ISAM algorithm with SA = 0.1. From the figure it can be seen that the ISAM algorithm can segment the sublingual veins accurately. As sublingual veins may be correlated with certain diseases (Pham & Cai, 2004), defining several quantitative features for classification in a computer-aided tongue disease diagnosis is necessary. According to the diagnostic standards of experienced doctors, two quantitative features can be selected after sublingual vein extraction, that is, the breadth feature and the chromatic feature. The breadth feature denotes the breadth measurement of the segmented sublingual veins, the value of which is the indicator of a special disease (Yan et al., 2009). The chromatic feature is another important pathological feature of sublingual veins. The colours used as diagnostic measurements in sublingual vein disease diagnoses are usually compounds of several colours due to the complex disorder caused by some pathological processes. The existing colour analysis mainly utilizes the RGB triple values or hue values of single pixels or the mean of the tongue texture block (C. H. Li & Yuen, 2002; B. Pang et al., 2004), which is difficult due to the limited information of these kinds of images. As presented in the previous section, we can use spectra to retrieve organism colours, as the wavelength range of the hyperspectral tongue imaging system covering the whole visible light includes the RGB colour spaces. Therefore, different colours of sublingual veins can be represented by the corresponding reflectance spectral curves. With these quantitative sublingual vein features, some classifiers, such as Bayesian networks, neural networks, and support vector machines, can be used to model the relationship between these quantitative features and diseases.

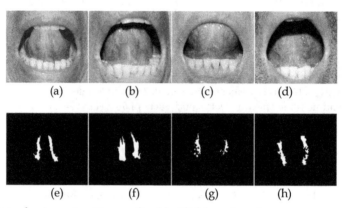

Fig. 12. Sublingual veins extraction results. (a)~(d) false colour images composed by single band images at 630 nm, 540 nm, and 430 nm as R, G, and B channels. (e)~(h) the extraction results by the ISAM algorithm.

8. Conclusion

Among the four diagnostic processes of TCM: inspection, auscultation and olfaction, inquiry, and pulse feeling and palpation, the examination of tongue is one of the most important approaches for getting significant evidences in diagnosing the patient's health conditions. However, owing to its drawbacks in quantification and standardization, the development of tongue diagnosis is stagnated (Zhang, Wang, Zhang et al., 2005). Computerized methods for TCM allow researchers to identify required information more efficiently, discover new relationships which are obscured by merely focusing on Western medicine, and bridge the gaps between Western Medicine and TCM (Lukman et al., 2007). Therefore, getting the overall information about tongue surface is very important for computerized tongue diagnosis system. In this chapter, an AOTF based HTIS which can capture hyperspectral images of human tongue at a series of wavelengths is developed and used in tongue diagnosis. The basic principles and instrumental systems of the new system, the data pre-processing method as well as some applications are presented. Compared with the pushbroom hyperspectral tongue imager used in our previous works (Q. Li et al., 2008; Q. L. Li et al., 2006), this new type of hyperspectral tongue imaging system has the advantage of having no moving parts and can be scanned at very high rates. As the hyperspectral tongue images can provide more information than the CCD based images, we can find some successful applications in computerized tongue diagnosis such as tongue body segmentation, tongue colour analysis and discrimination, tongue cracks extraction and classification, sublingual veins analysis, etc. Preliminary experiments show that the AOTF-based hyperspectral tongue imaging system is superior to the traditional CCD based methods because the hyperspectral images can provide more information about the tongue surface. In future studies, we will extract the quantitative features of the tongue surface and find some methods to model the relationship between these features and certain diseases.

9. Acknowledgment

This work is supported in part by the National Natural Science Foundation of China (NSFC) (grants 61177011, 60807035, 60976004)), the Specialized Research Fund for the Doctoral Program of Higher Education of China (grant 200802691006), the project supported by the Shanghai Commission of Science and Technology (SCST) China (grant 09JC1405300), the Fundamental Research Funds for the Central Universities, and the Project supported by the State Key Development Program for Basic Research of China(Grant No. 2011CB932903). We are grateful for the assistance and support provided by Mrs Ivona Lovric and the Editorial Board of this book.

10. References

Bakshi, D., & Pal, S. (2010, 16-18 Dec. 2010). *Introduction about traditional Tongue Diagnosis with scientific value addition*. Paper presented at the Systems in Medicine and Biology (ICSMB), 2010 International Conference on.

Ballard, D. H., & Brown, C. M. (1982). *Computer Vision*: Prentice Hall.

Chan, K. (1995). Progress in traditional Chinese medicine. *Trends in Pharmacological Sciences, 16*(6), 182-187.

Chaudhari, A. J., Darvas, F., Bading, J. R., Moats, R. A., Conti, P. S., Smith, D. J., et al. (2005). Hyperspectral and multispectral bioluminescence optical tomography for small animal imaging. *Physics in Medicine and Biology, 50*(23), 5421-5441.

Chiou, W. C. (1984). Dynamic descriptors for contextual classification of remotely sensed hyperspectral image data-analysis. *Applied Optics, 23*(21), 3889-3892.

Chiu, C.-C., Lan, C.-Y., & Chang, Y.-H. (2002). Objective assessment of blood stasis using computerized inspection of sublingual veins. *Computer Methods and Programs in Biomedicine, 69*(1), 1-12.

Crum, W. R., Hartkens, T., & Hill, D. L. G. (2004). Non-rigid image registration: theory and practice. *British Journal of Radiology, 77*, S140-S153.

Demos, S. G., & Ramsamooj, R. (2003). Hyperspectral imaging of cells: toward real-time pathological assessment. In K. M. Iftekharuddin & A. A. S. Awwal (Eds.), *Photonic Devices and Algorithms for Computing V, Proceedings of the SPIE* (Vol. 5021, pp. 133-137). San Diego, CA, USA.

Gupta, N. (2003). A no-moving-parts UV/visible hyperspectral imager. *Chemical and Biological Standoff Detection, 5268*, 89-95.

Hance, G. A., Umbaugh, S. E., & Moss, R. H. (1996). Unsupervised color image segmentation: with application to skin tumor borders. *IEEE Eng. Med. Biol. Mag., 15*(1), 104-111.

Hansen, G. L., Sparrow, E. M., & Kokate, J. Y. (1997). Wound status using color image processing. *IEEE Trans. Med. Imaging, 16*(1), 78-86.

Harsanyi, J. C., & Chang, C. I. (1994). Hyperspectral image classification and dimensionality reduction-an orthogonal subspace projection approach. *IEEE Transactions on Geoscience and Remote Sensing, 32*(4), 779-785.

He, Y., & Kundu, A. (1991). 2-D shape classification using hidden markov model. *IEEE Transactions on Pattern Analysis and Machine Intelligence, 13*(11), 1172-1184.

Hsing-Lin, L., Suzuki, S., Adachi, Y., & Umeno, M. (1993, 25-29 Oct. 1993). *Fuzzy theory in traditional Chinese pulse diagnosis.* Paper presented at the Neural Networks, 1993. IJCNN '93-Nagoya. Proceedings of 1993 International Joint Conference on.

Ikeda, N., Fujiwara, Y., & Yoshida, H. (2006, 18-21 Oct. 2006). *Tongue diagnosis support system.* Paper presented at the SICE-ICASE, 2006. International Joint Conference.

Inoue, Y., & Penuelas, J. (2001). An AOTF-based hyperspectral imaging system for field use in ecophysiological and agricultural applications. *International Journal of Remote Sensing, 22*(18), 3883-3888.

Irigoyen, J., & Herraez, J. (2003). *Electromagnetic spectrum and color vision.* Paper presented at the Proceedings of the 3rd International Symposium on Image and Signal Processing and Analysis, ISPA 2003.

Jiang, Y., Chen, J., & Zhang, H. (2000). Computerized system of diagnosis of tongue in Traditional Chinese Medicine. *Chinese Journal of Integrated Traditional and Western Medicine, 20*(2), 145-147.

Katagiri, S., Juang, B.-H., & Lee, C.-H. (1998). Pattern recognition using a family of design algorithms based upon the generalized probabilistic descent method. *Proceedings of the IEEE, 86*(11), 2345 - 2373.

Kim, K. H., Do, J. H., Ryu, H., & Kim, J. Y. (2008, 23-26 Nov. 2008). *Tongue diagnosis method for extraction of effective region and classification of tongue coating.* Paper presented at the Image Processing Theory, Tools and Applications, 2008. IPTA 2008. First Workshops on.

Kruse, F. A., Lefkoff, A. B., & Boardman, J. W. (1992). *The spectral image processing system (SIPS)-software for integrated analysis of AVIRIS data.* Paper presented at the Summaries of the 4th Annual JPL Airborne Geoscience Workshop, Pasadena.

Li, C. H., & Yuen, P. C. (2002). Tongue image matching using color content. *Pattern Recognition, 35*(2), 407-419.

Li, Q., Dai, C., Liu, H., & Liu, J. (2009). *Leukemic cells segmentation algorithm based on molecular spectral imaging technology* Paper presented at the International Symposium on Photoelectronic Detection and Imaging 2009: Advances in Infrared Imaging and Applications, Beijing, China.

Li, Q., Liu, J., Xiao, G., & Xue, Y. (2008). Hyperspectral tongue imaging system used in tongue diagnosis, *The 2nd International Conference on Bioinformatics and Biomedical Engineering, 2008. ICBBE 2008.* (pp. 2579-2581). Shanghai.

Li, Q., & Liu, Z. (2009). Tongue color analysis and discrimination based on hyperspectral images. *Computerized Medical Imaging and Graphics, 33*(3), 217-221.

Li, Q., Wang, Y., Zhang, J., Xu, G., & Xue, Y. (2010). Quantitative analysis of protective effect of Erythropoietin on diabetic retinal cells using molecular hyperspectral imaging technology. *IEEE Transactions on Biomedical Engineering, 57*(7), 1699-1706.

Li, Q., Wang, Y. T., Liu, H. Y., Guan, Y. N., & Xu, L. A. (2011). Sublingual vein extraction algorithm based on hyperspectral tongue imaging technology. *Computerized Medical Imaging and Graphics, 35*(3), 179-185.

Li, Q. L., Wang, Y. T., Liu, H. Y., Sun, Z., & Liu, Z. (2010). Tongue fissure extraction and classification using hyperspectral imaging technology. *Applied Optics, 49*(11), 2006-2013.

Li, Q. L., Xue, Y. Q., & Liu, Z. (2008). A novel system for tongue inspection based on hyperspectral imaging system. *Journal of Biomedical Engineering, 25*(2), 368-371.

Li, Q. L., Xue, Y. Q., Wang, J. Y., & Yue, X. Q. (2006). Application of hyperspectral imaging system in tongue analysis of traditional Chinese medicine. *Journal of Infrared and Millimeter Waves, 25*(6), 465-468.

Li, Q. L., Xue, Y. Q., Xiao, G. H., & Zhang, J. F. (2007). New microscopic pushbroom hyperspectral imaging system for application in diabetic retinopathy research. *Journal of Biomedical Optics, 12*(6), 1-4.

Li, W., Zhou, C., & Zhang, Z. (2004, June 15-19). *The segmentation of the body of tongue based on the improved snake algorithm in traditional chinese medicine.* Paper presented at the Proceedings of the 5th World Congress on Intelligent Control and Automation, Hangzhou.

Liu, L. L., & Zhang, D. (2007). Extracting tongue cracks using the wide line detector. In *Medical Biometrics* (Vol. 4901, pp. 49-56): Springer Berlin / Heidelberg.

Liu, L. L., Zhang, D., Kumar, A., & Wu, X. (2008). *Tongue line extraction.* Paper presented at the Pattern Recognition, 2008. ICPR 2008. 19th International Conference on, Tampa, FL.

Liu, Z., Jing-Qi, Y., Tao, Z., & Qun-Lin, T. (2006, 13-16 Aug. 2006). *Tongue Shape Detection Based on B-Spline.* Paper presented at the Machine Learning and Cybernetics, 2006 International Conference on.

Liu, Z., Yan, J. Q., Zhang, D., & Li, Q. L. (2007). Automated tongue segmentation in hyperspectral images for medicine. *Applied Optics, 46*(34), 1-7.

Lukman, S., He, Y. L., & Hui, S. C. (2007). Computational methods for Traditional Chinese Medicine: A survey. *Computer Methods and Programs in Biomedicine, 88*(3), 283-294.

Lun-chien, L., Hou, M. C. c., Ying-ling, C., Chiang, J. Y., & Cheng-chun, H. (2009, 17-19 Oct. 2009). *Automatic Tongue Diagnosis System.* Paper presented at the Biomedical Engineering and Informatics, 2009. BMEI '09. 2nd International Conference on.

Manolakis, D., & Shaw, G. (2002). Detection algorithms for hyperspectral Imaging applications. *Ieee Signal Processing Magazine, 19*(1), 29-43.

Melgani, F., & Bruzzone, L. (2002). Support vector machines for classification of hyperspectral remote-sensing images, *Geoscience and Remote Sensing Symposium, 2002. IGARSS '02. 2002 IEEE International* (Vol. 1, pp. 24-28).

Nenggan, Z., & Zhaohui, W. (2004, 10-13 Oct. 2004). *TCM-SIRD: an integrated aided system for traditional Chinese medicine Sizheng.* Paper presented at the Systems, Man and Cybernetics, 2004 IEEE International Conference on.

Nischik, M., & Forster, C. (1997). Analysis of skin erythema using true color images. *IEEE Trans. Med. Imaging, 16*(6), 711-716.

Ornberg, R. L., Woerner, B. M., & Edwards, D. A. (1999). Analysis of stained objects in histological sections by spectral imaging and differential absorption. *The Journal of Histochemistry & Cytochemistry, 47*(10), 1307-1331.

Pang, B., David, Z., & Wang, K. Q. (2005). Tongue image analysis for appendicitis diagnosis. *Inf. Sci., 175*(3), 160-176.

Pang, B., Wang, K., Zhang, D., & Zhang, F. (2002, 2002). *On automated tongue image segmentation in Chinese medicine.* Paper presented at the Pattern Recognition, 2002. Proceedings. 16th International Conference on.

Pang, B., Zhang, D., & Li, N. M. (2004). Computerized tongue diagnosis based on bayesian networks. *IEEE Trans. On Biomedical Eng., 51*(10), 1803-1810.

Pang, B., Zhang, D., & Wang, K. Q. (2005). The bi-elliptical deformable contour and its application to automated tongue segmentation in chinese medicine. *IEEE Transactions on Medical Imaging, 24*(8), 946-956.

Park, B., Windhama, W. R., Lawrencea, K. C., & Smitha, D. P. (2007). Contaminant Classification of Poultry Hyperspectral Imagery using a Spectral Angle Mapper Algorithm. *Biosystems Engineering, 96*(3), 323-333.

Pham, B. L., & Cai, Y. (2004). *Visualization techniques for tongue analysis in traditional Chinese medicine.* Paper presented at the roceedings of the SPIE.

Ren, H., & Chang, C. (2000). Target-constrained interference-minimized approach to subpixel target detection for hyperspectral images. *Optical Engineering, 39*(12), 3138-3145.

Resmini, R. G. (2004). Hyperspectral/spatial detection of edges (HySPADE): An algorithm for spatial and spectral analysis of hyperspectral information. *Algorithms and Technologies for Multispectral, Hyperspectral, and Ultraspectral Imagery X, 5425,* 433-442.

Shen, L., Wei, B., Cai, Y., Zhang, X., Wang, Y., Chen, J., et al. (2003). Image analysis for tongue characterization. *Chinese Journal of Electronics, 12*(3), 317-323.

Siu Cheung, H., Yulan, H., & Doan Thi Cam, T. (2007, 10-13 Dec. 2007). *Machine learning for tongue diagnosis.* Paper presented at the Information, Communications & Signal Processing, 2007 6th International Conference on.

Somosy, Z., Bognar, G., Thuroczy, G., & Koteles, G. J. (2002). Biological responses of tight junction to ionizing radiation and electromagnetic field exposition. *Cellular and Molecular Biology, 48*(5), 571-575.

Takeichi, M., & Sato, T. (1997). Computerized color analysis of "xue yu" (blood stasis) in the sublingual vein using a new technology. *Am J Chin Med, 25*(2), 213-219.

Thakoor, N., Gao, J., & Jung, S. (2007). Hidden markov model-Based weighted likelihood discriminant for 2-D shape classification. *IEEE Transactions on Image Peocessing, 16*(11), 2707-2719.

Timlin J A, S. M. B., Haaland D M, et al. (2004). Hyperspectral imaging of biological targets: the difference a high resolution spectral dimension and multivariate analysis can make. *IEEE International Symposium on Biomedical Imaging: Macro to Nano, 2,* 1529-1532.

Wang, K. Q., Zhang, D., & Li, N. M. (2001). *Tongue diagnosis based on biometric pattern recognition technology.* Singapore: The World Scientific Publishers.

Wang, S., Wang, P., & Wang, h. (2001). Tongue texture and hepatocirrhosis. *J. Gansu College of TCM, 18*(4), 36-38.

Wang, X., & Zhang, D. (2010). An Optimized Tongue Image Color Correction Scheme. *IEEE Transactions on Information Technology in Biomedicine,* 1355-1364.

Wang, Y. G., Yang, J., & Zhou, Y. (2007). Region partition and feature matching based color recognition of tongue image. *Pattern Recognition Letters, 28*(1), 11-19.

Watsuji, T., Arita, S., Shinohara, S., & Kitade, T. (1999, 1999). *Medical application of fuzzy theory to the diagnostic system of tongue inspection in traditional Chinese medicine.* Paper presented at the Fuzzy Systems Conference Proceedings, 1999. FUZZ-IEEE '99. 1999 IEEE International.

Wenshu, L., Shenning, H., Shuai, W., & Su, X. (2009, 3-5 Nov. 2009). *Towards the objectification of tongue diagnosis: Automatic segmentation of tongue image.* Paper presented at the Industrial Electronics, 2009. IECON '09. 35th Annual Conference of IEEE.

Wu, Z.-z., Zhang, X.-l., Li, Y.-h., Wang, J.-g., & Yang, M. (2008, 12-14 Dec. 2008). *Exploration of tongue coating protein based on proteomics assessment and bioinformatics analysis.* Paper presented at the IT in Medicine and Education, 2008. ITME 2008. IEEE International Symposium on.

Xu, J., Tu, L., Ren, H., & Zhang, Z. (2008, 16-18 May 2008). *A Diagnostic Method Based on Tongue Imaging Morphology.* Paper presented at the Bioinformatics and Biomedical Engineering, 2008. ICBBE 2008. The 2nd International Conference on.

Yan, Z., Wang, K., & Li, N. (2009). Computerized feature quantification of sublingual veins from color sublingual images. *computer methods and programs in biomedicine, 93*(2), 192-205.

Yan, Z., Yu, M., Wang, K., & Li, N. (2008). Sublingual vein segmentation from near infrared sublingual images. *Journal of Computer Aided Design & Computer Graphics 20*(12), 1569-1574.

Yang, C. (2002, 2002). *A novel imaging system for tongue inspection.* Paper presented at the Instrumentation and Measurement Technology Conference, 2002. IMTC/2002. Proceedings of the 19th IEEE.

Yu, S., Yang, J., Wang, Y., & Zhang, Y. (2007, 6-8 July 2007). *Color Active Contour Models Based Tongue Segmentation in Traditional Chinese Medicine.* Paper presented at the Bioinformatics and Biomedical Engineering, 2007. ICBBE 2007. The 1st International Conference on.

Yu, X., Tan, Y., Zhu, Z., Suo, Z., Jin, G., Weng, W., et al. (1994). Study on method of automatic diagnosis of tongue feature in Traditional Chinese Medicine. *Chinese Journal of Biomedical Engineering, 13*(4), 336-344.

Zhang, H. Z., Wang, K. Q., & Jin, X. S. (2005). *SVR based color calibration for tongue image.* Paper presented at the Proceedings of 2005 International Conference on Machine Learning and Cybernetics.

Zhang, H. Z., Wang, K. Q., Zhang, D., Pang, B., & Huang, B. (2005, 2005). *Computer Aided Tongue Diagnosis System.* Paper presented at the Engineering in Medicine and Biology Society, 2005. IEEE-EMBS 2005. 27th Annual International Conference of the.

Zheng, Y. J., Yang, J., Zhou, Y., & Wang, Y. Z. (2006). Color-texture based unsupervised segmentation using JSEG with fuzzy connectedness. *Journal of Systems Engineering and Electronics, 17*(1), 213-219.

Zhou, Y., Shen, L., & Yang, J. (2002). Feature analysis method of tongue image by Chinese medical diagnosis based on image processing. *Infrared and Laser Engineering, 31*(6), 490-494.

Zhou, Y., Shen, L., & Yang, J. (2002). Feature analysis method of tongue image for Chinese medical diagnosis based on image processing. *Infrared Laser Engineering, 31*(6), 490-494.

Zuo, W., Wang, K., Zhang, D., & Zhang, H. (2004, 18-20 Dec. 2004). *Combination of polar edge detection and active contour model for automated tongue segmentation.* Paper presented at the Image and Graphics, 2004. Proceedings. Third International Conference on.

6

Research on Medication Rules of Chronic Gastritis and Allergic Rhinitis Based on the Complex System Entropy Clustering Method

Renquan Liu[1], Yuhao Zhao[2], Chenghe Shi[3] and Guoyong Chen[1]

[1]*Beijing University of Chinese Medicine, Beijing,*
[2]*School of Traditional Chinese, Medicine, Capital Medical University, Beijing,*
[3]*Department of TCM,Peking University Third Hospital, Beijing,*
P.R. China

1. Introduction

1.1 Mining principle of herbal combinations

The highlight of this research is providing a appropriate statistical method to find out medication rules of chronic gastritis and allergic rhinitis, which will help us to guarantee clinical effects for this two diseases.

Five Viscera Tonifying Method (FVTM) was established by Prof. Gao Zhongying, a national prestigious and experienced practitioner of Traditional Chinese Medicine (TCM). This method extends the implication of tonfiying method while making a break-through in traditional TCM theory. With this featured method in pattern identification and herbal prescription, Prof. Gao is famed for his significant clinical effects by using well-prescribed formula. Modified Lung Tonifying Decoction (LTD), a representative formula of five viscera tonifying method, is indicated and effective for various lung diseases. We employed complex system entropy cluster technique to mine the data of prescriptions by this prestigious and experienced TCM practitioner. It is clinically significant to explore prescription rules of herbal medicine in the treatment of lung diseases to guarantee clinical effects.

According to statistics from World Health Organization (WHO), lung diseases have been one of the four leading diseases that pose great threatens to human health. Conventional treatment using western drugs proves to be advantageous yet its side-effects are hindering patient compliances and thus the clinical effects. There are over 1000 formula indicated for lung diseases, which have been developed in the 2000-year history of Traditional Chinese Medicine (TCM). Modern prestigious and experience TCM practitioners also have developed numerous their own effective formula based on inheriting the essence of prescription rules by ancient practitioners. To study the rules of these formulas is of great significance to facilitate the prescription rules of effective herbal treatment and to explore new formula for lung diseases.

There have been very few studies on prescription rules of herbal medicine for lung diseases by prestigious and experienced TCM practitioners. This study employed complex system entropy cluster technique to mine the data of prescriptions of the prestigious and experienced TCM practitioner and to explore prescription rules of herbal medicine in the treatment of lung diseases to guarantee clinical effects.

1.2 Data mining methods based symptoms clustering

The syndrome is the basic pathological unit and the key concept in traditional Chinese medicine (TCM), and the herbal remedy is prescribed according to the syndrome a patient catches. Nevertheless, few studies are dedicated to investigate the number of syndromes in chronic heart failure (CHF) patients and what these syndromes are. In this paper, we carry out a clinical epidemiology survey and obtain 317 CHF cases, including 62 symptoms in each report. Based on association delineated by mutual information, we employed a pattern discovery algorithm to discover syndromes, which probably have overlapped symptoms in TCM. A revised version of mutual information is presented here to discriminate positive and negative association. The algorithm self-organizedly discovers 15 effective patterns, each of which is verified manually by TCM physicians to recognize the syndrome it belongs to. Therefore, we conclude that the algorithm provides an excellent solution to chronic heart failure problem in the context of traditional Chinese medicine.

Heart failure (CHF) is the most terminal stages of cardiovascular disease to the clinical development of overall performance, with the improvement of living standards and the popularity of interventional cardiology techniques, the proportion of heart failure was increased gradually become a cause of coronary heart disease The main basis for heart failure (Lu&Zhong,2010). Activities by the degree of heart failure symptoms of impaired heart function status was assessed clinically NYHA classification is more commonly used by the patients cardiac function contribute to determine the extent of the disease Qing Qian and treatment options. At present, this area on TCM Syndrome research is still small. In this study, clinical epidemiology, collected coronary heart disease signs and symptoms of heart failure patients, through the heap of entropy together to compare the cardiac function in different situations and syndromes four diagnostic elements of the evolution of features, designed to further grasp the law of the disease syndromes, diagnosis and treatment for the disease to provide a basis for Chinese medicine.

Data mining is a systematic approach used not only to identify biomarkers for a disease but also to investigate the cellular interaction in the context of a disease to construct biological networks.

Data mining also has a crucial role to play in TCM-related research activities. By text mining, a branch of data mining approaches, the biological networks underlying cold and hot syndromes phenotypes are constructed by NEI specifications (Li et al.,2007).Similarly, through a combination of Chinese literatures on TCM and related English counterparts on most diseases on PubMed database, biological networks for a syndrome in TCM in the context of a disease can be automatically generated through text mining approaches (Zhou et al.,2007).In addition, several novel data mining approaches were presented to deal with various kinds of clinical or in vivo animal data. An unsupervised cluster algorithm called pattern discovery algorithm was developed to discover syndromes in TCM in the context of a disease,which provides the targets for formulae or prescriptions since they are prescribed based on syndromes diagnosed (Chen et al.,2007). Furthermore, animal models for syndrome in TCM in the context of diseases were built by using supervised data mining approach to'clone' diagnosis criterion from clinics to animals, which paves a way for in vivo experimental validation of a prescription.8 However, when applying data mining approach in TCM, few research efforts are made in research activities of TCM, it is important to investigate the role of data mining approaches in them.

In information theory, mutual information (MI) of two random variables is a measure that scales mutual dependence of the two variables. It has been applied in many fields, in which researchers treat as divergence or distance between two distributions.

Research on Medication Rules of Chronic Gastritis and Allergic Rhinitis Based on the
Complex System Entropy Clustering Method

139

2. Materials and methods

2.1 Mining principle of herbal combinations

2.1.1 Formula source

All the formula comes from clinical prescriptions by Prof. Gao Zhongying. Prof. Gao Zhongying is a national prestigious and experienced TCM practitioner. He was born in a TCM family of generations and has been working in the fields of TCM clinics, teaching and research for 55 years. He has worked as the director of TCM internal medicine department and herbs & formula department. He has studied TCM theories and applied them in clinic with care before establishing Five Viscera Tonifying Method (FVTM). This method is a breakthrough in traditional TCM theory. It extends the implication of tonifying method and represents featured pattern identification and herbal administration. His formulas are well-prescribed with significant clinical effects. LTD has proven to be effective as a representative of FVTM. To mine the data of formula by Prof. Gao is mainly to collect and categorize LTD prescriptions in this study.

2.1.2 Establishment of formula database

To meet the requirements of data mining and analysis, processing and categorizing the data is a perquisite. Standardized terms were used as 'Final Term' to code the symptoms, signs, tests in the case records. Independent 'Pattern Elements' were summarized or extracted from the cases after standardizing the diagnosis, patterns and treatment according to international and textbook criteria. Phrase databases of patterns and treatments were thus finally established. A database of the medicinal used in the formulas was categorized by their classes, functions, prosperities and meridian entry. The names of medicinals are consistent with those used in the current 21 century textbook.

A module of structured case records based on Access platform was established to collect the clinical data of Prof. Gao Zhongying. All the information about the patients were included using a national standard case record format and access database platform. Clinical data of the 389 cases were carefully recorded in details based on Systemic and Structured Data Entry Criteria in Collecting Clinical Information of Prestigious and Experienced TCM Practitioners. The structured clinical information and other data was included into the system and a Prof. Gao's clinical database was thus formed.

2.1.3 Data analysis method

Before introducing the algorithm, we give a rigorous definition to mutual information
The definition of mutual information

Suppose system $X = (X_1, X_2, \cdots, X_a, \cdots, X_p)^T$ is consisted of p variables, $p \in N$ (N set of natural number), where $X_a = (X_{a_i})$, $a = 1, 2, \cdots, p$; $i = 1, 2, \cdots, q$. Here our objective is to obtain some subsets which have some close properties from set X. Let $C_a(a = 1, \cdots, p)$ be set of classification of X_a, $C_{a_i} = i$ be i-th element of C_a, then we have $C_a = \{1, 2, \cdots, i \cdots, k\}$, $k \leq q$, and let n_i be quantity for X_a belong to i-th class, then entropy of X_a is defined as

$$H(X_a) = -\sum_{i=1}^{k} n_i / q \log n_i / q \qquad (1)$$

The joint entropy of X_a, X_b is similarly defined as

$$H(X_a \cup X_b) = -\sum_i \sum_j n_{ij} / q \log n_{ij} / q \tag{2}$$

where n_{ij} is quantity for X_a belong to i-th class of C_a simultaneously X_b belong to j-th class of C_b. For the convenience of application, expressions (1) and (2) can respectively be represented as

$$H(X_a) = \log q - \frac{1}{q} \sum_{i=1}^{k} n_i \log n_i \tag{3}$$

$$H(X_a \cup X_b) = \log q - \frac{1}{q} \sum_i \sum_j n_{ij} \log n_{ij} \tag{4}$$

Having had above-mentioned definition of entropy, in what follows, correlative measure by which statistical dependence between X_a and X_b is denoted is defined by their mutual information.

Definition 1. Correlative measure between two variables

For arbitrary $X_a \in X$, $X_b \in X$, suppose $X_a \cap X_b = \phi$, then entropy

$$H(X_a, X_b) = H(X_a) + H(X_b) - H(X_a \cup X_b) \tag{5}$$

is called correlative measure $\mu(X_a, X_b)$ between X_a and X_b.

Definition 2. Correlative measure among multi-variables

Suppose $X_a \cap X_b = \phi$ for arbitrary $a, b(a \ne b)$, $p \in N$ then

$$\mu(X_1, X_2, \cdots, X_p) \overset{\Delta}{=} \sum_{a=1}^{p} H(X_a) - H\left(\sum_{a=1}^{p} X_a\right) \tag{6}$$

is called correlative measure among X_1, X_2,...and X_p.

We can also extend the definitions of correlative measure among variables to that of subsets of complex system. In fact, the variable itself is also one particular subset.

Definition 3. Correlative measure among multi-subsystems

Suppose system X be partitioned into m subsystems $s_1, s_2, \cdots, s_m$, for arbitrary i, j $(i \ne j)$, $s_i \cap s_j = \phi$, $X = \sum_{i=1}^{m} s_i$, then

$$\mu(s_1, s_2, \cdots, s_m) \overset{\Delta}{=} \sum_{i=1}^{m} H(s_i) - H\left(\sum_{i=1}^{m} s_i\right) \tag{7}$$

is called correlative measure among $s_1, s_2, \cdots, s_m$.

Let us consider nonempty finite set X and set-family $E(X)$ consisted of its subsets, P is a set-function defined on $E(X)$ with properties:

i. $P(A) \ge 0$, $\forall A \in E(X)$,

ii. $P(\varnothing) = 0$

The complex entropy cluster algorithm

The algorithm is detailedly presented in (Chen et al.,2007), we also present it here.

Once association for each pair (every two variables) is acquired, we propose a self-organized algorithm to automatically discovery the patterns. The algorithm can not only cluster, but also realize some variables appear in some different patterns. In this section, we use three subsections to introduce the algorithm. The first introduce the concept of "Relative" set. Based on this, the pattern discovery algorithm is proposed in second subsection. The last subsection is devoted to presenting an n-class association concept to back up the idea of the algorithm.

For a specific variable X, a set, which is collected by mean of gathering N variables whose associations with X are larger than others with regard to X, is attached to it and is denoted as $R(X)$. Each variable in the set can be regarded as a "Relative" of X while other variables that not belong to the set are considered as irrelative to X, so we name $R(X)$ "Relative" set of X. The "Relative" sets of all 20 variables can be denoted by a $20 \times N$ matrix. Based on the matrix, the pattern discovery algorithm is proposed.

A pair (variable X and Y) is defined to be significantly associated if and only if X belongs to the "Relative" set of Y ($X \in R(Y)$) and vice versa ($Y \in R(X)$). It is convenient to extend this definition to a set with multiple variables. If and only if each pair of these variables is significantly associated, then we can call that the set is significant associated. A pattern is defined as a significantly associated set with maximal number of variables. All these kinds of sets constitute the hidden patterns in the data. Therefore, a pattern should follow three main criteria: (1) the number of variables within a set is no less than 2. (2) Each pair of the variables belong to a set is significantly associated. (3) Any variable outside a set can not make the set significantly associated. This means the number of variables within the set reaches maximum.

We defined that two variables X and Y are correlated if and only if they are inter-relative, i.e., X is a 'relative' of Y and vice versa. It is convenient to extend this definition to the case with multi-variables, if each pair between these variables is correlated, then we called that they are correlated. A set that is comprised of maximal variables in which each pair is correlated is defined as a pattern and all sets constitute the hidden patterns in the data acquired above.

2.2 Data mining methods based symptoms clustering
2.2.1 Clinical epidemiology
317 patients with coronary heart disease patients with heart failure were collected from May 2009 to March 2010 Dongzhimen Hospital, Beijing University of Chinese Medicine, Dongfang Hospital, Beijing University of Chinese Medicine, Department of Cardiology of the patients.

2.2.2 Diagnosis criteria
(1) coronary artery disease with reference to the International Society of Cardiology and the Society, named after the World Health Organization standardized clinical report of the Joint Task Team, "named after ischemic heart disease and diagnostic criteria"; (2) diagnosis of heart failure based on diagnosis of chronic heart failure in China in 2007 treatment guidelines; cardiac function with reference to the New York Heart Association (NYHA) 1928 annual standard.

2.2.3 Inclusion criteria
Coronary heart disease and chronic heart failure meet the above diagnostic criteria, older than 18 years of age and less than or equal to 80 years of age and informed consent, patients participated in this study.

2.2.4 Exclusion criteria

Exclusion criteria isBy the expansion of heart disease, pulmonary heart disease, rheumatic heart disease, cardiomyopathy, congenital heart disease and other heart disease due to heart failure patients; with acute myocardial infarction, cardiogenic shock, severe arrhythmias associated with hemodynamic changes in persons; concurrent infection : ① fever; ② blood increased, white blood cell count> 10 × 109 / L, neutrophils> 85%; ③ chest X-ray shadows suggestive of sheet; with severe hepatic insufficiency (liver function values> normal 2 times), renal insufficiency (Ccr> 20%, Scr> 3mg/dl or> 265μmol / L), blood system, the primary disease, malignant tumor; pregnancy or breast-feeding women; mental illness, infectious diseases

2.2.5 Survey methods

Survey methods of clinical epidemiology, screening results in the literature and two rounds of preliminary questionnaire was developed based on expert clinical four diagnostic information collection form, in patients with heart failure collect demographic data, present illness, symptoms and signs, and tongue, veins and other information.

2.2.6 Quality control

Clinical Hospital, prior to the survey of the designated person responsible for, the research group to develop the work of the researchers involved in the study manual for the doctor and unified training. Establish Epidate3.1 database, all cases investigated by double data entry.

3. Conclusion

3.1 Mining principle of herbal combinations

By using the following data analysis methods, the corresponding results are given in Table 1 to Table 3 as well as Figure 1.

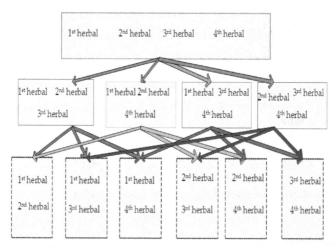

Fig. 1. The illustration of cluster process. Where 1st, 2nd ,3rd and 4th herbal represents milk-vetch root, rehmannia, heterophylly false satarwort root and Chinese magnolivine fruit respectively.

Herbal	Frequency	Usage	Herbal	Frequency	Usage
heterophylly false satarwort root	284	0.73008	scutellaria root	54	0.13882
milk-vetch root	270	0.69409	dwarf lilyturf tuber	52	0.13368
prepared rehmannia root	269	0.69152	common coltsfoot flower	46	0.11825
Chinese magnolivine fruit	265	0.68123	psoralea fruit	45	0.11568
tatarian aster root	222	0.57069	ephedra herb	43	0.11054
white mulberry root-bark	178	0.45758	Stir-baking bupleurum with vinegar	41	0.1054
pepperweed seed	136	0.34961	dried ginger rhizome	39	0.10026
snakegourd fruit; trichosanthes fruit	131	0.33676	Cassia twig	34	0.087404
pinellia rhizome	91	0.23393	great burdock achene	33	0.084833
platycodon root	91	0.23393	liquorice root	32	0.082262
rehmannia root	76	0.19537	heartleaf houttuynia herb	32	0.082262
tendrilled fritillaria bulb	64	0.16452	Chinese waxgourd seed	31	0.079692
stemona root	56	0.14396	smoked plum	31	0.079692
blackberry lily rhizome	55	0.14139	magnolia bark	30	0.077121
almond	55	0.14139			

Table 1. Commonly-used medicinal in the prescriptions of modified LTD for lung diseases

Herbal combination		Mutual information	Herbal combination		Mutual information
cockleburr fruit	blond magnolia flower	0.20823	euryale seed	pepperweed seed	0.07403
psoralea fruit	euryale seed	0.1568	perilla-seed	tatarian aster root	0.071148
blackberry lily rhizome	pepperwe ed seed	0.14528	snakegourd fruit	immature orange fruit	0.070149
ephedra herb	almond	0.1384	Stir-baking bupleurum with vinegar	blond magnolia flower	0.067455
platycodon root	pepperwe ed seed	0.13568	white atractylodes rhizome	ledebouriella root	0.064919
Indian bread	cassia twig	0.12965	common coltsfoot flower	pepperweed seed	0.063739
pinellia rhizome	red tangerine peel	0.1181	amur cork-tree bark	light yellow sophora root	0.06262
psoralea fruit	pepperwe ed seed	0.11559	stemona root	tatarian aster root	0.062125
prepared rehmannia root	Chinese magnolivi ne fruit	0.10894	Safflower	turmeric root tuber	0.061022
platycodon root	oroxylum seed	0.10519	atractylodes rhizome	light yellow sophora root	0.059596
platycodon root	great burdock achene	0.10188	tree peony bark	light yellow sophora root	0.059596
ephedra herb	great burdock achene	0.096925	donkey-hide gelatin pellets	dwarf lilyturf tuber	0.059468
bile arisaema	glabrous greenbrier rhizome	0.095717	pepperweed seed	tatarian aster root	0.05726
magnolia bark	almond	0.094751	light yellow sophora root	glabrous greenbrier rhizome	0.055996
platycodon root	white mulberry root-bark	0.088538	cassia twig	Safflower	0.055512
psoralea fruit	white mulberry root-bark	0.08771	kudzuvine root	Euonymi twig	0.055454

Research on Medication Rules of Chronic Gastritis and Allergic Rhinitis Based on the
Complex System Entropy Clustering Method

145

Herbal combination		Mutual information	Herbal combination		Mutual information
oldenlandia	bearded scutellaria	0.083543	snakegourd fruit	milk-vetch root	0.053697
suberect spatholobus stem	centipede	0.083543	common coltsfoot flower	blackberry lily rhizome	0.052638
rehmannia root	scutellaria root	0.083134	heterophylly false satarwort root	Chinese magnolivine fruit	0.052357
perilla-seed	pepperweed seed	0.082173	donkey-hide gelatin pellets	turmeric root tuber	0.052208
snakegourd fruit	scutellaria root	0.08126	great burdock achene	pepperweed seed	0.052098
cockleburr fruit	Stir-baking bupleurum with vinegar	0.079804	Indian bread	Euonymi twig	0.050529
curcumae rhizome	cassia twig	0.077009	cockleburr fruit	ledebouriella root	0.050329
cnidium fruit	glabrous greenbrier rhizome	0.076576			

Table 2. Commonly-used medicinal combinations and combining values in the prescriptions of modified LTD for lung diseases

pinellia rhizome	tendrilled fritillaria bulb	common coltsfoot flower	blackberry lily rhizome
cockleburr fruit	Stir-baking bupleurum with vinegar	Chinese magnolivine fruit	blond magnolia flower
common coltsfoot flower	blackberry lily rhizome	perilla-seed	pepperweed seed
blackberry lily rhizome	perilla-seed	pepperweed seed	tatarian aster root
donkey-hide gelatin pellets	white peony root	atractylodes rhizome	
donkey-hide gelatin pellets	atractylodes rhizome	light yellow sophora root	

pinellia rhizome	tendrilled fritillaria bulb	common coltsfoot flower	blackberry lily rhizome
donkey-hide gelatin pellets	atractylodes rhizome	dwarf lilyturf tuber	
donkey-hide gelatin pellets	liquorice root	turmeric root tuber	
donkey-hide gelatin pellets	Safflower	turmeric root tuber	
donkey-hide gelatin pellets	dwarf lilyturf tuber	turmeric root tuber	
white peony root; peony	suberect spatholobus stem	centipede	
white atractylodes rhizome	aged tangerine peel	liquorice root	
white atractylodes rhizome	prepared rehmannia root	Chinese magnolivine fruit	
stemona root	platycodon root	oroxylum seed	
stemona root	cassia bark	oroxylum seed	
pinellia rhizome	common coltsfoot flower	white mulberry root-bark	
thunberg fritillary bulb	liquorice root	hogfennel root	
thunberg fritillary bulb	great burdock achene	hogfennel root	
psoralea fruit	common coltsfoot flower	white mulberry root-bark	
psoralea fruit	common coltsfoot flower	pepperweed seed	
psoralea fruit	euryale seed	pepperweed seed	
cockleburr fruit	ephedra herb	blond magnolia flower	

Table 3. Core medicinal combinations in the prescriptions of modified LTD for lung diseases

The name of Lung Tonifying Decocction (LTD) has been found in several ancient literatures. The ingredients recorded in Yun QI Zi Bao Ming Ji (Yun Qi Zi's Collections of Life-saving Formula) are different from those in Bei Ji Qian Jin Yao Fang (Essential Prescriptions Worth a Thousand Gold for Emergiences) and San Yin Ji Yi Bing Zheng Fang Lun (Treatise on Three Categories of Pathogenic Factors and Prescriptions). Prof. Gao used the ingredients of former source. Some Scholars says this formula was originated from Yong Lei Qian Fang written by Li Zhongnan in 1331 and Jing Yue Quan Shu (Complete Works of Jingyue). Sang Bai Pi (Cortex Mori), Di Huang (Radix Rehmanniae), Ren Shen (Radix et Rhizoma Ginseng),

Zi Wan (Radix et Rhizoma Asteris), Huang Qi (Radix Astragali), Wu Wei Zi (Fructus Schisandrae Chinensis) formulates a representative formula for tonifying lung qi. It was originally indicated for Lao Sou (consumptive cough) due to five viscera deficiency pattern manifested as afternoon tidal fever, spontaneous sweating or nigh sweating, cough with sputum, dyspnea with panting. In the formula, Ren Shen and Huang Qi are sweet and warm in nature. They are used to tonify qi, supplement the defense aspect and secure the exterior. The two medicinals are targeted at deficiency of spleen and lung. Di Huang is to supplement kidney essence to supply qi, tonify the lower to supplement the upper part of the body. It is also used to supply water to moisten the lungs and remove the deficiency dryness in the upper source. Wu Wei Zi and Zi Wan can astringe the lungs and moisten the dryness to relieve dryness and coughing. Sang Bai Pi clears the heat and calms down the reverse qi to resolve phlegm and stop coughing. These medicinals used together are to tonify the spleen and kidneys, moisten the dryness and stop coughing. That's how it works in most cases in the clinic.

In terms of the number of medicinal, Prof.Gao tends to use a few medicinals with specific targets. On average there are around 12 medicinals in each of his formula. Table 1 shows that Prof. Gao sticks to the original ingredients of the formula. The commonly-used medicinals ranked in the first 6 places are originally used in the formula. Modification is often used for specific symptoms. For example Ban Xia (Rhizoma Pinelliae) and Gua Lou (Fructus Trichosanthis) are combined to strengthen the effects of phlegm resolving. Table 2 shows that Prof. Gao tends to use Xin Yi (Flos Magnoliae) combined with Cang Er (Fructus Xanthii) to open the nasal orifice, Wu Wei Zi (Fructus Schisandrae Chinensis) combined with vinegar processed Chai Hu (Radix Bupleuri) to antagonize allergy. The results indicate that it is significant to mine data of prescriptions by prestigious and experienced TCM practitioners by using complex system entropy cluster technique.

Modified LTD is effective for various lung diseases, yet it has not been included by the current formula textbook. There has been few literature and clinical studies on this formula as well. According to incomplete statistics, Prof. Gao has used the modified LTD to treat Chronic Obstructive Pulmonary Diseases (COPD), Idiopathic Pulmonary Fibrosis (IPF), anthrasilicosis, bronchiectasis, allergic asthma and rhinitis besides coughing and panting in the clinic. Most attention should be drawn to this formula by the clinicians to improve clinical effects.

3.2 Data mining methods based symptoms clustering

Information collection form will be provided by the signs and symptoms of each patient were statistically and found 317 cases of heart failure in patients with systemic symptoms Shenpi fatigue (100%), shortness of breath (93%), less gas lazy words (71 %), spontaneous (39%), chills (39%), five upset hot (27%) majority; head, face the common symptoms of dizziness (73%), lips cyanosis (58%), dark complexion (22%); mind and flank the chest symptoms (88%), palpitations (76%), wheezing (57%), chest pain (37%), expectoration (30%) were more; stomach and abdominal symptoms of bloating (48 %) was the most common; waist and limbs Yaoxisuanruan common symptoms (73%), limb trapped weight (51%), and edema (55%), hand, foot and not warm (39%); restaurants and taste of symptoms to loss of appetite (59%), dry mouth (48%), sticky mouth (27%) were more symptoms of sleep and the two will be to insomnia (65%), nocturia (38%) most common; tongue in order to sublingual vein abnormalities (61%), tongue dark (55%), crack the tongue (34%), tongue pink (24%), less or no moss moss (20%), fat large indentation tongue (19%) is more common; pulse late in the common pulse (49%), pulse astringent (21%), promoting Pulse (17%), pulse knot generation (10%).

By using pattern discovery algorithm, the 15 patterns were given in Table 4.

No.	Combination of symptoms	Syndrome diagnosed
1	Shortness of breath, asthma, fatigue, side limb edema	Qi Deficiency
2	Abdominal distention, gurgling, nausea, vomiting, mouth light thirsty	
3	Abdominal threatening pain, backache, headache, nausea expansion Xiong Xie	Qi stagnation
4	Subject to colds, cough, Long cough, sputum	
5	Shortness of breath, Shenpi, fatigue	Qi Deficiency
6	Shortness of breath, wheezing, sputum	
7	Shenpi, cough, bad air	
8	Fatigue, loss of appetite, shortness of breath	
9	Top-heavy, such as wrap, dizziness, limb paralysis Ma	
10	Ringing in the ears, knees soft, backache	
11	Tinnitus, backache, nausea expansion Xiong Xie	
12	Five upset hot, dry mouth, hot flushes and night sweats	Yin Deficiency
13	Five upset hot, constipation, hot flushes and night sweats	
14	Headache, nausea expansion Xiong Xie, channeling pain away	
15	Cough, Cough, the evil wind	

Table 4. 15 patterns for CHF

In heart failure have been recorded, including early, carved in Chinese medicine is a "heart palpitations", "Tan Yin" and "asthma card", "edema", "accumulation" and other areas. On the characteristics of the basic pathogenesis of heart failure, there are different points of view, Wong (Li et al.,2007) that the disease is mainly responsible for deficiency in the heart failure, falling seedlings lung, spleen, kidney all dirty and wet phlegm from each breeding Results from the heart Qi-oriented, blood stasis, water to drink as standard; Wang (Wang,2005) that the deficiency and yang-oriented virtual, blood stasis, water resistance, phlegm as the standard implementation of the levy; Chen (Li&Chen,2006) will be virtual, stasis, water summarized as the basic pathogenesis of the disease. 200 patients from four diagnostic methods of frequency analysis results, the heart failure patients often show the signs and False or True, false to qi deficiency, yang deficiency, yin deficiency is a common, real to stasis, water, sputum-based, I believe that deficiency may be associated with their hypertension, diabetes and other primary diseases related to each other based on the root theory of yin and yang, yang deficiency and yin, yang to a certain extent patients can occur when the signs of deficiency, it also Coronary Heart Yin decline in the basic pathogenesis of the important part.

Entropy algorithm for the clustering together of the heap in one, with the traditional method compared to non-supervised clustering, which is characterized by improved correlation between two variables method, effectively avoid the interference of negative data, through the calculate the two bivariate correlation coefficients between each variable designated the "friends group", after convergence, go to "friends group" within the limited number of variables, leaving the variables must be close to each other with higher levels of combination, this data extraction process and we are in the clinical symptoms and signs by a certain type of information gathering to designate property Panduan a similar card, therefore, become the method to explore between the clinical symptoms and Syndrome internal laws of the more common and objective mathematical method. In this study, patients with different cardiac function four diagnostic variables together elements of the heap after the analysis of the syndrome of basic and clinical match, but the law also has some defects, such as better together to make the variable into a class, we screened the raw data, which may lose some useful information. In conclusion, this study together after the data, while the heap is not fully reflect the clinical, but at least clinical symptoms of the disease trends in the evolution provide some reference.

4. References

Chen J, Xi G, Chen J et al., An unsupervised pattern (syndrome in traditional Chinese medicine) discovery algorithm based on association delineated by revised mutual information in chronic renal failure data, *J Biol Syst* 15(4):435–451, 2007.

LI Li-zhi. Chen Kej i'S Experience on the treatment of congestive heart failure. *Chinese Journal of Integrative Medicine on Cardio-/Cerebrovascular Disease*, 2006, 4(2): 136-138.

Li S, Zhang X, Wang Y et al., Understanding Zheng in traditional Chinese medicine in the context of neuro-endocrine immune network, *IET Syst Biol* 1(1):51–60, 2007.

LU Zai-ying, ZHONG Nan-shan. Internal Medicine. 7th ed. Beijing: People' s Medical Publishing House. 2010 : 170.

WANG Zhen-tao. Experience of syndrome differentiation and treatment on congestive heart failure. *Journal of Sichuan of Traditional Chinese Medicine* , 2005, 23(6): 9-10.

Zhou X, Liu B, Wu Z et al., Integrative mining of traditional Chinese medicine literature and MEDLINE for functional gene networks, *Artif Intell Med* 41(2):87–104,2007.

7

Advances in Chinese Medicine Diagnosis: From Traditional Methods to Computational Models

Arthur de Sá Ferreira
Centro Universitário Augusto Motta,
Brazil

1. Introduction

Ancient Chinese medicine practitioners deduced about 5,000 years ago that the exterior appearance of the body was closely related to the functions of the internal organs and viscera. They sought for explanations for this interior-exterior connection by establishing relationships between human beings and Nature. Other natural philosophers also applied such reasoning, *e.g.* Aristotle [384-322 BC], Leonardo Da Vinci [1452-1519], and René Descartes [1596-1650]. Although it is not possible to say that Chinese medicine practitioners were unique in this task, they organized those relationships in a pioneer manner long before their Western counterparts. Chinese and Western physicians were not distinct in their conceptual framework, but their respective medical practices evolved on different cultures and historical contexts. Therefore, it is expected that the advances on medical knowledge represent this cultural divergence.

Many efforts have been made to integrate the ancient, traditional knowledge of Chinese medicine into contemporary, Eastern medical practice. Diagnosis is a key element in this integration of medical systems since it links the patient's needs to the available therapeutic resources. The art of Chinese medicine diagnosis was enriched throughout history but it main traditional aspect remains unchanged: the exclusive use of information available to the naked senses. Clinical information provided by vision, hearing, smelling, and touching is interpreted in a framework of Chinese medicine theories of physiology. No equipment or instrument was developed with specific diagnostic purposes or based on Chinese medicine theories. However, advances in computation and biomedical instruments allowed more powerful analysis of clinical data and quantification of parameters otherwise assessed only in a qualitative fashion. As a consequence, computer models for diagnosis in Chinese medicine were developed and tested in the last few decades and are promising tools in the clinical environment.

This chapter introduces the traditional methods of diagnosis in Chinese medicine and introduces their evolution into computational models. Current methods for validation of computational model by the assessment of their diagnostic accuracy and possible sources of errors are also presented. Finally, perspectives on the issue of computational diagnosis are discussed.

2. Science and art in Chinese medicine diagnosis

Science may be understood as the common sense refinement through a prospective effort to transform sensorial impressions into sequential, logic facts with intra- and inter-experimental relationships subjected to verification and reproducibility at a certain level of confidence. Such relationships should minimize the quantity of basic principles while maximize the explained medical events. Such an organized knowledge has been guiding clinical practice in China since early times and may have interacted with other cultures on a reciprocal manner, either by knowledge transmission or acquisition. Ancient textbooks present extensive details regarding the empirical search for a cause-effect relationship, as well as the necessary training to become a physician. As a matter of fact, Chinese medicine practitioners held distinct positions in old China (Tao, 1953b). Systematization of Chinese medical knowledge allowed the accumulation of "positive" trial-and-error results, the discussion of "negative" results for therapy improvement, and the transmission of medical knowledge. Accordingly, new methods for diagnosis and intervention were developed in consonance with this systematization. In this sense, Chinese medicine is thus composed of scientific knowledge since its wide theoretical framework differentiates it from the popular knowledge.

Such scientific approach of medical theories is also reflected in the diagnostic field. From the historical point-of-view, diagnostic methods probably started with the simple need to answer dichotomous questions, such as "Is the subject dead or alive?". From this starting point, diagnostic methods evolved into more complex methods capable of identification of several constitutional aspects, different aetiologies and their relationships, as well as the differentiation of multiple morbid or comorbid states. Descriptions of prognosis based on the patient's examination reflect this high evolution of diagnostic methods since accurate prognosis depends on accurate diagnosis and extensive theory-based practice.

The main approach to scientific research on Chinese medicine has been to explain the observed phenomena by means of its experimental verification. By doing this, the validity of the Chinese medical knowledge is indirectly assessed by observing physiologic or therapeutic responses to acupuncture or herbs prescriptions. An interesting, alternative approach is to seek for the scientific evidence that corroborate or not data reported by Chinese medicine practitioners – ancient and contemporary ones included. Such an integrative approach is a very attractive strategy for development of robust methods in the diagnostic field.

3. Recognition of morbid states and the concept of pattern

Apparently, the first group of morbid conditions to be recognized were infections. As early as the Chin [221-207 BC] and Han [206 BC-219 AD] dynasties, outbreaks of epidemics led to the differentiation of infections and classification of their symptoms. In sequence, disorders of the digestive system were recognized and also named according to key-symptoms. Neurologic, metabolic, cardiovascular, and ophthalmic disorders are among the other early-recognized conditions (Tao, 1953a). Progressively, other morbid conditions were identified in the field of nutrition, paediatry, otorhinolaryngology, stomatology, dermatology, urologic obstetrics and gynaecology (Tao, 1958a; Tao, 1958b). The recognition of new diseases, as well as the improvement of information regarding manifestations, diagnosis and prognosis were continuous developed until nowadays.

The definition of morbid conditions in Chinese medicine differs from its counterpart in Western medicine. A pattern (or syndrome, *zheng*) is the morbid entity of Chinese medicine and can be derived from any physiologic theory: *Ba-gan, Zang-fu, Liu-jing, Wei-qi Ying-xue, San-jiao, Bing-yin, Qi-xue, Jin-ye, Wu-xing, Jing-luo* (Zaslawki, 2003). A pattern is a set of manifestations that are absent or present depending on individual, social and environmental conditions. This set of manifestations is similar to a "cluster of symptoms" in Western medicine (Dodd et al., 2001). Each pattern presents a wide description of manifestations including its onset, duration, location, progression and severity, collectively known as pattern dynamism (Zaslawki, 2003). Manifestations are not limited to signs and symptoms, but also body characteristics and shape, psychological statuses, personality, emotional conditions, interaction with environmental climate, and behaviours. The term "manifestation profile" describes a subset of all possible manifestations related to the pattern presented by a patient. Hence, different patients may present different manifestation profiles and yet get the same pattern as a diagnosis. As a corollary, the same manifestation profile exhibited by different patients may be related to different patterns.

Several types of patterns are distinguished, namely single, complex and multiple patterns. Single patterns are those related to a unique affected internal system (*zangfu*) or channel (*jingmai*). For instance, *Shen-yin* deficiency and *Gan-xue* deficiency are both single patterns. Complex patterns consist of two or more affected internal systems or channels and often share aetiologies or risk factors, being an example the *Gan-Dan* damp-heat. Multi-patterns are those in which several single patterns are observed due to either to pattern transmission or exposure to multiple aetiologies. For an example of multi-patterns, consider the following transmission, *Shen-yin* deficiency leading to *Gan-yang* rising.

Notice that the concept of pattern is not strictly related to diseases or syndromes in the Western medicine (Lu & Chen, 2009). In contemporary Chinese medicine literature, diseases were assigned to patterns based on matched 'signs and symptoms' to integrate both medical practices (O'Connor & Bensky, 1987; Auteroche & Navailh, 1992; Maciocia, 1996; Ross, 2003). Indeed, the scientific approach has been to assess the pair disease/pattern model. In this context, the same disease may be related to several patterns as well as the same pattern may be observed in several diseases. It is very important to observe this disease/pattern interaction because of the implications to statistical analysis and consequently data interpretation. Very often, a study sample is firstly selected from individuals with disease already diagnosed and secondly is subjected to the traditional Chinese medicine diagnostic procedure. Hence, statistical inference and data interpretation cannot be extrapolated to the overall population – implying limited external validity – but is limited to the disease under investigation.

4. Diagnosis as a pattern differentiation process

Ancient Chinese medicine literature does not to explicitly discuss diagnostic reasoning (Yang & Li, 1993; Luo, 1995; Yang, 2003; Flaws, 2004; Yang & Chase, 2004). Contemporary literature reports that Chinese medicine practitioners apply only the differentiation reasoning for decision-making (Maciocia, 1996; Zaslawki, 2003). The diagnosis in Chinese medicine is obtained through a process named "pattern differentiation" or "syndrome differentiation" (*bian zheng*). In such a process, the practitioner examines the patient to seek for meaningful manifestations that indicate a single, a complex or an even a multi-pattern condition. Recently, Chinese medicine diagnosis started to incorporate other strategies from Western medicine (Zhou & Zhang, 2006; Zhu et al., 2006; N.L. Zhang et al., 2008), such as the deductive-inductive reasoning, tests that confirm a target hypothesis, eliminate an alternative hypothesis, or discriminate among competing ones (McSherry, 1999).

Pattern differentiation is performed in a three-stage process, namely: information gathering, data interpretation, and decision-making:

- Information gathering: refers to the assessment of manifestations present or absent in patients using traditional examination, possibly in coadjutant with contemporary methods. It is highly dependent on the physician's ability to recognize manifestations and to consider those reported by the patient.
- Data interpretation: involves the understanding of the acquired clinical information and its consideration. Also, it encompasses the selection of the best physiologic theory to explain the patient's manifestation profile. If a particular theory does not explain the interaction among manifestations (and possibly patterns), another theory – more general or specific – can be selected in the next stage.
- Decision-making: is the process of identification of a pattern among other possible ones. If it was possible, practitioners should rely on pathognomonic manifestations to perform pattern differentiation. However, not all patterns exhibit such a feature, and many patterns share common manifestations. Moreover, patterns have several manifestations that can be present or not depending on individual constitution and environmental factors.

It is worth notice that pattern differentiation is "always possible" due to the wide concept of manifestation and the diversity of physiologic theories to better differentiate the true pattern (or patterns) from possible ones.

5. Traditional examination methods in Chinese medicine

In the medical diagnostic context, "traditional" refers to methods, knowledge, skills, and beliefs indigenous to different cultures applied to health obtainment, maintenance and restoration. Often, when adopted by different cultures it is termed "alternative" or "complimentary" medicine (WHO, 2008). For information gathering, the traditional methods are still applied nowadays and are essentially similar to those practiced by Western physicians (Peterson et al., 1992).

The traditional Chinese ontology of examination is named "Four Examinations" (sizhen). It consists of the sequential application of inspection (wang), auscultation and olfaction (wen), inquiry (wen), and palpation (qie) (Tao, 1958a). Several classic authors discussed detailed information regarding this sequence of examination and its impact on diagnostic errors and potential cure rates. For instance, a "superior" Chinese medicine practitioners collect data from patients according to the Four Examinations and interpret those manifestations using medical theories, obtaining a cure rate of 90%; "mediocre" and "inferior" doctors have cure rates of 70-80% and 60% patients, respectively (Yang & Li, 1993; Luo, 1995; Yang, 2003; Flaws, 2004; Yang & Chase, 2004). Recently, it was shown that individual examination methods provide diagnostic accuracies compatible with "inferior doctors" (Ferreira, 2008) and are significantly improved after cumulative application of all Four Examinations (Ferreira, 2009).

According to such ontology, the naked senses are considered sufficient to the trained, skilled practitioner to recognize and label patterns. While elaborated instrumentation was invented and developed for acupuncture and moxibustion treatment – including different types and shapes of needles, moxa presentations – not an instrument was developed for diagnostic purposes. This subjective, personal practice inputs an extremely high dependency in the examiner's knowledge and the applied procedures.

Several contemporary textbooks are devoted to the patient's examination following that ontology and will not be explored here. Some categories worth mention regarding each examination method (Zhou et al., 2004; Ferreira, 2008). Inspection is performed to collect information regarding the patient's: general aspect; face aspect; tongue body, fur, and movement; body constitution; gait; urine and stools aspect. Children under 2-3 years old must have their throat, orifices, finger veins, and *luo* channels inspected (S.C. Wang et al., 2002). Auscultation and olfaction are executed to collect information on the patient's: breath; speech; cough; secretion; and excretions. Inquiry is conducted to observe the patient's preferences; cold and fever; transpiration; head and body; chest and abdomen; pain; excretions; diet and appetite; sense organs; sleep; medical history; habits; and quality of life ("present dignity, past obscurity"). Palpation is performed to identify: painful areas; skin temperature; points; cubital skin; and pulse images.

Some criticism may arise from the sequence of the traditional ontology for examination. As a corollary of the holistic approach of Chinese medicine, the order in which Examination methods are applied does not change the pattern differentiation outcome. Assuming that practitioners always use the Four Examinations and are successful in this task, they conclude their screening procedure with the same manifestation profile no matter the applied order. This must not be confused with the timeline of onset of manifestations because when at screening, the patient presents simultaneously all manifestations. Although each Examination contributes differently for reducing pattern differentiation errors, it seems that the order in which the Four Examinations are used is just a matter of keeping a rigid routine to ensure that every aspect of screening was performed (Ferreira, 2011).

6. Introduction to computational models for pattern differentiation

With the advance in computing techniques and equipment, the pattern differentiation process is properly evolving into a computer-based procedure. The rapid evolution of mathematical methods based on computational algorithms allowed the implementation of diagnostic techniques derived from simple to complex routines. Additionally, study designs, statistical methods for data analysis, and guideline reports are also available for assessment of diagnostic accuracy and epidemiologic performance of automated methods. However, the computerization of Chinese medicine cannot overlook its theoretical foundation since it provides the basis for intervention.

6.1 Attributes of computational models for pattern differentiation

It is not difficult to build computational models for diagnostic purposes – the difficulty lies in making them good and reliable. An idealized pattern differentiation model should perform as a "superior" practitioner or even better. Thus, a computational model of pattern differentiation must present the following attributes:

- Respectful concerning the theoretical framework of Chinese medicine;
- Robust performance across a variety of suitable physiologic theories with minimal computational cost;
- Ability to perform despite having different amounts of manifestations in the manifestation profile;
- Ability to identify exams composed of single, complex and multi-patterns;
- Ability to merge manifestations that correspond to the same pattern;
- Ability to split manifestations that correspond to more than one pattern;
- Ability to decompose multiple patterns despite "noisy" manifestations and biological variability;

- Minimal use of arbitrary thresholds and minimal sensitivity to any required thresholds;
- Multi-pass algorithm to allow classification context to grow iteratively;
- Valid stopping criteria for iterative process;
- Ability to decouple low-assignment rate versus low-error rate trade-off as much as possible;
- Accuracy and completeness of pattern differentiation;
- Ability to supply some measurement of confidence regarding the pattern differentiation results.

6.2 Dataset of computational models for pattern differentiation

Despite the use of different approaches to perform pattern differentiation, some elements are common to those methods, such as the usage of knowledge datasets, training and testing databases, and questionnaires. As far as the manual insertion is the most frequent method applied, some discussion is needed on this topic.

Although many efforts have been made to standardize medical terms, currently there is no standard dataset for patterns and manifestations. In general, datasets have been generated by manual insertion of terms collected from literature (Ferreira, 2008; Ferreira, 2009, Ferreira, 2011) or by data mining algorithms (refer to Lukman et al., 2007 for a revision on mining methods applied to Chinese medicine; Zhou et al., 2010). Patterns on database must be mutually exclusive and collectively exhaustive (Harding, 1996), *i.e.*, for each manifestation there is at least one possible pattern, and there is no pattern without manifestations. Manual insertion leads datasets subjected to common errors of:

- Typography: typos, case-sensitive letters, and medical synonymous;
- Manifestation redundancy: for the same pattern, typing a manifestation twice or more in the same examination method or among different methods regarding the same pattern;
- Pattern label redundancy: typing the same pattern's label twice in the dataset, making such label not unique and possibly with different descriptions;
- Pattern description redundancy: typing the same pattern's description twice in the dataset yet with distinct labels, making their content not mutually exclusive (in this case, both patterns are indeed the same pattern).

The errors described above can be minimized or even eliminated with the use of simple routines for intra-pattern and inter-pattern exploratory analyses using common string search algorithms. It is strongly recommended running such routines for quality control of manually inserted datasets before model validation, especially when dealing with large datasets or even multiple datasets simultaneously. For instance, intra-pattern consistency can be obtained by excluding any repetitions of manifestations in the same examination method, as well as among the Four Examinations describing the respective pattern (Ferreira, 2008). Inter-pattern consistency can be obtained by ensuring that two patterns were not described with the same complete manifestation profile (Ferreira, 2008; Ferreira, 2009). Analysis of dual pattern similarity by means of the Jaccard coefficient (Jaccard, 1901) and associated confidence interval (Real, 1999) is an alternative to check for pattern redundancy (Ferreira, 2011). The use of a controlled vocabulary from dataset avoids the typos, eliminates language ambiguity and ensures that every one is using the same terms to mean the same attribute which limits the use of synonymous.

7. Computational models for pattern differentiation

The application of objective rules for pattern differentiation may help diminish diagnosis variability (G.G. Zhang et al., 2005; G.G. Zhang et al., 2008) dependent on the practitioner's expertise. A large amount of computational methods have been published, too many to list them all. Some of them were developed and tested against simulated and real cases, in different disease models, and are discussed here. In chronological sequence, this work includes the Traditional Chinese Medicine *Sizheng* Integrated Recorder and Aided Syndrome Differentiator (TCM-SIRD), modified Greedy Bayesian Pattern Search algorithm (GBPS*), Information Management System of Traditional Chinese Medicine Syndrome Project based on Prior Knowledge Support Vector Machine (P-SVM), Chinese Medical Diagnostic System (CMDS), Pattern Differentiation Algorithm (PDA), and Multi-Label k-Nearest Neighbour (ML-kNN).

7.1 Traditional Chinese Medicine *Sizheng* Integrated Recorder and Aided Syndrome Differentiator (TCM-SIRD)

Zheng and Wu (2004) developed the Traditional Chinese Medicine *Sizheng* Integrated Recorder and Aided Syndrome Differentiator (TCM-SIRD). This system performs information gathering based on sensors (image, pulse and odor signal acquisition) and text information. A computational routine, namely "Integrated *Sizheng* Information Application", merges the data transferred from sensors and provides assistant diagnosis service by means of data interpretation. The provided output (such as type of tongue coating, face image, and pulse) is used to form a primary differentiation of syndromes by the "*Sizheng* Expert Decision", the decision-making modulus based on rules extracted from Chinese medicine experts' experience. The objective rules extracted from expert practitioners were not described, neither their computational implementation.

The authors described methods to be implemented for an objective assessment of diagnostic with description of a single test case. Although the model for pattern differentiation was not detailed described, the authors advocated the use of the Four Examinations. No description was given on how the information was processed for diagnosis. No result regarding its diagnostic accuracy was reported.

7.2 Modified Greedy Bayesian Pattern Search algorithm (GBPS*)

X. Wang et al. (2004) designed a self-learning expert system with a novel hybrid learning algorithm based on Bayesian networks, called the modified greedy Bayesian pattern search algorithm (GBPS*). The proposed pattern differentiation model was based on the GBPS algorithm (Spirtes & Meek, 1995) with a modified version in the search procedure algorithm. The maximum accuracy of 88% obtained for pattern differentiation was estimated by pseudo-random generation of a sample. The authors discussed the high dimensionality of patient instances represented by multiple manifestations and diagnostic hypotheses. Their results suggested the use of most frequent attributes to reduce such dimensionality and consequently increase diagnostic accuracy.

The authors developed based on the "united system of syndrome differentiation" characterized by two characteristics. The first characteristic, the "key elements for syndrome differentiation", was abstracted from keywords in medical theories and grouped in two categories (the place where diseases occur; and the pathological state of the body or possible causes that make disease break out). As each key element usually exhibits a variable strength of association to manifestations, the pattern identification could be performed according to whether the key element is present or not. The second characteristic, the "standard syndrome-name database," was used to solve the problem that a pattern could be assigned with different labels by different practitioners. In the database, a standard pattern label includes at least one of the key elements described above. A dataset of 800 cases from real patients was used to train the Bayesian classifier.

The complete system for pattern differentiation is designed in modulus and its architecture consists of three parts: (1) input of the system, thereof one is sample database with attributes of symptoms and key elements, the other two are key-elements database and database of clinical observations to be diagnosed; (2) Analysis and diagnosis part, that is, the kernel part of the system, including: module for variable selection, module for discovering dependency relationship, module for learning classifiers, module for syndrome differentiation, module for mining frequent sets among key elements, and module for modification by experts; and (3) user interface, through which users and the system can interact with each other.

The computational model for pattern differentiation proceeds in two phases and its pseudo-code was provided (X. Wang et al., 2004). During the first phase, the key elements present by a patient are identified. The second phase searches the standard syndrome-name database, inquiring whether the corresponding patterns consist of these identified key elements. The algorithm considers all the attributes (including manifestations, key elements and patterns) as Boolean variables that take only two values: absent and present. The module for syndrome differentiation used the learned classifier to compute the posterior probability of every key element with Bayes theorem, and output those elements whose probability exceeds the threshold set by experts. Then the module queries and outputs the names of those patterns containing these key elements from standard pattern-name database. Furthermore, the module computes occurrence probability of each pattern by multiplying the probabilities of its corresponding key elements, under the assumption that these key elements are independent. Finally, the module selects the patterns with the probability excess diagnosis threshold.

7.3 Information Management System of Traditional Chinese Medicine Syndrome Project based on Prior Knowledge Support Vector Machine (P-SVM)

Yang et al. (2005) developed the Information Management System of Traditional Chinese Medicine Syndrome Project based on Prior Knowledge Support Vector Machine (P-SVM). SVM aims to process training and generalization with limited information provided by the sample data set without consideration of knowledge from application background. In the framework of limited sample data set learning, SVM makes maximum use of the information provided by sample data set theoretically regardless the application related knowledge. The authors reported an accuracy rate of 95% with the trained P-SVM to classify a sample set of 2,000 simulated records.

The general principle of the method is described here, and its pseudo-code was provided (Yang et al., 2005). A pattern dataset is used to train and test the P-SVM model. The test procedure consists of: a) generation of an expert knowledge dataset; b) description of the expert knowledge as rules to train the dataset to create the scale of confidence values; c) input data with confidence values to the Platt's Sequential Minimal Optimization (P-SMO) algorithm; d) comparison of the accuracy rates under different amount of training samples. The pattern dataset included the literature from 1978 to 2004 with approximately 400,000 entries and its ontology was organized with the entries: author, origin, title, subject heading, subheading, key word, and abstract. In the classification system of SVM with prior knowledge, the classifier will learn the traits of the certain thematic information from the corresponding prior knowledge. Therefore, based on the prior knowledge, the classifier is able to find out the appropriate literary information from the massive data.

No description of how the cases were simulated is available; thus, it is not possible to repeat the simulation procedure and to compare accuracy results. Moreover, the P-SVM theory was not discussed in light of the mode-of-thinking of Chinese medicine experts.

7.4 Chinese Medical Diagnostic System (CMDS)

Huang and Chen (2007) developed the Chinese Medical Diagnostic System (CMDS) for pattern differentiation of diseases related to the digestive system. It uses a Web interface and expert system technology in diagnosing 50 types of digestive system diseases. The authors compared the diagnosis of 20 simulated cases made by CMDS and diagnosticians and found the results satisfactory; however, they did not report either simulation procedures or statistical validity. The authors also stated that the Four Examinations were necessary for achieving a correct diagnosis. The authors reported 'high reliable and accurate diagnostic capabilities' in 95% of 50 simulated cases without any description of either how cases were simulated or possible sources and types of error.

The CMDs departed from an ontology-based model, in which the proposed ontology was derived from the traditional one but focused on digestive diseases and patterns. The whole system is composed by three main components: a) Java Expert System Shell (JESS); b) Database set; and c) knowledge extractor. The routine for pattern differentiation in depicted in the inference engine modulus of the JESS and automatically matches facts (user's entries) against patterns and concludes which rules are fired in CMDS. Two databases (general and knowledge databases) are used to store all information and rules necessary for pattern differentiation, respectively.

7.5 Pattern Differentiation Algorithm (PDA)

Ferreira (2008) proposed the pattern differentiation algorithm (PDA) based on an objective criterion developed to account for pattern holism (Guang, 2001). A second criterion was proposed and provided a significant increase in diagnostic accuracy of the model, being up to 94.7%(sensitivity = 89.8%; specificity = 99.5%) with the Four Examinations for *Zangfu* patterns (Ferreira, 2009). This method allowed testing the impact of different combinations of the Four Examinations and the amount of available information presented by patients on PDA's statistical performance. Also, it's associated method of model validation uncovered types of diagnostic errors otherwise not assessed by other computational models (Ferreira, 2011). Clinically, PDA was applied to patients with arterial hypertension and help understand that *Zangfu* patterns associated to this disease are indeed evidence of the progression of target-organ damage (Luiz et al., 2011).

PDA works in a three-stage schema and its pseudo-code was provided elsewhere (Ferreira, 2009). The first stage – data collection and dataset search – uses the data entry from patient's exam to search for free terms and quoted phrases, *e.g.*, *headache* and *"headache"*. The former term recalls patterns with *headache* within its manifestations profile (*ocular headache, occipital headache*, etc.); the latter term recalls patterns with the exact term. Combinatorial procedure (Zuzek et al., 2000) was used after data collection because the diagnosis does not depend on the sequence of the results obtained during the exam (Wolff, 2006). Manifestations were described as specifically as possible including onset ("palpitation in the morning", "palpitation in the evening"), duration ("acute headache", "chronic headache"), location ("occipital headache", "ocular headache") and severity ("dry tongue", "slight moist tongue", "moist tongue"), as well as any other characteristic that may be necessary to allow the pattern differentiation. Manifestations that co-occur in two or more patterns were assigned with the same term to increase the accuracy of string search algorithm.

At the second stage – selection of candidate patterns – a pattern is considered as a 'candidate' if it presents at least one manifestation collected at the exam. Patterns with no manifestations recognized were not used for further analysis. The "strength" of such indication of the candidate pattern is calculated as an objective criterion $F_{\%,K}$. This is an important stage since it recalls any possibility ($F_{\%,K}>0$) within the dataset and increases the sensitivity of the algorithm. Since patterns maybe described by different quantities of manifestations, the available information must be normalized to allow comparison among them and hence was used as a second objective criterion, $N_{\%,K,}$. It is expected that the occurrence of a successful pattern differentiation increases with decreasing $F_{\%,K}$. It is also expected that the occurrence of a successful pattern differentiation increases with increasing $N_{\%,K}$. However, as the accuracy of a diagnostic test is expected to decrease with either lower or higher cutoff values, it is appropriate to subtract a cutoff values from $N_{\%,K}$ to dislocate the accuracy curve to its optimum operating point. As such, the maximum accuracy is associated with the minimum $N_{\%-cutoff,K}$. Hence, the candidate patterns simultaneously ranked in descending order of $F_{\%,K}$ and ascending order of $N_{\%-cutoff,K}$ represent a list of diagnostic hypotheses.

The last stage – pattern differentiation – identifies the diagnosis. The diagnostic algorithm receives the manifestation profile and outputs for each tested profile: a) the identified diagnosis; b) the list of diagnostic hypotheses. Pattern differentiation is considered successful in either of two situations: 1) if PDA founds a unique diagnostic hypothesis that explains simultaneously all collected manifestations, i.e. $F_{\%,K}=100\%$; or 2) if there is one pattern among all diagnostic hypotheses with a highest, unique $F_{\%,K}$ value and lowest, unique $N_{\%-cutoff,K}$ value. Otherwise, if multiple diagnostic hypothesis were found with equal values of $F_{\%,K}$ and not unique values of $N_{\%,K}$ the procedure is considered unsuccessful since differentiation among competing patterns was not possible. In this case, physicians have access to the diagnostic hypotheses list and may want to revise the collected manifestations, continue examination of the patient to search for other manifestations, replace the collected symptoms/signs with more specific ones, or even subjectively chose a pattern.

PDA's average time for pattern differentiation of each case with the Four Examinations is estimated in less than 0.1s, which is suitable for clinical applications. There is no need to train PDA, which is a mathematical process already subject to bias. PDA's method is simple, and both criteria can be calculated even manually by a Chinese medicine practitioner (for a low number of candidate patterns). It's reasoning is entirely based on the actual process executed by Chinese medicine experts and thus reduces the error in data collection and analysis. PDA is more stable than other learning algorithms because the final diagnosis does not depend on the initial guess or sequence of manifestations used during the learning phase (Ferreira, 2009).

However, PDA is dependent on the pattern dataset. PDA's dataset was built in a form of open base, in which new information can be added (or modified) to the knowledge database to increase statistical performance of the criterion. As a corollary, the proposed methodology relies on human experts, not only to select the knowledge, but also to provide the database organization. To reduce the implications of the manual insertion of information, computational routines for inter-pattern and intra-pattern consistency were implemented. The major limitation of PDA is that it was tested only for *Zangfu* single patterns (Ferreira, 2008; Ferreira, 2009; Ferreira, 2011). Such case is the simplest one found in clinical practice for *Zangfu* patterns since the pathological process just begun to promote changes in homeostasis. The same subject may present several patterns simultaneously that are not mutually exclusive. Additionally, common etiologies and pattern transmissions among *Zangfu* are contributing factors to limit the model's performance. Finally, other theories are often used to perform diagnosis and were not yet evaluated (Maciocia, 1996).

7.6 Multi-Label k-Nearest Neighbour (ML-kNN)
Liu et al. (2010) obtained up to 78% accuracy using only the Inquiry method (n=185 manifestations) for identification of multi-patterns (based on 6 ZFSPs) related to coronary heart disease obtained from real cases. The pseudo-code of the ML-kNN was provided by the authors.

The kNN is an algorithm that searches for the nearest point in a training data set. This theory regards an instance as a point in synthesis space; thus, the label of a test instance is probably similar to those of several nearest points. The data set for pattern differentiation of coronary heart disease belongs to multi-label; whereas kNN only processes single label data sets, so the collected data set should be split into many groups of single label to be calculated. In the multi-label data, there is much relationship among each label, so simple splitting inevitably result in data loss. For this reason, multi-label learning algorithms are developed so as to better reveal the correlation of the labels, of which multi-label kNN (ML-kNN) is a popular technique. ML-kNN is a lazy multi-label learning algorithm developed on the basis of kNN. Based on the theory of kNN, ML-kNN aims to find k nearest instances for each test instance. In ML- kNN, the labels of test instances are judged directly by nearest instances, which is different from kNN.

8. Validation of computational models for diagnosis in Chinese medicine

For the model to be useful, expert practitioners must have confidence in the results and predictions that are inferred from it. Verifying or validating the model can provide such confidence. In principle, model validation is done by comparing the model's behaviour with the patient's and evaluating the difference. In the diagnostic field, the computational model is compared to either a gold-standard or a reference-standard method.

8.1 Model validation with "gold-standard" and "reference-standard"
The main issue related to diagnostic accuracy tests it he need for a "gold-standard" method or at least a "reference-standard" method to compare the results obtained with the model being tested. The gold-standard method for diagnosis is the one that provides the *true* health status of a person while the reference-standard method for diagnosis is the one that provide the health status *closest to the true one*. Obviously, gold-standard methods are preferred for model validation and assessment of a model's diagnostic accuracy. However, it is almost impossible to test clinical diagnostic models with gold-standard methods since the true

health status is unknown a priori. In this case, a diagnostic model with known statistical properties is applied to obtain a result that is used as the reference-standard.

Patterns identified by a panel of expert Chinese medicine practitioners has been used as the standard for diagnostic accuracy tests of computational models using data from population samples (Zhou & Zhang, 2006; Zhu et al., 2006; N.L. Zhang et al., 2008). This method presents a major drawback since the real diagnosis is not known and samples may be biased (hospital patients, community subjects, etc.). Moreover, the agreement in diagnosis among practitioners may be low (31.7%; 27.5–35%) (G.G. Zhang et al., 2005), despite some improvement after training (73%; 64.3–85.7%) (G.G. Zhang et al., 2008). The Standards for Reporting Interventions in Controlled Trials of Acupuncture (STRICTA) (MacPherson et al., 2010) recommend that the experience of Chinese medicine practitioners should be reported in clinical studies because such experience may influence diagnosis. As such, new diagnostic tests should not be compared to diagnoses made by Chinese medicine practitioners but with methods that guarantee correct diagnosis.

For the determination of the accuracy of Chinese medicine diagnostic tests, a large number of patients with possible combinations of the manifestations for each pattern must be generated. Thus, it is virtually impossible to estimate the diagnostic accuracy without computer methods. Stochastic simulation models have been used for research in health sciences. A well-known simulation method is the Monte Carlo (Metropolis & Ulam, 1949), in which the basic idea is to stochastically generate examples of a numerical variable and then evaluate the outcome of the model under evaluation. With stochastic methods, simulated patients can have their health status characterized by a computational model. The simulation of cases fixes both issues by randomly selecting manifestations only from the selected single pattern (Ferreira, 2009). Stochastic method allows a focus on the properties of manifestation profiles instead of individual manifestations. This procedure generates a large number of examples of any given pattern (stochastic process) and then examines the relative proportion of successes of the diagnostic test (deterministic process). Some modifications of the original Monte Carlo method are needed to enable stochastic methods to process nominal variables. Because cases are simulated from all possible manifestations of each pattern in the dataset, the output of the computational model can be compared to the actual name of the simulated pattern in the dataset. Thus, simulation of cases can be considered as a gold-standard method. Moreover, patient simulation models can be composed of independent algorithmic codes (i.e., there is no code sharing), so the results of the identification are blinded to the simulation parameters.

Currently, the computational model for simulating patients and testing diagnostic accuracy is the Manifestation Profile Simulation Algorithm (MPSA) (Ferreira, 2008; Ferreira, 2009, Ferreira, 2011). MPSA generates the study population according to different strategies to create case (true positive) and control (true negative) groups, as well as a proposal for identifying and handling missing cases. The inclusion criterion is the simulation of cases representing a single pattern in the knowledge dataset. For simulation purposes, MPSA assumes that the probability of each manifestation in the general population is given from previous studies or, if unknown, it is suggested to follow a uniform distribution (Ferreira, 2009). The comparison between the simulated pattern and the identified diagnosis yields the binary classification of the proposed method for pattern differentiation.

In MPSA, true positive (TP) cases of a pattern K are simulated by selecting from the dataset a random quantity of manifestations $N_{R,K}$. Each sorted manifestation is excluded from the set of possible manifestations to prevent multiple occurrences of the same manifestation at the respective simulated case. This iterative process continued until the $N_{R,K}$ manifestations were sorted to generate the manifestation profile. To obtain a true negative (TN) control for the same pattern K, two alternatives were proposed. In the first alternative, this respective pattern K is removed from the dataset and the same quantity $N_{R,K}$ is selected from the entire dataset and respective examination methods (Ferreira, 2008; Ferreira, 2009). The second alternative is to sort $N_{R,K}$ manifestations from another pattern pseudo-randomly chosen in the dataset after exclusion of pattern K (Ferreira, 2011). In both alternatives, the procedure allows a quantitative pair-wise comparison between TP and TN profiles with respect to the available information for pattern K, $N_{\%,K}$. Although the TP pattern was removed from the dataset, its manifestations that co-occur in other patterns are still present and could be selected to compose a TN manifestation profile. Since patterns may not present manifestations for some of the examination methods, empty manifestation profiles related to these examination methods represent missing cases and were excluded from analysis.

Despite the main advantage of knowing a priori the true pattern and methodological blinding, some limitations need to be mentioned. Manifestations may be sampled multiple times within the same run, resulting in less variation of manifestations profile than it would be expected to see in real patients. Also, manifestations may not be chosen at all, resulting in not tested data. However, large simulated samples from the dataset diminished these limitations (Ferreira, 2008). To assess the quality of the simulated cases and controls, a routine can be implemented to check if all manifestations were used for simulation of manifestations profiles. The algorithm performs a 'reverse engineering' by recreating the dataset from all simulated true positive cases. The algorithm searched among all manifestation profiles simulated for each pattern and grouped the manifestations present at least once among the simulated cases into a temporary dataset. After comparison with the original dataset, the algorithm reports whether the patterns that were completely simulated (*i.e.* all manifestations were used for analysis), partially simulated and not used for simulation (Ferreira, 2011).

8.2 Detection and classification problems

In general, the diagnostic process is designed to detect if the subject is healthy or ill. In this case, two groups of subjects with known true conditions are used: a group of individuals in which the condition to be tested is truly present; and a group o individuals in which the condition to be tested is truly absent. Adapted to Chinese medicine framework, a "healthy pattern" diagnosis must be described in the same manner as the "ill" patterns. For instance, the "liver-blood deficiency" pattern should have the mutually exclusive counterpart "liver-blood healthy" pattern. The description of such health-related patterns is possible because pattern differentiation process is not limited to assessing presence/absence of manifestations (e.g. asymptomatic individuals may be also have their patterns identified). A completely healthy person will present all healthy patterns simultaneously. However, in clinical practice it is difficult to find a patient that is completely healthy and thus the pattern differentiation process must be applied to patients. In this case, the diagnostic model must recognize the underlying pattern (or patterns) and not the healthy or ill statuses.

8.3 Sample sizes, participant recruitment and sampling

A important issue in diagnostic accuracy studies is the sample sizes determination, which can be estimated based on equations derived for detecting differences in accuracy tests using receiver operating characteristic (ROC) curves (Hanley & McNeil, 1982). For calculations, it is necessary the expected difference in accuracy between the reference and the index test, the level of significance (usually $\alpha=5\%$, $Z\alpha=1.645$, one-sided), and the power of the test (usually $\beta=90\%$, $Z\beta=1.28$). The equation designed to real cases can be used in simulated ones provided that the absolute consistency between original and recreated datasets is proved as described before. This is an important issue related to the quality control in this study and should not be omitted in other simulations studies were pattern differentiation outcomes are assessed (Ferreira, 2011).

8.4 Estimating the diagnostic accuracy of a diagnostic model

Diagnostic models present domains of validity, *i.e.* they should not be used outside the validation scope since there is no estimation concerning its performance. The implications range from underestimation to overestimation of the model's diagnostic accuracy. The Standards for Reporting of Diagnostic Accuracy (STARD) (Bossuyt et al., 2003) summarized the necessary steps for conducting scientific works to determine diagnostic accuracy of models. Although not specified in the STARD, such methodology can be also be adopted by studies in which computational models perform diagnosis, even in case of simulated patients. The validity of a new diagnostic model is obtained by comparison of the new model's results with the actual result. However, very often the actual value is not known most commonly due to absence of gold-standard diagnostic methods.

Accuracy, sensitivity, specificity, positive and negative predictive values are the most common measures of a model's performance. Accuracy is defined as the proportion of true results in the population. Sensitivity is the probability that the test is positive given that the patient is sick (Altman & Bland, 1994a), while specificity is the probability that the test is negative given that the patient is not sick (Altman & Bland, 1994a). Positive and negative predictive values are proportions of true positives and true negatives out of all positive results, respectively (Altman & Bland, 1994b). All those estimators are obtained from 2×2 confusion matrices (Table 1) made from classification of simulated and identified diagnosis (Jekel, 1999; Altman & Bland, 1994a; Altman & Blend, 1994b). Departing from Table 1 and adapting the epidemiological concepts to Chinese medicine framework, computational models can be evaluated with estimations of:

		Gold-standard test result	
		Simulated pattern (Case)	Other pattern (Control)
New test result	Identified pattern	True positive (TP)	False positive (FP)
	Other pattern	False negative (FN)	True negative (TN)

Table 1. Confusion 2×2 matrix for assessment of diagnostic accuracy between the reference test and pattern differentiation algorithm.

a. Accuracy: proportion of successful pattern differentiation (true results) in the population (equation 1). Diagnostic accuracy indicates the total sum of corrected assigned cases.

$$Accuracy = \frac{TP+TN}{TP+FN+TN+FP} \times 100\% ; \qquad (1)$$

b. Sensitivity: proportion of successful pattern differentiations correctly predicted by PDA in cases (equation 2).

$$Sensitivity = \frac{TP}{TP+FN} \times 100\%; \tag{2}$$

c. Specificity: proportion of successful pattern differentiations correctly predicted by PDA in controls (equation 3);

$$Specificity = \frac{TN}{TN+FP} \times 100\%; \tag{3}$$

d. Negative predictive values: proportion of unsuccessful pattern differentiation correctly predicted by PDA (equation 4).

$$Negative \quad predictive \quad value = \frac{TN}{TN+FN} \times 100\%; \tag{4}$$

e. Positive predictive values: proportion of successful pattern differentiation correctly predicted by PDA (equation 5).

$$Positive \quad predictive \quad value = \frac{TP}{TP+FP} \times 100\%. \tag{5}$$

ROC plots are used to visualize and estimate accuracy of the model's classification. Those estimators are readily available from 2x2 crosstabs obtained from simultaneous classification of the results regarding the "gold-standard" and the new model under evaluation. In ROC plots, the smallest cutoff value is the minimum observed test value minus 1, and the largest cutoff value is the maximum observed test value plus 1. All the other tested cutoff values were the averages of two consecutive ordered observed test values (Hanley & McNeil, 1982; Hanley & McNeil, 1983; Altman & Bland, 1994c).

8.5 Comparing diagnostic accuracy of two computational models

Consider now the situation where two computational models can be used. It is of interest to select the best model in terms of diagnostic accuracy. Such a comparison can be performed based on a pair of 2x2 confusion matrices (Table 2) made from classification of simulated and identified diagnosis simultaneously by the two computational models.

	True negative				True positive		
	Model 1	-	+		Model 1	+	-
Model 2	-	A	B	Model 2	+	a	b
	+	C	D		-	c	d

Table 2. Confusion 2x2 matrices for comparison of binomial proportions between the two diagnostic tests. (+) and (-) indicate positive and negative test results respectively. B is the number of TN cases classified correctly by test 2 and falsely by test 1 and conversely for C cases and analogously for the TP group.

The 95% confidence interval (95%CI) for the binomial proportions p (accuracy, sensitivity, specificity, negative predictive value, positive predictive value; equations 1-5) can be calculated with Wilson's method (Agresti & Coull, 1998). If both models are to be evaluated on the same samples of TP and TN cases, an adaptation of McNemar's test for correlated proportions is applied (Linnet & Brandt, 1986). The TP and the TN profiles are divided into four parts according to their test responses (Table 2). Estimations related to ROC curves (AUC and respective 95%CI) can be obtained with the nonparametric Wilcoxon statistic (Hanley & McNeil, 1982; Hanley & McNeil, 1983).

Since the Four Examinations provide the basic ontology for pattern differentiation, it is of interest to study the partial contribution of each Examination as well as their cumulative, sequential application. Hence, the diagnostic accuracy may be studied in terms of the following sets of the Four Examinations:

1.   Inspection;
2.   Auscultation & Olfaction;
3.   Inquiry;
4.   Palpation;
5.   Inspection, Auscultation & Olfaction;
6.   Inspection, Auscultation & Olfaction, Inquiry;
7.   Inspection, Auscultation & Olfaction, Inquiry, Palpation.

Indeed, as manifestations are closely related to the interdependent internal organs, combined Examination methods are preferable since they cover several forms of presentation of the same pattern.

8.6 Recognition of diagnostic errors in pattern differentiation

All models have a certain domain of validity. This may determine how exactly they are able to describe the system's behavior. It is hazardous to use a model outside the area it has been validated for. Reports of errors for Chinese medicine practitioners are available from ancient literature (Yang & Li, 1993; Luo, 1995; Yang, 2003; Flaws, 2004; Yang & Chase, 2004) including non-skilled practice, misdiagnosis and mistreatment; however, little contemporary literature is available on this subject. Evidence shows that subjectivity of manifestations or limited detection of clinical features is the major causes of unreliable pattern differentiation made by Chinese medicine practitioners (Kim et al., 2008; O'Brien et al., 2009). While diagnostic errors can never be eliminated, they can be minimised through understanding factors related to the pattern differentiation process.

Recognition of factors related to the performance of diagnostic methods is relevant to the development of reliable methods that can be implemented for clinical and research purposes. The first limitation to pattern differentiation algorithms is that the user must possess a certain level of knowledge to discriminate or interpret the patient's complains (Harding, 1996). Therefore, an implicit assumption to all current computational models is that the patients are capable of reporting their symptoms and that the Chinese medicine practitioners are able to correctly identify manifestations.

Pattern similarity is intrinsic to Chinese medical knowledge. Pattern similarity introduces errors in the pattern differentiation process, as the patient's true pattern may not be properly assigned. Dual pattern similarity has moderate, statistically significant effect on pattern differentiation outcome but cumulative application of the Four Examinations progressively reduces the strength of significant association between pattern similarity and diagnostic errors (Ferreira, 2011).

Currently three pattern differentiation outcomes can be distinguished, namely (a) identification of the true pattern (correct diagnosis), (b) identification of a pattern that is not the true pattern (misdiagnosis) and (c) no identification of pattern at all (undiagnosis). For discrimination of those types of diagnostic errors, 2x3 crosstabs (Table 3) are used to differentiate among correct diagnosis, misdiagnosis and undiagnosis.

		Gold-standard test result	
		Simulated pattern (Case)	Other pattern (Control)
New test result	Identified pattern	Correct (TP)	Erroneous (FP)
	Other pattern	Erroneous (FN)	Correct (TN)
	No pattern identified	Absent	Absent

Table 3. Crosstabs (2x3) for investigation of diagnostic errors of computational models.

The distinction of error types in this study is possible if the manifestation profiles of true negative controls are any other true pattern that was not its true positive counterpart, and not just random manifestations from all patterns in dataset as in other studies. This modification expands the interpretation of false negative cases from one wide option ('it can be any other pattern, no pattern at all, or it was not possible to uniquely identify any pattern K') into two separate options ('it is pattern K' or 'it was not possible to uniquely identify any pattern in dataset'). With this true condition made known a priori it is possible to distinguish misidentification from no identification among unsuccessful outcomes (Ferreira, 2011).

9. Future directions

Although validated diagnostic models are available, several issues limit their application in patient care. For instance, almost all computational models deal with single patterns – a condition rarely seen in clinical practice – or a single disease. Complex and multiple patterns present additional difficulties in the diagnostic task since there are several combinations of two or more patterns that could result in the same diagnosis. Multiple patterns decomposition is then an open field of research with direct clinical applications and should be investigated.

Standardization of treatment prescription is possible since well-defined, consistent diagnosis can be achieved with computational models. Current trends focus in computer-aid to perform diagnosis and treatment. It is believed that the combination of traditional methods and modern resources may improve the efficacy of Chinese medicine intervention.

Suggested topics for future research on computational models for pattern differentiation:

- Construction of an internationally available Chinese medicine ontology and web-based knowledge dataset with patterns and manifestations.
- Use of qualitative, "fuzzy-like" scales developed in Eastern medicine. Ex.: tongue fur.
- Discovery of which subsets of manifestations lead to a more accurate diagnosis Determination of the distribution of manifestations in each pattern (and patterns in the dataset) to improve the simulation of manifestation profiles.
- Incorporation of common etiologies and pattern transmissions into computational models to extend its application in general clinical practice.

10. References

Agresti, A.; & Coull, B.A. Approximate is better than "exact" for interval estimation of binomial proportions. *The American Statistician*, Vol. 52, No. 2, (May 1998), (119-126), ISSN 0003-1305.

Altman, D.G.; & Bland, J.M. Diagnostic tests 1: Sensitivity and Specificity. *British Medical Journal*, Vol. 308, (June 1994a), (1552), ISSN 0959-535X.

Altman, D.G.; & Bland, J.M. Diagnostic tests 2: predictive values. *British Medical Journal*, Vol. 309 (July 1994b), (102), ISSN 0959-535X.

Altman, D.G.; & Bland, J.M. Diagnostic tests 3: receiver operating characteristic plots. *British Medical Journal*, Vol. 309 (July 1994c), (188), ISSN 0959-535X.

Auteroche, B.; Navailh, P. (1992). *O Diagnóstico na Medicina Chinesa*. Andrei, ISBN 978-85-747-6070-6, São Paulo, Brazil.

Bossuyt, P.M.; Reitsma. J.B.; Bruns, D.E.; Gatsonis, C.A.; Glasziou, P.P.; Irwig, L.M.; Moher, D.; Rennie, D.; de Vet, H.C.W.; & Lijmer, J.G. The STARD statement for reporting studies of diagnostic accuracy: explanation and elaboration. *Annals of Internal Medicine*, Vol. 138, No 1, (January 2003), (W1-W12), ISSN 0003-4819.

Dodd, M.; Janson, S.; Facione, N.; Faucett, J.; Froelicher, E.S.; Humphreys, J.; Lee, K.; Miaskowski, C.; Puntillo, K.; Rankin, S.; & Taylor, D. Advancing the science of symptom management. *Journal of Advanced Nursing*, Vol. 33, No. 5, (March 2001), (668-676), ISSN 0309-2402.

Ferreira, Ade. S. Statistical validation of strategies for Zang-Fu single pattern differentiation. *Zhong Xi Yi Jie He Xue Bao*, Vol. 6, No. 11, (November 2008), (1109-1116), ISSN 1672-1977.

Ferreira, A.S. Diagnostic accuracy of pattern differentiation algorithm based on traditional Chinese medicine theory: a stochastic simulation study. *Chinese Medicine*, Vol. 4, (December 2009), (24), ISSN 1749-8546.

Ferreira, A.S. Misdiagnosis and undiagnosis due to pattern similarity in Chinese medicine: a stochastic simulation study using pattern differentiation algorithm. *Chinese Medicine*, Vol. 6, (January 2011), (1), ISSN 1749-8546.

Flaws, B. (translator). (2004) *Nán Jīng (The Classic of Difficulties)*. Blue Poppy Press, ISBN 1-891845-07-1, Denver, United States of America.

Guang, J.Y. The mode of thinking in Chinese clinical medicine: characteristics, steps and forms. *Clinical Acupuncture and Oriental Medicine*, Vol. 2, No. 1, (March 2001), (23-28), ISSN 1461-1449.

Hanley, J.A.; & McNeil, B.J. The meaning and use of the area under a receiver operating characteristic (ROC) curve. *Radiology*, Vol. 143, (April 1982), (29-36), ISSN 0033-8419.

Hanley, J.A.; & McNeil, B.J. A method of comparing the areas under receiver operating characteristic curves derived from the same cases. *Radiology*, Vol. 148, (September 1983), (839-843), ISSN 0033-8419.

Harding, W.T. Compilers and Knowledge Dictionaries for Expert Systems: Inference Engines of the Future. *Expert Systems with Applications*, Vol. 10, No. 1, (1996), (91-98), ISSN 0957-4174.

Huang, M.J.; & Chen, M.Y. Integrated design of the intelligent web-based Chinese Medical Diagnostic System (CMDS): systematic development for digestive health. *Expert Systems with Application*, Vol. 32, No. 2, (February 2007), (658-673), ISSN 0957-4174.

Jaccard, P. Étude comparative de la distribution florale dans une portion des Alpes et des Jura. *Bulletin del la Société Vaudoise des Sciences Naturelles*, Vol. 37, (1901), (547-579).

Jekel, J.F.; Elmore, J.G.; & Katz, D.L. (1999). *Epidemiologia, Bioestatística e Medicina Preventiva*, Artmed, ISBN 8536302968, Porto Alegre, Brazil.

Kim, M.; Cobbin, D.; & Zaslawski, C. Traditional Chinese medicine tongue inspection: an examination of the inter- and intrapractitioner reliability for specific tongue characteristics. *The Journal of Alternative and Complementary Medicine*, Vol. 14, No. 5, (June 2008), (527-536), ISSN 1075-5535.

Linnet, K., & Brandt, E. Assessing diagnostic tests once an optimal cutoff point has been selected. *Clinical Chemistry*, Vol. 32, (July 1986), (1341-1346), ISSN 0009-9147.

Liu, G.P.; Li, G.Z.; Wang, Y.L.; & Wang, Y.Q. Modelling of inquiry diagnosis for coronary heart disease in traditional Chinese medicine by using multi-label learning. *BMC Complementary Alternative Medicine*, Vol. 10, (2010), (37), ISSN 1472-6882.

Lu, A.P.; & Chen, K.J. Integrative Medicine in Clinical Practice: From Pattern Differentiation in Traditional Chinese Medicine to Disease Treatment. *Chinese Journal of Integrative Medicine*, Vol. 15, No. 2, (April 2009), (152), ISSN 1993-0402.

Luiz, A.B.; Cordovil, L.; Barbosa Filho, J.; & Ferreira, A.S. Zangfu zheng (patterns) are associated with clinical manifestations of zang shang (target-organ damage) in arterial hypertension. *Chinese Medicine*, Vol. 6 (June 2011), (23), ISSN 1749-8546.

Lukman, S.; He, Y., & Hui, S.C. Computational methods for Traditional Chinese Medicine: A survey. *Computer Methods and Programs in Biomedicine*, Vol. 88, No. 3, (December 2007), (283-294), ISSN 0169-2607.

Maciocia, G. (1996). *Fundamentos da Medicina Tradicional Chinesa: Um texto abrangente para acupunturistas e fitoterapeutas*. Roca, ISBN 85-7241-150-X, Rio de Janeiro, Brazil.

MacPherson, H.; Altman, D.G.; Hammerschlag, R.; Youping, L.; Taixiang, W.; White, A.; Moher D; & STRICTA Revision Group. Revised STandards for Reporting Interventions in Clinical Trials of Acupuncture (STRICTA): extending the CONSORT statement. *PLoS Medicine*, Vol 7, No. 6, (June 2010), (e1000261), ISSN 1549-1277.

McSherry, D. Strategic induction of decision trees. *Knowledge-Based Systems*, Vol. 12, No. 5, (October 1999), (269-275), ISSN 0950-7051.

Metropolis, N.; & Ulam, S. The Monte Carlo method. *Journal of the American Statistical Association*, Vol 44, No. 247, (September 1949), (335-341), ISSN 0162-1459.

O'Brien, K.A.; Abbas, E.; Zhang, J.; Guo, Z.X.; Luo, R.; Bensoussan, A.; & Komesaroff, P.A. Understanding the reliability of diagnostic variables in a Chinese medicine examination. *The Journal of Alternative and Complementary Medicine*, Vol. 15, No. 7, (July 2009), (727-734), ISSN 1075-5535.

O'Connor, J. & Bensky, D. (1987). *Acupuncture a Comprehensive Text*. Eastland Press, ISBN 0-939616-00-9, Seattle, United States of America.

Peterson, M.C.; Holbrook, J.H.; Von Hales, D.; Smith, N.L.; & Staker, L.V. Contributions of the history, physical examination, and laboratory investigation in making medical diagnoses. *Western Journal of Medicine*, Vol. 156, No. 2, (February 1992), (163-165), ISSN 1476-2978.

Real, R. Tables of significant values of Jaccard's index of similarity. *Miscellània Zoològica*, Vol. 22, No. 1, (June 1999), (29-40), ISSN 0211-6529.

Ross, J. (2003). *Combinação Dos Pontos de Acupuntura: a Chave para o Êxito Clínico*, Roca, ISBN 85-7241-417-7, São Paulo, Brazil.

Spirtes, P., & Meek, C. (1995). Learning Bayesian networks with discrete variables from data. *Proceedings of the First International Conference on Knowledge Discovery and Data Mining*, pp. 294–299, ISBN 978-0-929280-82-0, Menlo Park, California, USA, August 20-21, 1995.

Tao, L. Achievements of Chinese medicine in the Chin (221-207 BC) and Han (206 BC-219 AD) dynasties. *Chinese Medical Journal*, Vol. 71, No. 5, (September-October 1953a), (380-386), ISSN 0366-6999.

Tao, L. Achievements of Chinese medicine in the Sui (598-617 A.D.) and Tang (618-907 A.D.) dynasties. *Chinese Medical Journal*, Vol. 71, No., (July-August 1953b), (801-820), ISSN 0366-6999.

Tao, L. Achievements of Chinese medicine during the Ming (1368-1644 A.D.) dynasty. *Chinese Medical Journal*, Vol. 76, No. 2, (February 1958a), (178-198), ISSN 0366-6999.

Tao, L. Chinese medicine during the Ming dynasty. *Chinese Medical Journal*, Vol. 76, No. 3, (March 1958b), (285-301), ISSN 0366-6999.

Wang, S.C., Li, Y.G., & Guo, X.M. (2002). *Pediatrics of Traditional Chinese Medicine - A Newly Compiled Practical English-Chinese Library of Traditional Chinese Medicine*, Shanghai University of Traditional Chinese Medicine, ISBN 7-81010-653-8, Shanghai, China.

Wang, X.; Qu, H.; Liu, P.; & Cheng, Y. A self-learning expert system for diagnosis in traditional Chinese medicine. *Expert Systems with Applications*, Vol. 26, No. 4, (May 2004), (557-566), ISSN 0957-4174.

Wolff, J.G. Medical diagnosis as pattern recognition in a framework of information compression by multiple alignment, unification and search. *Decision Support Systems*, Vol. 42, No. 2, (November 2006), (608-625), ISSN 0167-9236.

World Health Organization. Traditional medicine. Fact sheet nº 134. Revised November 2008. Available from http: //www.who.int/mediacentre/factsheets/fs134/en/

Luo, X.W. (translator). (1995) *Jīnkuì Yàoluè (Synopsis of Prescriptions of the Golden Chamber with 300 Cases)*. New World Press, ISBN 7-80005-291-5, Beijing, China.

Yang, S.Z.; & Li, J.Y. (translators). (1993). *Pí Wèi Lún (Treatise on the Spleen & Stomach)*, Blue Poppy, ISBN 0-936185-41-4, Denver, United States of America.

Yang S.Z. (translator). (2003). *Zhōng Zàng Jīng (Master Hua's Classic of the Central Viscera)*, Blue Poppy, ISBN 0-936185-43-0, Denver, United States of America.

Yang, S.Z.; & Chace, C. (translators). (2004). *Zhēn Jiŭ Jiă Yǐ Jīng (The Systematic Classic of Acupuncture & Moxibustion)*, Blue Poppy, ISBN 0-936185-29-5, Denver, United States of America.

Yang, X.B.; Liang, Z.H.; Zhang, G.; Luo, Y.J.; & Yin, J. (2005). A classification algorithm for TCM syndromes based on P-SVM. *Proceedings of 2005 International Conference on Machine Learning and Cybernetics*, pp. 3692-3697, ISBN 0-7803-9091-1, Piscataway, New Jersey, USA, August 18-21, 2005.

Zaslawki C. Clinical reasoning in traditional Chinese medicine: implications for clinical research. *Clinical Acupuncture and Oriental Medicine*, Vol. 4, No. 2-3, (2003), (94-101), ISSN 1461-1449.

Zhang, G.G.; Lee, W.; Bausell, B.; Lao, L.; Handwerger, B.; & Berman, B. Variability in the Traditional Chinese Medicine (TCM) Diagnoses and Herbal Prescriptions Provided by Three TCM Practitioners for 40 Patients with Rheumatoid Arthritis. *The Journal of Alternative and Complementary Medicine*, Vol. 11, No. 3, (July 2005), (415-421), ISSN 1075-5535.

Zhang, G.G.; Singh, B.; Lee, W.; Handwerger, B.; Lao, L.; & Berman, B. Improvement of Agreement in TCM Diagnosis Among TCM Practitioners for Persons with the Conventional Diagnosis of Rheumatoid Arthritis: Effect of Training. *The Journal of Alternative and Complementary Medicine*, Vol. 14, No. 4, (May 2008), (381-386), ISSN 1075-5535.

Zhang, N.L.; Yuan, S.; Chen, T.; & Wang, Y. Statistical Validation of Traditional Chinese Medicine Theories. *The Journal of Alternative and Complementary Medicine*, Vol. 14, No. 5, (June 2008), (583-587), ISSN 1075-5535.

Zheng, N.; & Wu, Z. (2004). TCM-SIRD: an integrated aided system for traditional Chinese medicine Sizheng. *Proceedings of 2004 IEEE International Conference on Systems, Man and Cybernetics*, pp. 3864-3868, ISBN 0-7803-8566-7, The Hague, The Netherlands, October 10-13, 2004.

Zhou, C.L; & Zhang, Z.F. Progress and prospects of research on information processing techniques for intelligent diagnosis of traditional Chinese medicine. *Zhong Xi Yi Jie He Xue Bao*, Vol. 4, No. 6, (November 2006), (560-566), ISSN 1672-1977.

Zhou, X.; Chen, S.; Liu, B.; Zhang, R.; Wang, Y.; Li, P.; Guo, Y.; Zhang, H.; Gao, Z.; & Yan, X. Development of traditional Chinese medicine clinical data warehouse for medical knowledge discovery and decision support. *Artificial Intelligence in Medicine*, Vol. 48, No. 2-3, (February-March 2010), (139-152), ISSN 0933-3657.

Zhou, X.Z.; Wu, Z.H.; Yin, A.N.; Wu, L.C.; & Fan, W.Y.; Zhang, R. Ontology development for unified traditional Chinese medical language system. *Artificial Intelligence in Medicine*, Vol. 32, No. 1, (September 2004), (15-27), ISSN 0933-3657.

Zhu, W.F.; Yan, J.F.; & Huang, B.Q. Application of Bayesian network in syndrome differentiation system of traditional Chinese medicine. *Zhong Xi Yi Jie He Xue Bao*, Vol. 4, No. 6, (November 2006), (567-571), ISSN 1672-1977.

Zuzek, A.; Biasizzo, A.; Novak, F. Sequential diagnosis tool. *Microprocessors and Microsystems*, Vol. 24, (2000), (191-197), ISSN 0141-9331.

8

Effectiveness of Traditional Chinese Medicine in Primary Care

Wendy Wong[1], Cindy Lam Lo Kuen[1],
Jonathan Sham Shun Tong[2] and Daniel Fong Yee Tak[3]
[1]Department of Family Medicine and Primary Care, LKS Faculty of Medicine,
[2]Department of Clinical Oncology, LKS Faculty of Medicine,
[3]Department of Nursing Studies, LKS Faculty of Medicine,
The University of Hong Kong
Hong Kong

1. Introduction

This chapter first describes the role of Traditional Chinese Medicine (TCM) in health care. It then reviews the literature on the effectiveness of TCM with a special focus on primary care. An appraisal of the outcome measures in the context of TCM is made. The relationship between TCM and the concept of health-related quality of life (HRQOL) is discussed. The current applications and limitations of the HRQOL measures derived from Western culture to TCM are identified. The chapter ends with an overview of Chinese culture specific measures for evaluating the effectiveness of TCM in primary care.

2. The role of Traditional Chinese Medicine (TCM) in health services

In China, it was estimated that there were 3.1 billion TCM outpatient visits per year for the 1.3 billion population [1]. Currently, TCM accounts for 40% of all health services delivered in China, and it has been part of the formal Chinese healthcare system since 1950 under the political directives of Mao Tse Tung [2]. However, the development of TCM in Hong Kong followed a different path as it was not recognized by the Government as part of the formal healthcare system until 1997 when Hong Kong was reunited with China. The Hong Kong Special Administrative Region (SAR) government tried to re-integrate TCM into the health care system in the past decade by the establishment of the Chinese Medicine Council of Hong Kong (CMCHK) as a statutory body under the Chinese Medicine Ordinance to regulate and register Chinese Medicine Practitioners (CMP) in 1999 [3]. Although TCM in Hong Kong is still mostly a private service, piloting outpatient TCM clinics and limited inpatient services have started in public hospitals. Subsidized TCM primary care outpatient services have been provided by the Tung Wah Group Hospitals for nearly half a century in Hong Kong [4].

Even though Western Medicine consultation is the most commonly used type of primary care, 50 to 60% of people have consulted TCM in Hong Kong and 13.5% of the people have consulted TCM frequently or occasionally [5, 6]. There are 5604 registered CMP serving a population of 6.8 million in Hong Kong [3] and most of them provide primary care. A recent survey found that 19% of all private outpatient services were provided by Chinese Medicine Practitioners (CMP) [7] suggesting that many people find TCM helpful enough to be willing to pay for the service. Users of TCM were found to be more likely to be women, older persons, chronic disease patients with lower quality of life, and the lower socioeconomic group [8]. With its whole person approach, TCM may have a role in primary care to enhance the quality of life and health of people especially the elderly and those with chronic diseases.

TCM is regarded as a form of complementary and alternative medicines (CAM) in most countries other than China. CAM refers to a broad set of health practices that are not part of the country's own tradition and are not integrated into the dominant health care system [9]. The number of CAM visits exceeded the number of visits to all primary care physicians, and the estimated total out-of-pocket expenditure on CAM was US$27 billions in 1997 which was comparable to that for all primary care physician services for the same year [10]. TCM, especially acupuncture and bone-setting, is one of the most popular CAM globally being practiced widely in Asia, the United States (US), Canada, Europe and Australia [10]. TCM makes up a major proportion of the CAM services in the US [10] increasing from 34% in 1989 to 42% in 1997 [11]. Many of these patients reported improvement with their illnesses that Western Medicine failed to help [12]. In Denmark, the proportion of patients who had used TCM at least once annually increased from 23% in 1987 to 43.7% in 2007 [13]. TCM consultations accounts for a total expenditure of £580 million in the United Kingdom (UK) [14].

The increasing use of TCM has caused a profound impact on the global health care services. The National Centre of Complementary and Alternative Medicine (NCCAM) and the National Health Service (NHS) have been established in the US and the UK respectively, to allocate national budget for TCM services in primary care. Other European countries also have provided public financing for TCM [10]. The global increase use of TCM has called for more information on its function and outcomes to guide medical resource allocation.

3. Effectiveness of Traditional Chinese Medicine

The effectiveness of acupuncture in pain control was first demonstrated by an expert panel systematic review in the NIH conference in 1997 [15], which attracted the world's attention to TCM. This has established the place of TCM in health care. Artemisia annua was proved to be effective in against resistant malaria and gave hope of preventing more than 800 thousand deaths from malaria among children each year [16, 17]. In Geriatrics, TCM has been shown to not only improve health-related quality of life (HRQOL) in the treatment of illnesses, but also to promote healthy aging [18]. Wesnes and Ward et al. found Panax ginseng significantly improved an index of memory quality by 7.5% and this effect persisted for the whole treatment period until 2 weeks after washout [19]. TCM has also been studied for the prevention of acute severe respiratory syndrome (SARS) in hospital workers [20]. None of the health workers who took the supplement had contracted SARS compared to 0.4% of health care workers who did not (p=0.014). Improvement in influenza-like symptoms and quality of life were also observed among herbal supplement users. A remarkable effectiveness of TCM was found in patients with irritable bowel syndrome in a randomized controlled trial that showed an improvement measured by the total bowel symptoms scale and global improvement scores assessed by both patients and gastroenterologists [21]. Many studies in Europe were carried out in recent years to evaluate TCM treatments for specific conditions with variable results. In the UK, a daily decoction containing 10 herbs was found to be more effective than placebo in improving patients with chronic atopic dermatitis in erythema, surface damage, patients' subjective feeling on itching and sleep in a randomized, double-blind placebo-controlled trial [22, 23]. In Nerthlands, the effectiveness of Chinese herbal medicine (CHM) integrated with TCM diagnosis was confirmed for the treatment of postmenopausal symptoms when compared with hormone replacement therapy (HRT) or placebo in a randomized placebo-controlled trial [24]. It was found that CHM could significantly improve the amount of hot flushes than placebo. In addition, quality of care research in a TCM hospital in German found that TCM care could reduce the intensity of complaints, improve quality of life (in terms of both mental and physical-related HRQOL scores of SF-36) and subjective and objective global rating of conditions of inpatients subjects [25]. However, there were few research data on the effectiveness of TCM in primary care even though it is most commonly used for this purpose.

The National Health Service (NHS) of the UK conducted 4 large-scale population studies on the impact of CAM in reorganization of primary care services in 1999 [14, 26, 27]. Results showed that patients not only had their health outcomes significantly improved or expectation met after the consultation but also had significantly decreased in the use of medication and general practitioner time. A limitation of these surveys was that they did not differentiate between the different types of CAM.

A study by the Swiss Federal Department of Home Affairs evaluated and compared the health status and health care utilization rates of users of complementary and alternative medicine (CAM) clinics found that patients attending CAM clinics had higher consultation rates and more severe illnesses than patients in conventional primary care clinics [28]. This study gave evidence on poorer self-perced health status of CAM patients which need for a more physician-based medical services provided by CAM practitioners in primary care. The need for evaluating Chinese medicine and assure the quality of care was revealed by a population survey in Beijing [29] and a qualitative study in the UK [30]. Before this study, there were no data available on the effectiveness of TCM in primary care yet. The effectiveness of TCM primary care service as a whole remained unknown and that for the treatment of common problems were limited. Such information is needed to inform policy makers and the public how TCM is best utilized in our health care system [31, 32].

3.1 Evaluating the effectiveness of Traditional Chinese Medicine (TCM)

Despite the fact that TCM is popular globally and national institutes have been established for the integration of TCM into their health care systems, scientific evidence to support its use is not sufficient. The effectiveness of a highly individualized treatment made by a Chinese Medicine Practitioner (CMP) is usually subject to only the CMP's assessment and patients' subjective perception. The lack of a standardized outcome measurement method limits its scientific evaluation and generalizability of the results. The requirement of the paradigm of evidence based practice in using randomized controlled trials (RCT) as the 'gold standard' for the evaluation of treatment effectiveness has led to the denigration of non-experimental studies. A major conference held in 1993 concluded that only RCT was capable to confirm the benefit brought by TCM, and recommendation should not be made from evidence gathered in observational or case-control studies. However, only a few

Chinese herbal remedies and acupuncture have been proven by RCT [15]. Most claims on the effectiveness of TCM were based on empirical experience, leading to some people concluding that TCM was mostly not effective or even harmful [33]. Nevertheless, the debate on the most appropriate study designs for evaluating the effectiveness of TCM continues.

Unfortunately, most randomized controlled trials (RCT) conducted on TCM were rated to be poor in quality [34, 35] but RCT is not the only research study design and has its limitation. Classical RCT enforced the evaluation of TCM by the conventional Western medicine model, which can be impractical and inappropriate [36]. Black pointed out that not every intervention can be evaluated by a randomized trial and most importantly the rigorous random allocation may reduce the effectivenss of the intervention by not considering the subject's active participation, beliefs and preference [37]. We need observational or cohort studies to evaluate some interventions while others should be tested by RCT. Studies conducted by Thomas and Fitter showed the impossibilities of blinding Chinese Medicine Practitioners or patients during acupuncture interventions or giving individualized TCM treatments according to patients preference [38]. The realization of the inappropriateness of classical RCT to evaluate TCM led to the development of two alternative clinical trial methods: (1) the partial randomization design; and (2) the pragmatic design with prior randomization by Fitter [39] to evaluate the effectiveness of TCM. The partial randomization design takes patients' preference into account before they are randomized into treatment or placebo groups. Upon recruitment, patients are asked whether they have a preference for certain treatments, and if they do, they are assigned to the preferred treatment. If not, they are randomly assigned into either the study or the control treatments. The pragmatic design with prior randomization classifies eligible patients into syndrome groups by TCM practitioners before they are randomized to receive the appropriate treatment or placebo.

The study by Zaslawshi showed the pragmatic design with the integration of the CMP's syndrome differentiation based on TCM theory into a randomizd controlled trial was feasible in an acupuncture clinical trial [40]. This model was also used successfully in a RCT on the treatment of Irritable bowel syndrome (IBS) with Chinese herbal medicine showing better improvement in patients treated with individualized Chinese herbal formulae than standard TCM treatment and placebo groups [21].

The Medical Research Council in the UK [41], the NIH in the US [42] and WHO [43] have established guidelines on the research methodology for evaluating the effectiveness of CAM. All these recognize that conventional research methodology may not be applicable and recommended syndrome differenitaion in clinical trials. The pragmatic design of applying TCM syndrome differentiation to guide the formulation of the treatment before randomization is recommended to be a clinical trial model for attainining evidence-based TCM [44, 45].

4. Health outcome measures in the context of Traditional Chinese Medicine

Clinical outcomes can be categorized into four types (1) clinician-reported outcomes; (2) physiological outcomes; (3) caregiver-reported outcomes and (4) patient-reported outcomes (PROs) [46]. Clinician-reported outcomes are the observation, global impression or functional assessment made by professionals including doctors and nurses. Physiological outcomes include results from different laboratory tests (e.g. blood test, ultrasonic examination, X-ray etc). Caregiver-reported outcomes include the patient's behavior dependency and functional status observed by the caregiver. Patient reported outcomes (PROs) represent the patients' own perception of the changes in their own health condition, response to treatment and feelings, which include but not limited to general health status, symptoms, functional status and health-related quality of life (HRQOL). The first two types of outcomes used to be the main measures of efficacy or effectiveness of treatments but they are no longer adequate or sensitive enough for modern health care that aims at improving quality of life [47]. PROs started to gain popularity especially in the field of oncology. WHO defined the concept of 'health' as 'a state of complete physical, mental and social well-being and not merely the absence of disease or infirmity.'[48]. This definition has changed the conventional use of morbidity and mortality to measure health outcomes. Health care has become more concerned with the impact of health on social behavior and psychological well-being. In 1970s, quality of life began to be applied as an outcome to the medical field [49-53]. In 1975, the word 'quality of life' started to be used as a keyword in medical journals such as Annals of Surgery or Health Educaiton [54]. In 1977, 'quality of life' became indexed in the Index Medicus (Medline) database. In 1966, only four quality of life related articles published in Medline, 511 articles were published in 1998 and 4872 were published in 2008. The number of articles increased to a total of 72989 from 1966 to 2008 reflecting the increasing applications of QOL in medicine.   The Oncologic Drugs Advisory Committee of the Food and Drug Administration (FDA) announced the beneficial effects on quality of life (QOL) as an endpoint and it could serve as the basis for approval of new oncology drugs [55]. Health-related quality of life (HRQOL) has become a standard outcome indicator in many clinical trials, population studies and health services in Western Medicine. There is potential for it to be used as a primary outcome measure for TCM.

5. The philosophy and conceptual base of Traditional Chinese Medicine

To evaluate the effectiveness of Traditional Chinese Medicine (TCM) its underlying philosophy and concepts of health must be defined. Dating back to the 8th century BC, Chinese defined the health by the concepts of the Yin and Yang which formed the theoretical base of TCM. Chinese Medicine practitioners (CMP) consider patients' symptoms in the context of an imbalance between Yin and Yang, In TCM, the equilibrium of Yin and Yang is best described in the earliest book on TCM, Internal Classic of Medicine [56].

"If the Yin and Yang energies of a man are kept in a state of equilibrium, his body will be strong and his spirit sound, if his Yin and Yang energies are dissociated, his vital energy will be declined and finally exhausted." and *"A healthy man is one whose physique, muscle, blood and Qi are harmonious and appropriate with each other."*

A perfect equilibrium between Yin and Yang indicates a perfect health state and implies good life quality. Disease is the result of a break down of the equilibrium between Yin and Yang with an excess or deficiency of either Yin or Yang. Symptoms develop as a result of the imbalance between Yin and Yang, which can be assessed by Chinese Medicine Practitioners (CMP) with the four diagnostic methods which are "Inspection", "auscultation-olfaction", "inquiry" and "palpation". A TCM treatment regimen aims at regulating and re-establishing the balance between Yin and Yang within the individual. This may involve reducing the redundancy of Yin or Yang or reinforcing the deficiency of Yin or Yang through the process of "planning treatment according to the individualized diagnosis called Bianzheng and lunzhi". By this principle, even though two patients presenting different symptoms/

illnesses, if the underlying TCM syndrome differentiation is the same, the treatments are still the same. This is known as different illnesses same treatment. On the other hand, two patients with the same presentation of symptoms/illness, if the underlying TCM syndrome differentiations are different, the treatments should be different. The main TCM treatments modalities include herbal medicines, acupuncture, moxibustion, exercises, breathing techniques and diets.

The health concept in TCM also emphasizes the importance of diet, daily activities, physical functioning and emotion, which conincides with that defined by the World Health Organization. In promoting health, Internal Classic of Medicine [56] described that:

"Those who knew the way of keeping good health in ancient times lived in accordance with nature, followed the principle of Yin and Yang, conformed with the art of prophecy, modulated their food and drinks, worked and rested in regular times and avoided overwork; therefore, they could maintain both the body and spirit to live to the natural old age of more than one hundred years."

6. Outcome indicators of TCM

As mentioned above, Traditional Chinese Medicine (TCM) has long been criticized for the lack of standardized outcome measures. The individualized prescription made by the Chinese Medicine Practitioner (CMP) is usually based on the CMP's subjective assessment. Particularly, the assessments between different CMP for the same patient can be greatly different, a lack of consistency in the assessment methods and outcome limits the generalizability of TCM and makes its evaluation difficult. Some researchers have tried to develop measures to standardize TCM syndrome differentiation diagnosis but it has been criticized that this method is limiting the strength of TCM in individualized treatment [57] and forcing TCM to adopt the classification of Western Medicine. In fact, the evaluation of TCM has little about measuring outcomes [58]. To evaluate the effectiveness of TCM, conventional outcome indicators such as laboratory or physical examination developed from Western Medicine have been applied in TCM research but there are great doubts on their appropriateness in the context of TCM. Some aspects such as complexion, spirit and vitality improvement cannot be captured by these indicators but they are very important indicators of health in TCM.

7. Traditional Chinese Medicine (TCM) and Health-related Quality of Life (HRQOL)

Health-related quality of life shares the same concepts and objectives as TCM. It should theoretically be the most appropriate outcome measure of the effectiveness of TCM. A paper by Lai et al [59] published in 2000 discussed and established the relationship between TCM and HRQOL. They pointed out that Chinese Medicine Practitioners (CMP) mainly rely on patients' reported symptoms and daily activities in their diagnostic process. The assessment of disease progression greatly depends on patients' feedback. Patients' subjective perception of the effect of their illness and treatment could be captured more scientifically by standardized HRQOL measures. To evaluate the effectiveness of TCM more scientifically, they suggested three directions: (1) Applying international generic HRQOL measures to evaluate the clinical effect of TCM; (2) Using standard methods to develop generic HRQOL measures for TCM, and (3) Developing TCM-condition specific HRQOL measures. Many other practitioners and researchers also agreed that HRQOL should be used as an important outcome of TCM because it can capture the latter's emphasis on the balance in physical, social and psychological well being [60, 61]. This outcome measure should complement conventional methods such as CMP assessment or laboratory results in the evaluation of TCM.

7.1 The concepts of health-related quality of life

The term Quality of life (QOL) is difficult to be defined. It summarizes a wide range of life events [62] and is a subjective appraisal of an individual of his/her life as a whole in various aspects. These aspects may range from the perception of well-being, satisfaction with one's life, achievement of personal goal, social usefulness, normalcy to duration of life, impairment, functional status (social, psychological, and physical), health perceptions, and opportunity. The definition of quality of life in fact depends on subjective perception which is greatly influenced by the environment, social, political and economic situations and cultures. Cummins had identified more than 100 definitions of QOL in the literature [63]. In general, QOL refers to a global state of satisfaction with life as a whole and the presence of positive feelings and the absence of negative ones. The broad and inclusive definitions of QOL go far beyond the medical model and only those aspects related to health are relevant to Medicine.

The term Health-related quality of life (HRQOL) is an attempt to quantify the net consequence of a disease and its treatment on the patients' perception of his ability to live a useful and fulfilling life [64]. It aims at measuring the effect of health by using a defined number of dimensions that are relevant to the person. These dimensions are structured firstly according to the WHO definitions of health to include the physical, psychological and social well-being [48]. Some authors extended the dimensions by adding spirituality. The purpose of HRQOL assessment is not only on measuring the presence and severity of illnesses but also on showing how an illness or treatment is experienced by an individual [65]. It has been used extensively in clinical trials [66-68], health economic research [69-72] and quality of care evaluations [73-76].

Although HRQOL has been criticized as too 'soft' or less reliable than conventional physiologic indicators, HRQOL can detect important clinical changes in many chronic conditions that other clinical outcome measures cannot. HRQOL differentiated patient adherence between three anti-hypertensive agents (captopril, methyldopa, and propranolol) that had similar efficacy in lowering blood pressure but different effects on quality of life [77]. Brown et al. found that a SF-36 physical functioning socre and role limitation score lower than the UK norm by 20 and 23, respectively, predicted a need for coronary revascularisation, the use of anxiolytics and the need for two or more angina drugs in patients who had acute myocardial infarctions [78]. Spertus et al. was able to show the benefit of a special angina clinic in that patients had greater improvements in quality of life measured by the Seattle Angina Questionnaire (SAQ) than those receiving usual care from a general medicine clinic [79]. Goodwin et al's systematic review concluded that HRQOL targeting specific symptoms could guide treatment decisions and was often the only significant outcome measure in breast cancer drug trials [80]. HRQOL is now regarded as the most important outcome indicator to guide medical decisions on the optimal treatment for breast cancer in the US [80].

7.2 HRQOL in measuring effectiveness of primary care

If HRQOL is to be used as an outcome measure of the effectiveness of TCM in primary care, it has to be valid and applicable to this setting. Primary care practitioners have always relied very much on patients' subjective symptoms in making diagnoses and evaluating treatment outcomes. A recent review on outcome measures for primary care showed the evolution and recognition of the importance of function and health-related quality of life as indicators of subjective health [81]. The accumulating evidence that HRQOL measures are valid and reliable has facilitated its increasing use in clinical service and research in primary care [82-84]. Before a HRQOL measure can be considered as applicable to primary care, it should [85],

- *Measure the aspects and effects of the illness that the patient decides are most important (relevant)*
- *Enable the patient to score the chosen variables (subjective)*
- *Be a sensitive measure of within person change over time (responsive)*
- *Be applicable to the whole spectrum of illness seen in primary care (generic)*
- *Be capable of measuring the effects of a wide variety of care (generic)*
- *Be brief and simple enough to complete in a 7-10 minute consultation.*

The first HRQOL that was applied to primary care was the COOP Charts, which was later adopted by the World Organization of Family Doctors (WONCA) and modified into the COOP/WONCA Charts for internatinal application in primary care [86]. It was translated and validated for the Chinese population in Hong Kong in 1994 [87, 88]. It demonstrated the negative impacts on the life of patients from common chronic diseases such as depression, diabetes mellitus, osteoarthritis and asthma in primary care (Lam and Lauder 2000). The MOS Short-form 36-item (SF-36) Health Survey has become a popular HRQOL measure worldwide since its first publication in 1992. Studies have shown that SF-36 can predict the utilization of primary care services [89], and low HRQOL in community-dwelling elderly had higher mortality rates [90]. Patients with gouts were found to have poorer HRQOL (lower functional limitation scores of the SF-36 Health Survey) and higher rates of inpatient utilization and mortality among all US veterans [91]. The Chinese (HK) version of the SF-36 Health Survey was validated and normed on the Hong Kong population in 1998. It was found to be a sensitive measure of the impact of chronic disease and determinant of primary care service utilization in the Chinese adult population in Hong Kong [88, 89, 92].

7.3 Application of health-related quality of life measures in Traditional Chinese Medicine

Since health-related quality of life (HRQOL) measures were recommended as an important outcome measures in clinical research by the World Health Organization and China Department of Health [93, 94], there has been a surge of HRQOL studies in TCM in the last two decades. Most of the applications were in the fields of cancer, cardiovascular diseases, pain management, geriatrics and respiratory diseases, but very few in primary care.

7.4 Application of HRQOL measures in TCM for the treatment of cancer

The first paper applying HRQOL measurement to TCM was published in 1986 on liver cancer patients [95]. The Karnofsky Performance Scale Index (KPSI) [96] was used as a pre-treatment assessment tool to predict the prognosis of liver cancer patients treated by Chinese herbs and radio-therapy. After this publication, HRQOL measures were used more often to assess the effectiveness of TCM after chemo- or radio therapy in liver and lung cancer patients [97-100]. The KPSI was the most commonly used in these early studies. The KPSI was found to be responsive to improvement after TCM interventions. It was reported that 67.7% of stage II or III liver cancer patients [98] and 32 liver cancer patients who did not respond to chemo-therapy [99] had improved KPSI scores after TCM treatment. The KPSI scores was able to show in a cohort study on gastric, liver and esophagus cancer patients that the combination of Chinese herbs with chemotherapy was better than chemo-therapy alone [101]. Ma et al's meta-analysis further confirmed the sensitivity of KPSI in 7 randomized controlled clinical trials in showing TCM integrated with chemo-therapy was better than chemotherapy alone (OR = 3.4; 95% CI = 2.5 - 4.6, p<0.05) in the treatment of non-small cell lung cancer [102].

In recent years, more HRQOL measures have become available and being used in clinical trials on TCM. The European Organization for Research and Treatment of Cancer (EORTC QLQ-C30) questionnaire [103] was applied to evaluate the effect of medical qigong in cancer patients with or without chemotherapy [104]. It was found that EORTC QLQ-C 30 scores were significantly improved in both groups and medical qigong could also reduce the side effects of patients who underwent chemotherapy. Other HRQOL measures specific for cancer like Functional Assessment of Cancer Therapy-Prostate (FACT) have also been used. FACT-Prostate (FACT-P) [105] was used in assessing the effect of a dietary supplement containing eight herbal extracts (PC-SPES) on prostate cancer patients and reported a significant improvement in functional, emotional and physical well-being in the treatment group [106]. The FACT-Lung (FACT-L) [107] was used to asses the benefit of Chinese herbal medicine treatment on non-small cell lung cancer patient showing that integration of TCM with Western Medicine (WM) or TCM treatment alone were associated with better improvement in terms of total, physical and emotional status than WM alone [108].

7.5 Applications of HRQOL measures in TCM treatments of other conditions

Other than oncology, HRQOL measures have been applied to many studies on cardiovascular disease, pain management, geriatrics and respiratory diseases. A number of widely used international generic and disease-specific HRQOL measures have been used to assess the effectiveness of TCM treatment of cardiovascular diseases. The quality of life index (QLI) [109] and the Activities Daily Living Scale (ADL) [110] had been applied to cerebral hemorrhage patients to show that TCM was more beneficial than Western medicine in improving the cognitive function and the activities of daily living [111]. Wang et al. and Siu et al. found that TCM was equally effective as an antihypertensive drug, Norvasc, in improving all domains of SF-36 Health Survey in patients with hypertension [61, 112]. The Seattle Angina Questionnaire (SAQ) [113] was used in coronary artery bypass grafting patients and found that combining TCM with conventional Western care can significantly improve the domains of angina stability, angina frequency, treatment satisfaction and disease perception measured by the SAQ when compared with conventional Western care [114].

In evaluating the effectiveness of TCM treatment on patients with osteoarthritis, the SF-36 Health Survey, SF-12 Health Survey, Visual Analog Scale (VAS), Western Ontario and McMaster University osteoarthritis index (WOMAC), Lequesne Index and Global Satisfaction Scale have all been used [115-117]. The effectiveness of Complementary and Alternative Medicine (CAM) clinic in relieving pain of OA patients by the combination usage of herbs, chiropractice and acupuncture was detected by the SF-12v2 Health Survey [117]. Another study using the SF-36 v2 Health Survey showed that TCM could enhance social functioning and mental health in the elderly population [118]. The efficacy of willow bark extract was confirmed by a statistically significant difference of 14% in the WOMAC pain dimension between the treatment and placebo groups [116]. Ginger extracts were associated with a reduction of pain on a VAS and the Lequesne Index in a randomized placebo-controlled clinical trial [115, 119].

In evaluating the effectiveness of TCM in respiratory diseases [120], Xue et al. used a combination of symptoms scores diaries, the Rhinoconjunctvitis and Rhinitis Quality of Life Questionnaire (RQLQ), patient's global evaluations of improvement and physician's objective evaluation in a multi-center randomized double-blind, placebo-controlled clinical trials on allergic rhinitis. The RQLQ indicated significant beneficial effects of TCM treatment with an improvement in categorical items by 60.7% against an improvement by 29.6% from placebo. Their study also cross-validated improvement in quality of life by patients' global evaluation and practitioners' objective assessments.

HRQOL assessment of the effectiveness and efficacy of TCM have also been applied to studies on HIV[121] , hepatitis C virus [122, 123], vomiting and nausea in pregnant women [124], chronic alcoholism [125] and somatoform disorders [126].

7.6 Limitation of existing health-related quality of life measures in evaluation of Traditional Chinese Medicine

Despite the increasing applications of HRQOL measures developed from Western culture to the evaluation of TCM, their validity has been questioned. Song et al. stressed out that such applications should be only a transitional state [127] since the cultural context of Western HRQOL measures may not fully match the health concepts in the Chinese culture. Wu et al. pointed out that health concept from the Western culture may neglect the important Chinese concepts of the relationship between health and the seasonal changes or the importance of syndrome differentiation in TCM, which may hinder the development of TCM [128, 129].

Outcome measures of TCM should be coherent with its underlying philosophy and theory so that they could be sensitive and responsive to the changes brought about by TCM treatments [45, 130, 131]. For example, the commonly used Karnofsky Performance Scale Index (KPSI) [96] only focuses on objective assessment of the patient's ability to perform daily activities, work or self-care, it is not sufficient in describing other changes brought by TCM intervention such as the abilities to adapat to climatic changes or dinunal changes [132]. The domains measured by Western HRQOL measures may not be valid to TCM. Therefore it is uncertain whether the results truly reflect those related to TCM. This had called for the development of HRQOL measures specific for TCM.

7.7 Development of Chinese culture specific HRQOL measure for TCM

To develop HRQOL measures applicable to TCM, the Chinese health concepts must be first explored [133]. Cheung et al conducted a qualitative survey on TCM experts in their study on the content validity of a liver syndrome measure commented that the importance of meaning of health from the Chinese culture is unique and need further investigation [134].

Several TCM condition-specific HRQOL measures have been developed. The Emotion scale for Ganzangxiang of TCM was developed to measure HRQOL specific to the anxiety and depression syndrome that are classified under the liver-syndrome by the TCM theory [135,

136]. PiWei-syndrome differentiation measure [137] and the Liver-Fire Ascending Syndrome Scale [138, 139] were developed with similar principles to capture specific physical symptoms, psychological states changes related to specific TCM diagnosis. TCM syndrome differentiation indicators were included in the IBS-TCM differentiation measure for patients with irritable bowel syndrome [140].

While TCM-syndrome specific measures may be relevant and sensitive for a particular condition, there is doubt on the rationale and feasibility of developing a measure for each of the thousands TCM syndromes [141]. Others have urged the need for a generic TCM measure that should include the basic principles of TCM such as the balance of Yin and Yang or cold and heat, deficiency and excess. A generic HRQOL measure not only can evaluate the clinical effectiveness of different TCM treatments, it can also allow evaluation of health of the general population and comparison of patients with different illnesses [142]. A generic HRQOL measure applicable to TCM could also provide a common standard tool for the validation of the TCM syndromes specific measures to enhance research of TCM in clinical practice [143].

The Yin and Yang Scale was the first generic TCM measure developed based on the Yin and Yang principles. Although it was originally intended only for research purpose and not for clinical assessment, it was found that yin and yang scores could be used to differentiate groups of patients effectively in clinical practice. The Yin and Yang scale was also found to be easier to endorse than the detailed syndrome evaluation making it more useful in the research setting [144]. The Yin and Yang Scales served as a preliminary model of generic TCM measures, but it does not really measure HRQOL.

8. The Chinese Quality of Life instrument (ChQOL)

Leung et al. developed the first and probably the only generic TCM HRQOL measure, the Chinese Quality of Life (ChQOL) instrument in Mainland China in 2005 [145]. The initial model was developed from a review of the literature on TCM, which included the equilibrium of Yin Yang in four dimensions: (1) Physical form and Vitality & Spirit, (2) harmonization of man and society and (3) harmonization of man and nature and (4) Seven emotions. Based on these 4 dimensions, four TCM scholars generated 13 facets that were grouped into two domains: 1. Physical form and Vitatlity & Spirit, and 2. emotion. No facet could be identified for the dimensions on harmonization of man and society or the harmonization of man and nature because CMP rarely ask patients about these two dimensions, which were then excluded from the final Chinese Quality of Life instrument.

Items were then generated for the 13 identified facets and drafted in wordings that were used in the communication between Chinese Medicine Practitioners (CMP) and patients. Response options on intensity, frequency or capacity appropriate to the items were adopted from previously validated response options of the WHOQOL-100, The initial draft Chinese Quality of Life Instrument (ChQOL) had a 3-domain structure with 69 items. Each item was rated on a 5-point Likert scale and the scale scores were transformed to a range of 100, with higher scores indicating better HRQOL. The draft was reviewed by 100 CMP who added more items resulting in an 80-item instrument. The second draft was evaluated by a convenient sample of 15 subjects including both healthy and patients consulting a TCM clinic by cognitive debriefing interviews to confirm the linguistic and semantic clarity of the items. Two items were dropped and revisions were made to 78 items. These 78 items were then field tested on 273 subjects including in-patients and out-patients of a TCM hospital and healthy subjects conveniently recruited from the community of Southern Mainland China. Psychometric testing and factor analyses eliminated items that were below the standards of the respective psychometric properties resulting in the final ChQOL with a 3-domain structure and 50 items. The domains are namely physical form (20 items), vitality and spirit (12 items) and emotion (18 items). The three domain scores can be summarized into an overall score. The conceptual structure and the ChQOL are described in other published journal [146].

8.1 Validity and psychometric properties of the ChQOL

Construct validity of the 50-item ChQOL was confirmed by factor analysis and item-scale correlations. The facet-domain correlations ranged from 0.71-0.89 and domain-overall score correlations ranged from 0.56-0.78, supporting the scaling structure. Factor analysis also confirmed the 3-domain structure. The reliability of the ChQOL was supported by internal consistency with Cronbach's alpha ranging from 0.71-0.90 at the facet level and 0.80-0.89 at the domain level. Test-retest reliability was tested on 56 healthy subjects at 2-day interval, giving an intra-class correlations (ICC) ranging from 0.68-0.84 at the facet level and 0.83-0.87 at the domain level. Convergent construct validity was confirmed by moderate correlations between ChQOL scores and SF-36 or WHOQOL-100 scores. Responsiveness of the ChQOL had been examined on 32 subjects with congenital heart diseases showing effect size changes in the three ChQOL domain scores ranging from 0.25 to 0.93.

The ChQOL was adapted into a HK version and pilot tested on 122 Cantonese speaking people (69 patients with chronic diseases who consulted TCM clinic and 53 healthy subjects conveniently recruited in the community) in Hong Kong [132]. The ChQOL (HK version) scales showed good construct validity with the facet-domain correlations ranging from 0.64-0.89 and domain-overall score correlations ranging from 0.79-0.81. Internal consistency was supported by Cronbach's alpha ranged from 0.73-0.90 at the facet level and 0.73-0.83 at the domain level. Test-retest reliability tested in a 2-day interval was good with intra-class correlations (ICC) ranging from 0.77-0.88 at the facet level and 0.89-0.90 at the domain level. Convergent construct validity was confirmed by moderate correlations between the ChQOL (HK version) and the Hong Kong WHOQOL-100. In addition, the ChQOL (HK version) scores were able to discriminate between patients and healthy subjects.

Results from these pilot studies of the ChQOL and its HK version are encouraging. It can become a standard HRQOL measure for the evaluation of the effectiveness of TCM if further studies can confirm its acceptability, feasibility, validity, reliability, sensitivity and responsiveness in different Chinese populations and clinical settings.

8.2 Potential applications of the ChQOL

Over the past 50 years, molecular, cellular and pharmacological research have dominated the research in TCM, but clinical trials on effectiveness have been largely neglected [147]. The few TCM clinical studies evaluated effectiveness of TCM by conventional physical examination or laboratory tests [148] often showed only modest benefits. The use of a validated HRQOL measure can expand the scientific evidence on the effectiveness of TCM by capturing the improvement in HRQOL of patients. The Chinese Quality of Life instrument (ChQOL), if further proven to be responsive to changes related to TCM, can help to solve a major deficiency in evidence-based TCM practice. The ChQOL is generic so that it can be applied to people with different health status or illnesses. This is most suitable for evaluating the effectiveness of primary care that manages a wide spectrum of patients and conditions. Evidence on the effectiveness of TCM in primary care is important to establish its role in our health care system and to inform the public in their choice of service.

9. Summary

There is evidence supporting the role of Traditional Chinese Medicine (TCM) in primary care with increasing use, resources allocation, regulations, research and education. This trend is not only limited to China but also occurring in Western countries. Health-related quality of life (HRQOL) shares the same concepts and objectives as TCM, which should be a most appropriate outcome measure for assessing the effectiveness of TCM. As HRQOL has already been established as a standard outcome measure in Western medical care, it could be used for scientific evaluation of the effectiveness of TCM in primary care. HRQOL measures developed in the Western culture have been applied to oncology and other areas such as cardiovascular disease, pain management, and geriatrics with variable success. However, these Western measures cannot capture all the health benefits of TCM, which hinders further development and clinical research of TCM. The Chinese quality of life instrument (ChQOL), based on the Chinese cultural concepts of health, is a promising HRQOL measure that can become a scientific outcome measurement tool for TCM. The ChQOL is generic making it applicable to all types of patients and particularly suitable for primary care that manages a wide spectrum of illnesses.

10. References

[1] Dong, H. and X. Zhang, *An overview of traditional Chinese medicine. In: Traditional Medicine in Asia.*, World Health Organization Regional Office for South-East Asia, Editor. 2002, SEARO Regional Publication No. 39: New Delhi. p. 17-29.

[2] Xu, J. and Y. Yang, *Traditional Chinese medicine in the Chinese health care system.* Health Policy, 2008.

[3] CMCHK. *Chinese Medicine Council of Hong Kong.* 2008; Available from: http://www.cmchk.org.hk.

[4] Tung Wah Group of Hospitals. *Chinese Medicine Services.* 2008.

[5] Lau, J.T.F., E.M.F. Leung, and H.Y. Tsui, *Predicting traditional Chinese medicine's use and the marginalization of medical care in Hong Kong.* American Journal of Chinese Medicine, 2001. 29: p. 547-558.

[6] Lau, J.T.F. and A. Yu, *The choice between Chinese Medicine and Western Medicine practitioners by Hong Kong adolescents.* American Journal of Chinese Medicine, 2000. 28: p. 131-139.

[7] Leung, G.M., I.O.L. Wong, W.S. Chan, S. Choi, and S.V. Lo, *The ecology of health care in Hong Kong.* Social Science & Medicine, 2005. 61: p. 577-590.

[8] Chung, V., E. Wong, J. Woo, S.V. Lo, and S. Griffiths, *Use of Traditional Chinese medicine in the Hong Kong Special Administrative Region of China.* The Journal of Alternative and Complementary Medicine, 2007. 3: p. 361-367.

[9] WHO. *Traditional Medicine - Growing needs and potential.* in *WHO Policy Perspectives on Medicine.* 2002. Geneva.

[10] WHO, *WHO global atlas of traditional, complementary and alternative medicine,* WHO Centre for Health Development, Editor. 2005: Kobe, Japan.

[11] Eisenberg, D.M., *Trends in alternative medicine use in the United States, 1990 -1997: results of a follow-up national survey.* Journal of the American Medical Association, 1998. 280: p. 1569-1575.

[12] Fisher, P. and R. van Haselen, *Effectiveness gaps: a new concept for evaluating health service and research needs applied to complementary and alternative medicine.* Journal of Alternative and Complementary Medicine, 2004. 10(4): p. 627-632.

[13] Dateshidze, L. and N.K. Rasmussen, *Health and morbidity in Denmark 2000 - and the development since 1987,* National Institute of Public Health, Editor. 1987: Cophenhagen.

[14] Thomas, K.J., J.P. Nicholl, and P. Coleman, *Use and expenditure on complementary medicine in England: a population based survey.* Complementary Therapies in Medicine, 2001. 9: p. 2-11.

[15] National Institute of Health, *Acupuncture,* in *National Institute of Health Consensus Development Conference Statement.* 1997.

[16] Mueller, M.S., N. Runyambo, I. Wagner, S. Borrmann, K. Dietz, and L. Heide, *Randomized controlled trial of a traditional preparation of Artemisia annua L. (Annual Wormwood) in the treatment of malaria.* Transactions of the Royal Society of Tropical Medicine and Hygiene, 2004. 98: p. 318-321.

[17] WHO, *Assessment of therapeutic effect of antimalarial drugs for uncomplicated falciparum malaria in areas with intense trasmission,* in *World Health Orgaization.* 1996: Geneva.

[18] Bent, S., L. Xu, L.-Y. Lui, M. Nevitt, E. Schneider, G. Tian, s. Guo, and S. Cummings, *A randomized controlled trial of a Chinese herbal remedy to increase energy, memory, sexual function, and quality of life in elderly adults in Beijing, China.* The American Journal of Medicine, 2003. 115: p. 441-446.

[19] Wesnes, K.A., T. Ward, A. McGinty, and O. Petrini, *The memory enhancing effects of a Ginkgo biloba/Panax ginseng combination in healthy middle-aged volunteers.* Psychopharmacology, 2000. 152: p. 353-361.

[20] Lau, J.T.F., P.C. Leung, E.L.Y. Wong, C. Fong, K.F. Cheng, S.C. Zhang, C.W.K. Lam, V. Wong, K.M. Choy, and W.M. Ko, *The use of herbal formula by hospital care workers during the Severe Acute Respiratory Syndrome Epidemic in Hong Kong to prevent Severe Acute Respiratory Syndrome transmission, relieve Influenza-related symptoms, and improve quality of life: a prospective cohort study.* The Journal of Alternative and Complementary Medicine, 2005. 11: p. 49-55.

[21] Bensoussan, A., N.J. Talley, M. Hing, R. Menzies, A. Guo, and M. Ngu, *Treatment of irritable bowel syndrome with Chinese herbal medicine.* JAMA, 1998. 280: p. 1585-1589.

[22] Sheehan, M.P., M.H. Rustin, D.J. Atherton, C. Buckley, D.W. Harris, J. Brostoff, L. Ostlere, and A. Dawson, *Efficacy of traditional Chinese herbal therapy in Adult Atopic Dermatitis.* Lancet, 1992. 340: p. 13-17.

[23] Latchman, Y., B. Whittle, M. Rustin, D.J. Atherton, and J. Brostoff, *The efficacy of traditional Chinese herbal therapy in atopic eczema.* International Archives of Allergy and Immunology, 1994. 104(3): p. 222-226.

[24] Kwee, S.H., H.H. Tan, A. Marsman, and C. Wauters, *The effect of Chinese herbal medicines (CHM) on menopausal symptoms compared to horomone replacement therapy (HRT) and placebo.* Maturitas - The European Menopause Journal, 2007. 58: p. 83-90.

[25] Melchart, D., W. Weidenhammer, K. Linde, and R. Saller, *"Quality profiling" for complementary medicine: the example of a hospital for Traditional Chinese Medicine* The Journal of Alternative and Complementary Medicine, 2003. 9: p. 193-206.

[26] Ong, C.K., *Health status of people using complementary and alternative medical practitioner services in four English counties.* American Journal of Public Health, 2002. 92: p. 1653-1656.

[27] Ernst, E. and A. White, *The BBC survey of complementary medicine use in the UK.* Complementary Therapies in Medicine, 2000. 8: p. 32-36.

[28] Busato, A., A. Donges, S. Herren, M. Widmer, and F. Marian, *Health status and health care utilisation of patients in complementary and conventional primary care in Switzerland - an observational study.* Family Practice, 2006. 23: p. 116-124.

[29] Xie, Y.G., *The research on the needs and utilization of Chinese Medicine Service in Beijing.* Beijing Journal of Traditional Chinese Medicine, 2004. 3: p. 135-138.

[30] Frenkel, M.A. and J.M. Borkan, *An approach for integrating complemnetary alternative medicine into primary care.* Family Practice, 2003. 20(3): p. 324-332.

[31] Tang, J.L. and T.W. Wong, *The need to evaluate the clinical effectiveness of traditional Chinese medicine.* HKMJ, 1998. 4: p. 208-210.

[32] Kelner, M.J., H. Boon, B. Wellman, and S. Welsh, *Complementary and alternative groups contemplate the need for effectiveness, safety and cost-effectiveness research.* Complementary Therapies in Medicine, 2002. 10: p. 235-239.

[33] Ernst, E., *Complementary medicine - doing more good than harm?* British Journal of General Prcatice, 1996. 46: p. 60-61.

[34] Tang, J.L., S.-Y. Zhan, and E. Ernst, *Review of randomized controlled trials of traditional Chinese medicine.* British Medical Journal, 1999. 319: p. 160-161.

[35] Leung, P.C. and M.W.N. Wong, *A critical analysis of professional and academic publications on traditional Chinese medicine in China.* The American Journal of Chinese Medicine, 2001. 30: p. 177-181.

[36] Kaptchuk, T.J., *The double-blind, randomized, placebo-controlled trial: gold standard or golden calf?* Journal of Clinical Epidemiology, 2001. 54: p. 541-549.

[37] Black, N., *Why we need observational studies to evaluate the effectiveness of health care.* BMJ, 1996. 312: p. 1215-1218.

[38] Thomas, K.J. and M.J. Fitter, *Evaluating complementary therapies for use in the national health service: 'horses for courses'. part 2: alternative research strategies.* Complementary Therapies in Medicine, 1997. 5: p. 94-98.

[39] Fitter, M.J. and K.J. Thomas, *Evaluating complementary therapies for use in the national health service: 'horses for courses'. part 1: the design challenge.* Complementary Therapies in Medicine, 1997. 5: p. 90-93.

[40] Zaslawski, C., *Clinical reasoning in traditional Chinese medicine: implications for clinical research.* Clinical Acupuncture and Oriental Medicine, 2003. 4: p. 94-101.

[41] Medical Research Council. *A framework for development and evaluation of RCTs for complex interventions to improve health.* 2000 [cited 2005 8-8-2005]; Available from: http://www.mrc.ac.uk/pdf-mrc_cpr.pdf.

[42] Levin, J.S., T.A. Glass, L.H. Kushi, J.R. Schuck, L. Steele, and W.B. Jonas, *Quantitative methods in research on complementary and alternative medicine: a methodological manifesto.* Medical Care, 1997. 35: p. 1079-1094.

[43] WHO, *General guidelines for methodologies on research and evaluation of traditional medicine.* 2000. p. 1-74.

[44] Critchley, J.A.J.H., Y. Zhang, C.C. Suthisisang, T.Y.K. Chan, and B. Tomlinson, *Alternative therapies and medical science: designing clinical trials of alternative/complementary*

medicines - is evidence-based traditional Chinese medicine attainable? Journal of Clinical Pharmacology, 2000. 40: p. 462-467.

[45] Tonelli, M.R. and T.C. Callahan, *Why alternative medicine cannot be evidence-based.* Academic Medicine, 2001. 76: p. 1213-1220.

[46] Acquadro, C., R. Berzon, D. Dubois, N. Leidy, P. Marquis, D. Revicki, M. Rothman, and PRO Harmonization Group, *Incoporating the patient's perspective into drug development and communication: an ad hoc task force report of the Patient-Reported Outcomes (PRO) Harmonization Group meeting at the Food and Drug Administration, February 16, 2001.* Value in Health, 2003. 6(5): p. 503-504.

[47] Donald, L.P., *Patients-Reported Outcomes (PROs): An Organizing Tool for Concepts, Measures, and Applications.* Quality of Life Newsletter, 2003. 31: p. 1-5.

[48] WHO, *The first ten years of the World Health Organization, WHO.* 1985: Genevq.

[49] Crowne, D.P., *A new scale of social desirability independent of psychopathology.* J Consult Psychol, 1960. 24: p. 349-354.

[50] Seiler, L.H., *The 22-item scale used in field studies of mental illness: a question of method, a question of substance and a question of theory.* J Health Soc Behav, 1973. 14: p. 252-264.

[51] Chapman, C.R., *Measurement of pain: problems and issues.* , in *Advanced in pain research and therapy*, Bonica JJ and A. DG, Editors. 1976, Raven Press. p. 345-353.

[52] Clark, W.C., *Pain sensitivity and the report of pain: an introduction to sensory decision theory*, in *Pain new perspectives in therapy and research*, Weisenberg M and Tursky B, Editors. 1976, Plenum Press: New York. p. 195-222.

[53] Rosser, R.M., *Recent studies using a global approach to measuring illness.* Med Care, 1976. 14 (suppl): p. 138-147.

[54] Hu, X.J., B.L. Zhang, and G.X. Cai, *The application and research of health-related quality of life instruments in Chinese Medicine.* Gianjin Journal of Traditional Chinese Medicine, 2002. 19: p. 72-74.

[55] Johnson, J. and R. Temple, *Food and drug administration requirements for approval of new anticancer drugs.* Cancer Treatment Reports, 1985. 69(10): p. 1155-1159.

[56] Wu, L.N. and Q.A. Wu, *Yellow Empeor's canon of internal medicine.* 1997, Beijing: Zhongguo ke xue ji shu chu ban she.

[57] Yang, W.Y., *Chinese Medicine: Macroscopical coordination of functional Medicine.* 2001. 416.

[58] Lai, S.L., *The clinical efficacy of Traditional Chinese Medicine.* Chinese Journal of Information on TCM, 2000. 7: p. 88-89.

[59] Lai, S.L., J.Q. Hu, and X.F. Guo, *Evidence-based Medicine and clinical studies of Traditional Chinese Medicine.* Journal of Guangzhou University of Traditional Chinese Medicine, 2000. 17: p. 1-8.

[60] Liu, F.B., J.H. Wang, and W.W. Chen, *Investigation of application of health-related quality of life instruments in Traditional Chinese Medicine.* Traditional Chinese Drug Research and Clinical Pharmacology, 1997. 8: p. 179-181.

[61] Xiao, J.F. and J.Z. Cai, *Impact of the health-related quality of life of type-II hypertension elderly by treatment of integration of Chinese and Western Medicine* Fujian Journal of Traditional Chinese Medicine, 2002. 33(1): p. 10-11.

[62] Fayers, P.M. and D. Machin, *Quality of life: assessment, analysis, and interpretation.* 2000.

[63] Cummins, R.A. *Quality of life definition and terminology: a discussion document from the International Society for Quality of Life studies.* 1998. Virginia: Blackburg.

[64] Schipper, H., J.J. Clinch, and C.L.M. Olweny, *Quality of life studies. Definition and conceptual issues*, in *Quality of life and Pharmaeconomics in Clinical Trials*, B. Spiker, Editor. 1996, Lippincott-Raven: Philadelphia. p. 11-24.

[65] Bullinger, M., *Assessing health related quality of life in medicine. An overview over concepts, methods and applications in international research*. Restorative Neurology and Neuroscience, 2003. 20: p. 93-101.

[66] Lourander, L., I. Ruikka, and J. Rautakorpi, *Psychological methods applied to evaluate symptomatic geratric treatment*. Geriatrics, 1970. 25(8): p. 124.

[67] Morgan, W.P. and D.H. Horstman, *Psychometric correlates of pain perception*. Perceptual & Motor Skills, 1978. 47(1): p. 27-39.

[68] Edelstyn, G.A., K.D. MacRae, and F.M. MacDonald, *Improvement of life quality in cancer patients undergoing chemotherapy*. Clinical Oncology, 1979. 43-49.

[69] Weinstein, M.C. and W.B. Stason, *Foundations of cost-effectiveness analysis for health and medical practices*. New England Journal of Medicine, 1977. 296(13): p. 716-21.

[70] Jean, G.L., *Day care: cost effectiveness vs. quality of life*. Aging & Leisure Living, 1978. 1(1): p. 8-10.

[71] Mathias, C.M.J., *Improving the quality of life for the elderly*. Journal of the American Geriatrics Society, 1979. 27(9): p. 385-388.

[72] Kriedel, T., *Cost-benefit analysis of epilepsy clinics*. Social Science & Medicine - Medical Economics, 1980. 14(1): p. 35-39.

[73] Cattell, R.B., *Evaluating therapy as total personality change: theory and available instruments*. American Journal of Psychotherapy, 1966. 20(1): p. 69-88.

[74] Salzberg, H.C. and D.R. Bidus, *Development of a group psychotherapy screening scale: an attempt to select suitable candidates and predict successful outcome*. Journal of Clinical Psychology, 1966. 22(4): p. 478-481.

[75] Barrett, G.V., T.R. Williamson, and C.L. Thornton, *Perception of depth as measured by magnitude estimation*. Perceptual & Motor Skills, 1967. 25(3): p. 905-908.

[76] Cattell, R.B. and L.R. Killian, *The pattern of objective test personality factor differences in schizophrenia and the character disorders*. Journal of Clinical Psychology, 1967. 23(3): p. 342-348.

[77] Croog, S.H., S. Levine, and M.A. Testa, *The effects of antihypertensive therapy on the quality of life*. New England Journal of Medicine, 1986. 314: p. 1657-1664.

[78] Brown, N., M. Melville, D. Gray, T. Young, J. Munro, A.M. Skene, and J.R. Hampton, *Quality of life four years after acute acute myocardial infarction: shor form 36 scores compared with a normal population*. Heart, 1999. 1999(81): p. 352-358.

[79] Spertus, J.A., T.A. Dewhurst, C.M. Dougherty, P. Nichol, M. McDonell, B. Bliven, and S.D. Fihn, *Benefits of an "angina clinic" for patients with coronary artery disease: A demostration of health status measures as markers of health care quality*. American Heart Journal, 2002. 143: p. 145-150.

[80] Goodwin, P.J., J.T. Black, L.J. Bordeleau, and P.A. Ganz, *Health-related quality-of-life measurement in randomized clinical trials in breast cancer--taking stock*. Journal of the National Cancer Institute, 2003. 95: p. 263-281.

[81] Wilkin, D., I. Hallan, and M. Doggett, eds. *Measures of need and outcome for primary health care*. 1992, Oxford University Press: Oxford.

[82] Mossey, J.M. and E. Shapiro, *Self-rated health: a predictor of mortality among the elderly*. American Journal of Public Health, 1982. 72: p. 800-808.

[83] McDowell, I. and C. Newell, eds. *Measuring health: a guide to rating scales and questionnaires.* 2nd ed. ed. 1996, Oxford University Press.

[84] Spertus, J.A., P. Jones, M. McDonell, V. Fan, and S.D. Fihn, *Health status predicts long-term outcome in outpatients with coronary disease.* Circulation, 2002. 106: p. 43-49.

[85] Ruta, D.A., A.M. Garratt, M. Leng, and I.T. Russell, *A new approach to quality of life: the patient-generated index.* Medical Care, 1994. 32: p. 1109-1126.

[86] Landgraf, J.M.N., E C, *Summary of the WONCA/COOP International health assessment field trial. The Dartmouth COOP primary care network.* Australian Family Physicians, 1992. 21(3): p. 255-257, 260-262, 266-269.

[87] Lam, C.L.K., C. Van Weel, and I.J. Lauder, *Can the Dartmouth COOP/WONCA charts be used to assess the functional status of Chinese patients?* Family Practice, 1994. 11: p. 85-94.

[88] Lam, C.L.K. and I.J. Lauder, *The impact of chronic diseases on the health-related quality of life (HRQOL) of Chinese patients in primary care.* Family Practice, 2000. 17(2): p. 159-66.

[89] Lam, C.L.K., D.Y.T. Fong, I.J. Launder, and T.P. Lam, *The effect of health-related quality of life (HRQOL) on health service utilisation of a Chinese population.* Social Science & Medicine, 2002. 55(9): p. 1635-1646.

[90] Tsai, S.Y., L.Y. Chi, L.C. Hsen, and P. Chou, *Health-related quality ofe life as a predictor of mortality among community-dwelling older persons.* European Journal of Epidemiology, 2007. 19-26.

[91] Singh, J.A. and V. Strand, *Gout is associated with more comorbidities, poorer health-related quality of life and higher healthcare utilisation in US veterans.* Annals of the Rheumatic Diseases, 2008. 67(9): p. 1310-1316.

[92] Lam, C.L.K., I.J. Launder, T.P. Lam, and B. Gandek, *Population based norming of the Chinese (HK) version of the SF-36 health survey.* The Hong Kong Practitioner, 1999. 21: p. 460-470.

[93] Ministry of Health of the People's Republic of China, *Guidelines of the Prevention and Treatment of Cancers,* Ministry of Health of the People's Republic of China, Editor. 1986-2000.

[94] WHO, *The development of the WHO quality of life assessment instrument.* WHO, 1993.

[95] Yu, E.X., *Radiotherapy of hepatic carcinoma.* Chinese Journal of Practical Surgery, 1986. 3: p. 157-158.

[96] Grieco, A. and C.J. Long, *Investigation of the Karnofsky Performance Status as a measure of quality of life.* Health Psychology, 1984. 3: p. 129-142.

[97] Pu, B.K., W.X. Tang, Z.Q. Zhang, and H.S. Lin, *The clinical observation of Fei Liu Ping Gao in treating late stage primary lung cancer.* Journal of Traditional Chinese Medicine, 1991. 4: p. 21-23.

[98] Huang, L.Z., S.L. Ceng, Y.L. Jian, Y.H. Wu, Y.B. Sun, and M.Q. Pan, *Clinical obversation of 31 cases of primary liver cancer treated by Gan Fu Lei Pian.* Hunan Journal of Traditional Chinese Medicine, 1997. 13: p. 4-5, 12.

[99] Zhou, L.M., J.J. Zhu, J.Y. Hong, X.C. Fu, G.M. Cheng, and L. Wu, *Injection of Kang Lai Te in treating post-radiotherapy failure of non small cell pulmonary carcinoma.* Journal of Practical Oncology, 1999. 14: p. 313-314.

[100] Cai, Z.R., *The impact of Yan Su on the quality of life of late stage liver cancer patients.* Heilongjiang Journal of Traditional Chinese Medicine, 1999. 6: p. 62.

[101] Tan, L.X. and J.F. Ji, *Clinical efficacy of new cancer drugs of Lan Xiang Xi Ru in treating late stage carcinoma.* Chinese Journal of Information on TCM, 1997. 4: p. 11-12.

[102] Ma, L., Y.N. Weng, and X. Xiao, *Intergration of Traditional Chinese Medicine and chemotherapy for the treatment of non-small cell lung cancer - meta analysis of the impact on clinical efficacy and health-related quality of life.* Chinese Journal of Practical Chinese with Modern Medicine, 2004. 4: p. 709-712.

[103] King, M.T., *The interpretation of scores from the EORTC quality of life questionnaire QLQ-C30.* Quality of Life Research, 1996. 5(6): p. 555-567.

[104] Oh, B., P. Butow, and B. Mullan, *Medical qigong for cancer patients: pilot study of impact on quality of life, side effects of treatment and inflammation.* The American Journal of Chinese Medicine, 2006. 36(3): p. 459-472.

[105] Esper, P., F. Mo, G. Chodak, M. Sinner, D. Cella, and K.J. Pienta, *Measuring Quality of life in men with prostate cancer using the Functional Assessment of Cancer Therapy-Prostate (FACT-P) instrument.* Urology, 1997. 50(6): p. 920-928.

[106] Pfeifer, B.L., J.F. Pirani, S.R. Hamann, and K.F. Klippel, *PC-SPES, a dietary supplement for the treatment of horomone-refractory prostate cancer.* BJU International, 2000. 85: p. 481-485.

[107] Cella, D.F., A.E. Bonomi, S.R. Lloyd, D.S. Tulsky, E. Kaplan, and P. Bonomi, *Reliability and validity of the Functional Assessment of Cancer Therapy - Lung (FACT-L) quality of life instrument.* Lung Cancer, 1995. 12: p. 199-220.

[108] Li, L.N., W.S. Liu, K. Xu, W.Y. Wu, Y.L. Liu, D.Y. Zhu, H.Y. Luo, and C.Y. Chen, *Clinical efficacy and health-related quality of life of Chinese Medicine Syndrome differentiation for the treatment of stage III and IV non-small cell lung carcinoma.* Chinese Journal of Lung Cancer, 2003. 6: p. 216-219.

[109] Spitzer, W.O., *Measuring the quality of life of cancer patients. A concise QL-index for use by physicians.* Journal of Chronic Diseases, 1981. 34(12): p. 585-597.

[110] Mahoney, F.I. and D.W. Baarthel, *Functional evaluation: The Barthel index.* Maryland State Medical Journal, 1965. 14: p. 61-65.

[111] Liang, Q., X. Li, and G. He, *The observation of the quality of life on cerebral hemorrhage treated with decotion of Ping Gan Xi Feng.* Bulletin of Hunan Medical University, 1996. 21(5): p. 403-406.

[112] Wang, Y., R.B. Zhang, and B.R. He, *The impact of health-related quality of life of Chinese and Western medication on hypertension patients.* Zhejiang Journal of Integrated Traditional Chinese and Western Medicine, 1999. 9: p. 86-88.

[113] Spertus, J.A., J.A. Winder, T.A. Dewhurst, R.A. Deyo, J. Prodzinski, M. McDonnell, and S.D. Fihn, *Development and evaluation of the Seattle Angina Questionnaire: A new functional status measure for coronary artery disease.* Journal of the American College of Cardiology, 1995. 25(2): p. 333-341.

[114] Ruan, X.M., Y. Lin, W. Jiang, J.X. Hu, Q.X. Chen, H.L. Wu, Z.J. Chen, H.C. Zhou, and C.L. Huang, *Clinical observation on quality of life in coronary artery bypass grafting patients treated according to syndrom differentiation of TCM.* Chinese Journal of Integrated Traditional and Western Medicine, 2003. 23(11): p. P. 804-807.

[115] Bliddal, H., A. Rosetzsky, P. Schlichting, M.S. Weidnet, L.A. Andersen, H.-H. Ibfelt, K. Christensen, O.N. Jensen, and J. Barslev, *A randomized, placebo-controlled, cross-over study of ginger extracts and Ibuprofen in osteoarthritis.* Osteoarthritis and Cartilage, 2000. 8: p. 9-12.

[116] Schmid, B., R. Ludtke, H.-K. Selbmann, I. Kotter, B. Tshidewahn, W. Schaffner, and L. Heide, *Efficacy and tolerability of a standardized Willow Bark Extract in patients with Osteoarthritis: randomized Placebo-controlled, double blind clinical trial.* Phytotherapy Research, 2001. 15: p. 344-350.

[117] Secor, E.R.J., J.H. Blumberg, M.J. Markow, J. MacKenzie, and R.S. Thrall, *Implementation of outcome measure in a complementary and alternative medicine clinic: evidence of decreased pain and improved quality of life.* The Journal of Alternative and Complementary Medicine, 2004. 10: p. 506-513.

[118] Cicero, A.F.G., G. Derosa, R. Brillante, R. Bernardi, S. Nascetti, and A. Gaddi, *Effects of Siberian Ginseng (Eleutherococcus senticosus maxim.) on elderly quality of life: a randomized clinical trial.* Arch. Gerontol. Geriatr. Suppl., 2004. 9: p. 69-73.

[119] Altman, R.D. and K.C. Marcussen, *Effects of a Ginger extract on knee pain in patients with osteoarthritis.* Arthritis and Rheumatism, 2001. 44: p. 2531-2538.

[120] Xue, C., F. Thien, J. Zhang, W. Yang, C.D. Costa, and C. Li, *Effects of adding a Chinese herbal preparartion to acupuncture for seasonal allergic rhinitis: randomised double-blind controlled trial.* Hong Kong Medical Journal, 2003. 9: p. 427-434.

[121] Weber, R., L. Christen, M. Loy, S. Schaller, S. Christen, R.B. Joyce, U. Ledermann, B. Ledergerber, R. Cone, R. Luthy, and M.R. Cohen, *Randomized, placebo-controlled trial of Chinese herb therapy for HIV-1-infected individuals.* Journal of Acquired Immune Deficiency Syndromes, 1999. 22(1): p. 56.

[122] Kainuma, M., J. Hayashi, S. Sakai, K. Imai, N. Mantani, K. Kohta, T. Mitsuma, Y. Shimada, S. Kashiwagi, and K. Terasawa, *The efficacy of herbal medicine (Kampo) in reducing the adverse effects of IFN-B in Chronic Hepatitis C.* The American Journal of Chinese Medicine, 2002. 30: p. 355-367.

[123] Jakkula, M., T.A. Boucher, U. Beyendorff, S.M. Conn, J.E. Johnson, C.J. Nolan, J.p. Craig, and J.H. Albrech, *A randomized trial of Chinese herbal medicines for the treatment of symptomatic hepatitis C.* Archives of Internal Medicine, 2004. 164: p. 1341-1346.

[124] Vutyavanich, T., T. Kraisarin, and R. Ruangsri, *Ginger for nausea and vomiting in pregnancy: randomized, double-masked, placebo-controlled trial.* Obstetrics and Gynecology, 2001. 97: p. 577-582.

[125] Shebek, J. and J.P. Rindone, *A pilot study exploring the effect of Kudzu Root on the drinking habits of patients with Chronic Alcoholism.* The Journal of Alternative and Complementary Medicine, 2000. 6: p. 45-48.

[126] Yamada, K., R. Den, K. Ohnishi, and S. Kanba, *Effectiveness of herbal medicine (Kampo) and changes of quality of life in patients with Somatoform Disorders.* Journal of Clinical Psychopharmacology, 2005. 25: p. 199-201.

[127] Song, J. and K.J. Chen, *Several critical questions needed to be asked for clinical observation of Traditional Chinese Medicine.* Chinese Journal of Integrated Traditional and Western Medicine, 2003. 23: p. 564-565.

[128] Hu, S.Y., Z. Wang, T.S. Cai, J.S. You, and Q. Yao, *Preliminary Development of Emotion rating scale for Ganzangxiang of Traditional Chinese Medicine.* Chinese Journal of Clinical Psychology, 2001. 9: p. 84-89.

[129] Hu, S.Y., Z. Wang, C.Y. Yu, and J.S. You, *Researching thoughts and methods of emotion scale for Gangzangxiang of Traditional Chinese Medicine.* China Journal of Basic Medicine in Traditional Chinese Medicine, 2001. 7: p. 9-11.

[130] Edwards, R.A., *Our research approaches must meet the goal of improving patient care.* Alternative Therapies in Health and Medicine, 1997. 3: p. 99.

[131] Matko, M., *"Complementary and alternative" medicine - a measure of crisis in academic medicine* Croatian Medical Journal, 2004. 45: p. 684-688.

[132] Zhao, L., K.F. Leung, and K. Chan, *The Chinese Quality of Life instrument: reliability and validity of the Hong Kong Chinese version (ChQOL-HK).* The Hong Kong Practitioner, 2007. 29: p. 220-232.

[133] Yang, X.B., J.Q. Hu, and S.L. Lai, *Thoughts on the Standardization of Syndrome differentiation of Chinese Medicine.* Chinese Journal of Information on TCM, 2001. 8: p. 10-11.

[134] Zhang, H.N., S.Y. Hu, Z.Q. Chen, and J.Q. Luo, *An analysis on the first questionnaires for the syndrome standard of hepatic stagnation causing phlegm retention among cases with depression.* Journal of Hunan College of Traditional Chinese Medicine, 2002. 27: p. 519-521.

[135] Wang, Z., S.Y. Hu, T.S. Cai, and D.S. Xia, *Development of emotion rating scale for Ganzangxiang of Traditional Chinese Medicine (ERSG).* Chinese Journal of Behavioral Medical Science, 2004. 13: p. 104-106.

[136] Wang, Z., S.Y. Hu, and T.S. Cai, *Factor analysis of emotion rating scale for ganzangxiang of Traditional Chinese Medicine.* Chinese Mental Health Journal, 2003. 17: p. 306-308.

[137] Liu, F.B., J.Q. Fang, Z.H. Pan, Q. Li, X.L. Liu, and Y.T. Hao, *The development of syndrom differential scale of the spleen-stomach disease used for computer aided expert diagnosis system.* Academic Journal of Sun Yat-Sen University of Medical Sciences, 2000. 21(4S): p. 112-116.

[138] Liu, Z.Z., Z.Q. Chen, and Q. Guo, *Study on syndrome scale for Liver-qi stagnation syndrome.* Journal of Traditional Chinese Medicine University of Hunan, 2007. 27: p. 48-51.

[139] Liu, X.Z., Z.Q. Chen, and Q. Guo, *Primary compilation of a scale for Liver-fire ascending syndrome.* Chinese Journal of Clinical Rehabilitation, 2006. 10: p. 1-3.

[140] Quan, K.X. and W.J. Wu, *Establishment and evaluation of irritable bowel syndrome instruments for TCM.* Journal of Traditional Chinese Medicine and Chinese Materia Medica of Jilin, 2004. 24: p. 6-8.

[141] Zhao, L., K.T. Chan, K.F. Leung, and F.B. Liu. *Quality of Life and Chinese Medicine - The development of health status measures for Chinese Medicine.* in *The 2nd World Integrative Medicine Congress.* 2004. Beijing.

[142] Li, F.L. and R. Liang, *Application and thoughts of TCM syndrome differentiation in questionnaire development.* Journal of Beijing Univeristy of Traditional Chinese Medicine, 2006. 29: p. 162-164.

[143] Li, G.C., W.K. Chen, X.Y. Mei, C.X. Peng, and L. Zou, *Discussion on quantitative analysis method about variable of macroscopical differentiation of syndromes of TCM.* China Journal of Basic Medicine in Traditional Chinese Medicine, 2005. 11: p. 650-652.

[144] Langevin, H.M., G.J. Badger, B.K. Povolny, R.T. Davis, A.C. Johnston, K.J. Sherman, J.R. Kahn, and T.J. Kaptchuk, *Yin scores and Yang scores: a new method for quantitative diagnostic evaluation in traditional Chinese medicine research.* The Journal of Alternative and Complementary Medicine, 2004. 10: p. 389-395.

[145] Leung, K.F., F.B. Liu, L. Zhao, J.Q. Fang, K. Chan, and L.Z. Lin, *Development and validation of the Chinese quality of life instrument* Health and quality of life Outcomes, 2005. 3: p. 26.

[146] Wong, W., C.L.K. Lam, K.F. Leung, and L. Zhao, *Is the Content of the Chinese Quality of Life Instrument (ChQOL) Really Valid in the Context of Traditional Chinese Medicine in Hong Kong?* Complementary Therapies in Medicine, 2009. 17(1): p. 29-36.

[147] Tang, J.L. and P.C. Leung, *An efficacy-driven approach to the research and development of traditional Chinese medicine.* Hong Kong Medical Journal, 2001. 7: p. 375-380.

[148] Guo, X.F., S.L. Lai, and W.X. Liang, *Choice and application of the outcome indexes for clinical effectivenesss assessment of Traditional Chinese Medicine.* Journal of Guangzhou University of Traditional Chinese Medicine, 2002. 19: p. 251-255.

9

Application and Effect of Acupuncture and Moxibustion for Analgesia in Perioperative Period of Total Knee Arthroplasty

Bang Jian He and Peijian Tong
*Zhejiang Traditional Chinese Medicine University,
China*

1. Introduction

As patients going to take total knee arthroplasty(TKA) lying in bed for a long time, eating less, bowel movements Slowing down, then influencing defecation.And they will come up with tension and fearness.At the same time, their lifestyle is changing. Epidemiological survey of constipation displaying: tension, anxiety and depression are the dangerous factors of constipation. Eating less, Diet low in fiber content are easily leading to constipation. In addition, lots of patients aren't used to defecate in bed for a long time, which will also making the defecation difficult. While constipation may cause whole body and partial illness, we should pay more attention to it.

Total knee replacement surgery has become the ultimate effective treatment for the disease. However, this surgical method is associated with severe postoperative pain, including severe pain 60%, 30% moderate pain, not only to patients with pain, but also to varying degrees, affect the circulatory, respiratory, digestive, endocrine, immune and other function of each system that may lead to various postoperative complications, serious impact on early postoperative functional rehabilitation and treatment. Postoperative pain not due to early exercise, active physical therapy, so prone to deep vein thrombosis, pulmonary embolism, infection and other complications. Patients within the environment can also lead to disorder, anxiety is not conducive to sleep and rest, short-term deterioration in the quality of life of patients. Severe pain due to joint dysfunction caused by anxiety, depression, most patients need a year of health care in order to get the final improveing. Almost all patients are expected to be their smallest incision, postoperative pain and satisfaction with the lightest of functional recovery. Therefore, adequate postoperative analgesia, especially for sports is not just pain relief, but also to help patients get out of bed early, active physical therapy, as much as possible to restore knee activity and the prevention of deep vein thrombosis formation and other complications. In addition, effective postoperative analgesia reduces stress response, so that patients in a stable environment, and reduce patient anxiety, sleep and rest help to improve the quality of life in patients with short-term..

Early postoperative pain caused by stress response, significantly increased the secretion of stress-quality alcohol, so that myocardial contractility, heart rate, cardiac output increased, liver and kidney blood vessels and gastrointestinal vasoconstriction, myocardial oxygen consumption significantly increase induced myocardial oxygen supply/oxygen ratio disorders, but also make the body insulin sensitivity, glucose uptake and utilization of energy for the oxidation of reduced capacity. These will affect the perioperative and postoperative quality of life of patients recovered as soon as possible. Therefore, postoperative pain and reduce the body's stress response, the promotion of early postoperative recovery has a positive effect.

2. Mechanism of acupuncture analgesia in the perioperative period of total knee arthroplasty

The current total knee arthroplasty analgesia strategies, mainly compound of preemptive analgesia and multimodal analgesia. Postoperative analgesia with epidural administration, intravenous, intra-articular administration, local continuous joint cryotherapy, oral drug therapy. Today, we discuss mainly the total knee replacement surgery perioperative analgesic mechanism of acupuncture, as follows:

2.1 Nerve
2.1.1 Central mechanism
Signal is acupuncture acupuncture analgesia and pain signals in the central nervous system interactions, processing and integration of the results. Studies have shown that the central nervous system from spinal cord to the cerebral cortex at all levels are involved in this interaction. Acupuncture analgesia is a multi-channel, multi-level synthesis process. Spinal cord of the central segment of the downstream modulation and high modulation is the main mechanism of acupuncture analgesia.

2.1.1.1 Spinal cord injury is acupuncture signal and primary signal integration hub. Acupuncture both hyperalgesia induced by dorsal horn neurons produce inhibitory postsynaptic potentials (IPSP), but also caused depolarization of the spinal cord and peripheral transmission occurs presynaptic inhibition. Therefore, the level of acupuncture in the spinal cord can produce analgesia, the mechanism involves both presynaptic inhibition, postsynaptic inhibition is also involved.

2.1.1.2 The structure of the spinal cord above the mechanism of acupuncture analgesia in the spinal cord above the central thalamic structures including nuclear-forebrain loop-the loop parafascicular nucleus, the brain-the edge of pain loop, descending inhibitory system under the central nucleus and thalamus-ventrolateral orbital cortex-in the periaqueductal gray pathway. ① central thalamus in the nucleus-forebrain loop-the loop parafascicular nucleus: acupuncture causes the central nuclear signals resulting from the impulse may be excited by forebrain circuits (caudate nucleus, pillow core, cortex and thalamic reticular nucleus) to reach the parafascicular nucleus, activity of pain-sensitive neurons produce inhibitory modulation.② in the brain-the edge of pain loop: the limbic system in the midbrain periaqueductal gray (PAG), nucleus accumbens, amygdala and habenula, these neural pathways between nuclei with each other to form a circular path. The loop to 5-HT and enkephalin as neurotransmitters. Acupuncture to the releasing of brain 5-HT and enkephalin, promote analgesic effects loop rotation. ③ descending inhibitory system: Acupuncture information can be passed from brain PAG nucleus raphe magnus (NRM) to reach the spinal cord or trigeminal plexus, the information produced inhibition of pain modulation. (Liu Xiang, 1996) The following line suppression system, the main initiation site, the medullary NRM neurons, and one of the seam - spinal neurons as an indicator of unit discharge was observed acupoint electric stimulation PAG, nucleus accumbens and caudate nucleus can activate NRM neurons inhibition of spontaneous discharge and damage response; and electrolysis damage to these brain areas are able to block the analgesic effect of EA. Prompt the activation of descending inhibitory systems in play a major role in acupuncture analgesia. ④under the central thalamic nucleus - ventral lateral orbital cortex - in the periaqueductal gray matter: Teachers (Tang, Jing-shi &Yuanbing, 2002) research group studies have shown that the hypothalamus under the central nucleus (Sm)-ventrolateral orbital cortex (VLO)-PAG is not only a central feeling pain, but also constitute an important in pain modulation negative feedback loop, through the activation of the brainstem descending inhibitory system, the level of modulation in the spinal cord and trigeminal nociceptive transmission. The fine fiber loop in the excitement generated by acupuncture analgesia play an important role. Sm neurons they observed the response to acupuncture, as well as damage to Sm or VLO, or Sm injection of local anesthetic effect of acupuncture. The results show that acupuncture can activate neurons in rat Sm activity, these neurons respond to noxious mechanical stimulation was not found on non-noxious stimulation of neurons. Further studies have shown, bilateral electrolytic damage can be significantly reduced Sm or VLO strong electro-acupuncture (5.0 mA) on rat tail flick reflex inhibition, while the weak-pin (0.5mA) of the inhibitory effect no significant effect. Tip strong electro-acupuncture analgesia produced fine fibers excited by activation of Sm-VLO-PAG pathway. Sm microinjection in the local anesthetic lidocaine can significantly weaken the strong EA (5-6 mA) of the rat spinal dorsal horn nociceptive neurons in response to the inhibitory effect, while the weak-pin (1mA) had no effect on the effects of. The results for the Sm-VLO-PAG pathway involved in the fine fibers provides further proof of the analgesic.

2.1.2 Peripheral mechanisms

Peripheral nerve needle nerve signal transmission, the types of acupuncture by or to the types of fiber conduction problems, had long been in dispute. After a large number of experiments, now that: electric acupuncture(EA) of varying intensity, a different transmission fibers can be excited. Low-intensity electro-acupuncture (2 V) major excitatory I, II class and some III (Aδ) class crude fiber transmission through the integration of the role of pain in spinal cord segments to achieve analgesia, but also on the mechanism involved in the spinal cord, the analgesic effect showed limited of the specificity; and high-intensity electric acupuncture(EA) 18 V (over C fiber threshold, equivalent to noxious stimulation) is mainly excited III (Aδ), especially IV (C) class small transmission fibers, the spinal cord through the activation of negative feedback on the NRM pain adjustment mechanism to play a wide range of effects long after the analgesic effect of this analgesic effect without showing broad specificity. These facts prove that acupuncture is a noxious stimulus, transmission of C fibers in acupuncture analgesia play an important role. Capsaicin (Cap) effective selective damage to a descendant of C fibers, in recent years to use it in a sense of electric acupuncture(EA)-human transmission have done a lot of research. (Fangzong Ren, et al 1992 & Liu Xiang, et al, 1997) observed that after peripheral nerve with capsaicin treatment, significantly reduced the analgesic effect of EA, clear that the peripheral nerve C fibers are the main ingredients involved in acupuncture analgesia.(Xu Rong et al, 1993) will be a direct effect of capsaicin in the rat sciatic nerve, its pain threshold was significantly higher; electric acupuncture(EA) capsaicin treatment side of the "ring dance" of the analgesic effect, significantly lower than prior to treatment and control side effects Tip a capsaicin-sensitive C fiber transmission of information not only involved in pain transmission, but also involved in acupuncture analgesia an essential component of information transmission.

2.1.3 Neurotransmitters

Acupuncture analgesia by the brain to complete a number of neurotransmitters in the joint, and neurotransmitters in acupuncture analgesia mechanisms of acupuncture analgesia is the most extensive and deep areas.

2.1.3.1 Endogenous opioid peptides (EOP) acupuncture is mainly dominated by activating the endogenous opioid peptides in pain modulation system and analgesic effects, so the EOP is an important material basis for acupuncture analgesia.

(Wang Hongbei et al, 1998) at different frequencies of electroacupuncture on acute adjuvant arthritis (AA) in rats with pain and tissue reaction of β-endorphin (β-EP) Content of the study, observed two 5 Hz and 100 Hz frequencies for the AA rats were significantly power analgesic effect, but also significantly increased the hypothalamic content of β-EP, the two frequency electroacupuncture analgesia are related to hypothalamic β-EP levels were significantly elevated positive correlation, but both the frequency and electro-acupuncture analgesia between elevated β-EP levels in the hypothalamus no significant difference in the role. (Chen et al, 2004) further found that acupuncture can promote β-EP precursor POMC original (POMC) mRNA expression increased to further enhance the β-EP levels to analgesic effect. This not only immediate effect of acupuncture analgesia, there are more significant after-effects,. (Wang Sheng Xu et al, 1999) studies have shown that acupuncture can Jiaji AA levels in rat spinal cord dorsal horn of the original before dynorphin (PPD) mRNA expression was significantly increased, suggesting that EA may activate the dynorphin system resistant to injury, the level of inflammation in the spinal cord and hyperalgesia is modulated. (Huang Yong, 2004)A method of acupuncture in the study satisfied leucine enkephalin on the AA effects in rabbits, and found that satisfied a method and routine acupuncture can significantly improve the AA rabbit serum in the hypothalamus and brain leucine enkephalin (LEK) level of analgesic effect. LEK for the regulation of serum, Na A is better than routine acupuncture

Acupuncture can not only promote the release of central EOP can also make local EOP inflammation increases the synthesis and release, to achieve peripheral analgesia. (Zhao chang huan &Zhou jun, 2002)positions AA rats in the study of electricity for local opioid peptide gene expression observed when the EA in the AA rats increased the pain threshold, but also promote inflammation in local immune cells POMC and preproenkephalin (PENK) mRNA expression increased, to achieve peripheral pain modulation. Inflammation in AA rats while local injection of β-EP and LEK antisera may antagonize the analgesic effect of electro-acupuncture, in which β-EP antiserum stronger effect, suggesting that β-EP and LEK are involved in EA's peripheral towns pain in the process (Yangjie Bin et al, 1999), different acupuncture on peripheral analgesic mechanism of AA rats in the study, using electro-acupuncture, moxibustion, Bloodletting and four methods of acupoint-injection can increase the pain threshold of AA rats to electro-acupuncture, point injection is excellent, its peripheral analgesic mechanism may promote inflammation in local analgesic substances by β-EP and LEK increased, causing physical pain prostaglandin E2 (PGE2), histamine, 5 - hydroxytryptamine (5-HT), norepinephrine (NE) reduction achieved.

2.1.3.2 Monoamine neurotransmitter monoamine neurotransmitters are important bioactive substances in vivo, the relationship with acupuncture analgesia, the study is more 5-HT, NE and dopamine (DA). (Wang Sheng Xu et al, 1999) were observed in the EA Jiaji of AA in peripheral blood and the spinal cord content of monoamine neurotransmitters, studies show that: EA AA rats after the platelet 5-HT, and plasma 5-- HIAA (5-HIAA, 5-HT, the end product of catabolism) were significantly increased, indicating that acupuncture in the promotion of platelet 5-HT increased absorption, but also the blood of free accelerated catabolism of 5-HT involved in analgesia, electro-acupuncture to peripheral NE and DA were significantly decreased, which may be respectively enhanced sympathetic activity and inhibition of autonomic nervous activity. In the spinal cord, EA Jiaji AA rats significantly increased spinal 5-HT and 5-HIAA levels, while 5-HIAA increased significantly more than the 5-HT, indicating that electro-acupuncture analgesia Jiaji mechanism downstream activation of 5-HT, 5-HT on pain control system synthesis, release and use also increased, but synthesis faster than the speed of the release and use, so 5-HT content increased, indicating that 5-HT, is involved in spinal pain modulation important neurotransmitter; EA Jiaji spinal cord NE and DA content were significantly decreased, indicating that the NA and DA are involved in the mechanism of electroacupuncture analgesia in the spinal cord. These results suggest that peripheral and spinal cord monoamine neurotransmitters are involved in inflammatory pain modulation in rats during electroacupuncture analgesia. (Liang fan long et al 2001)prosperity AA rats in the study of electricity for local inflammation in 5-HT, NE, DA content in, they get the same results, and show some of the after-effects.

2.1.3.3 Substance P(SP), (Wang Sheng Xu et al, 2000), electro-acupuncture in the study of AA Jiaji effect of substance P in rat spinal cord found that EA can make the AA rat spinal cord lumbar enlargement of SP-positive cells in the immune response to a further increase in Tip EA Jiaji inhibit adjuvant-induced spinal cord dorsal horn release of SP, the SP storage increases, the mechanism through the spinal cord and spinal analgesic effect.

2.1.3.4 Nitrogen monoxidum(NO) is a neurotransmitter of new neurons found at different levels play an important role in pain modulation. (Tian Jin Hua et al, 1996) confirmed that NO can not only promote the formation of the spinal cord level and development of hyperalgesia, and pain in the brain caused by the role. （Pan Huijuan et al, 2002） also experiment found that acupuncture can significantly increase the pain threshold of AA rats, and has obvious after-effects; AA rats while significantly reducing the NO content in brain tissue, resulting in analgesia.

2.2 Psychology

2.2.1 Release of endorphins within the brown skin is a neuromodulator class of chemicals that can alter or adjust the postsynaptic neuron function, sexual and emotional pain control has an important role. Because of its role in pleasure and pain regulation and control, known as the "key to enter heaven." Researchers have checked out the course of acupuncture in reducing pain, endorphins at least part of the role (Fields & Levine, 1984; Murray, 1995; Watkins & Mayer, 1982), which is similar to opium and coffee, with the same receptors in the brain

2.2.2 Distracting mental process of the importance of the pain experience can be used to illustrate two extreme examples: First, do not feel physical pain stimulus, and second, when stimulated by a strong pain did not feel pain. Feelings of pain that occur will be pain response scenarios and habits of the impact of acquisition, so by distracting, resulting in appropriate information to enhance the contrast stimuli ability to overcome pain. Mel Zach (Ronald Melzack, 1973, 1980) proposed gated background theory that describes the psychological impact of pain perception, the theory that the cells in the spinal cord, as cut off as the door and prevent some of the pain signals into the brain, while allowing other signals into the brain and spinal cord to receptors in the skin send information to open or closed, the information provided from the brain of pain experienced by the background scene. Acupuncture treatment by applying an external stimulus, distracted the attention of patients, pain in the affected area so that it no longer focus on the scene. Psychology from the Chinese point of view, this should be easy to therapy empathy through the spirit of the transfer, change the patient's point of Love within the guilty to distraction emotions, changes in aspirations, in order to treat pain caused by emotional factors.

2.2.3 Since the perceived control of pain experience and decided on the physiological and psychological factors, to successfully deal with the pain factor is the establishment of another major source of stress, perceived control, that can change the event or experience for the process or result of faith. If you believe you can influence some of the symptoms of discomfort or pain of the daily process, you may better adapt to the symptoms of these disorders. Good results of acupuncture analgesia trust the doctor before administering treatment to give patients confidence so that patients have to reduce or cure the pain beliefs, and thus affect the perceived control of pain through the process. Therefore, the confidence of patients and doctors who stress indoctrination is extremely important. Chinese psychology to love wins love with this therapy or a fit of the Department.

2.2.4 Social and environmental support to provide social support is a resource for others to tell someone he is loved, cared for and respected, he lives in contact with each other and help each other a social network (Cohen & Syme, 1985). Acupuncture analgesia in the treatment of this social support mainly from doctors and family members, doctors information support, such as on the cause of the disease, information, recommendations on the effects of uncertainty, as well as doctors and their families emotional support, etc. Many researchers have pointed out that social support's role in mitigating damage when given to patients can rely on a sense, they are better able to cope with stress, pain and suffering, it can promote the individual has been diagnosed with the disease from rehabilitation. For pain patients, acupuncturists and differentiation before administering treatment information and emotional support in the treatment of the point of the eye. At the same time when the clinic environment, differentiation, treatment of mental quiet position also helps patients self-control and regulation. Enlighten the language of psychology, medicine therapies, including delight joyful way, way clear up doubts, and doubts therapy is also suggested that social support. But rather God Seishi therapy is a supportive environment, through meditation or repose, to achieve "without thinking of the suffering inside and outside workers are not shaped at all" to a read on behalf of the Wan study results.

2.2.5 Catharsis chronic pain damage to human health, its immune function, neurotransmitter, autonomic nervous system, mental and psychological adverse effects will be, it allows patients with physical pain, mental distress, reduce outdoor activities and social interaction, and gradually form a "sleep a fatigue, insomnia and a pain in a troubled one, "the vicious circle of pain in patients with enlarged and somatization. Therefore, so that patients get the emotional drain should have a good health benefits. Doctor to listen to on the one hand, and the course of treatment by acupuncture to relieve tension and calm the mind the body can have a relaxation response, which is an effective response to combat stress, muscle tension, cortical excitability, heart rate and blood pressure have decreased, the pain eased. This was reflected in the Chinese psychology along the intelligence from For therapy, the patient's compliance ideas, emotions, mind and body to meet the needs of patients, but the patient's psychological interpretation of the cause

In summary, the psychological mechanism of acupuncture analgesia can not be questioned. And the role of acupuncture analgesia in acupuncture, in place of a body from the outside and thoughtful hub at all levels, involving the nervous, endocrine and immune interactions of multiple factors, including anti-pain and pain caused by two aspects of the unity of opposites complex dynamic integration process. In this process, the nervous system and neurotransmitters as well as between various neurotransmitters, nerve, endocrine and immune systems are not isolated individual, but rather complement each other, interact, participate in the modulation of acupuncture on pain role. Although the mechanism of acupuncture analgesia in recent years made great progress in the study, but the mechanism of acupuncture analgesia has still not clear, need from multi-disciplinary, multi-level, multi-angle in-depth study in order to promote the town of acupuncture mechanism of pain and to promote the wider use of acupuncture in clinical.

3. Preoperative eletroacupuncture for postoperative pain

The clinical practice of acupuncture is growing in popularity world-wide. In parallel, interest in the scientific basis of acupuncture has been increasing, as reflected by a dramatic rise in the number of scientific publicationson acupuncture and related techniques (ART) in the recent decade. After 40 years of extensive studies, compelling evidence has been obtained to support acupuncture as a useful tool for treating a spectrum of diseases.In fact, more than 40 disorders have been endorsed by the World Health Organization (WHO) as conditions that can benefit from acupuncture treatment. Pain is particularly sensitive to acupuncture. Postoperative pain management remains a significant challenge for healthcare providers. Many patients experience pain after surgery, with about 86% reporting moderate, severe, or extreme pain. Opioids remain the mainstay for postoperative pain control. However, opioid analgesics are associated with undesirable side-effects, including nausea, vomiting, pruritus, sedation, dizziness, and decreased gut motility which can lead to delayed post-operative recovery. The use of adjunct analgesics that provide opioid-sparing effects and decrease the incidence of opioid-related side-effects is therefore useful. Acupuncture, a component of traditional Chinese medicine, is a well-known and widely used treatment for pain and other conditions that has been employed in China for more than 3000 yr. There have been increasing numbers of clinical trials evaluating the efficacy of acupuncture and related techniques as an adjuvant method for postoperative analgesia. Paul F, et al. designed a randomized, double-blind, sham-controlled study, which was used to compare three prophylactic acustimulation treatment schedules: preoperative—an active device was applied for 30 min before and a sham device for 72h after surgery;postoperative—a sham device was applied for 30 min before and an active device for 72h after surgery;and peri-operative—an active device was applied for 30 min before and 72 h after surgery (n 35 per group). All patients received a standardized general anesthetic, and on dansetron 4mg IV was administered at the end of surgery.The incidence of vomiting/retching and the need for rescue antiemetics were determined at specific time in tervals for up to 72 h after surgery. Nausea scores were recorded with an 11-point verbalrating scale.Other out come vari-ablesassessed included discharge times(for outpatients), resumption of nor malactivities of daily living, complete antiemetic response rate, and patient satisfaction with

Antiemetic therapy and quality of recovery.Perioperative use of the Relief Band significantly increased complete responses(68%)compared with use of the device before surgery only(43%).Median postoperative nausea scores were significantly reduced in the peri- and post-operative (versus preoperative) treatment groups.Finally, patient satisfaction with the quality of recovery (83± 16 and 85± 13 vs 72± 18) and antiemetic management (96± 9 and 94± 10 vs 86±13) on an arbitrary scale from 0 worst to 100 best was significantly higher in the groups receiving peri- or postoperative (versus preoperative) acustimulation therapy. For patients discharged on the day of surgery, the time to home readiness was significantly reduced (114± 41 min versus 164±50 min; P< 0.05) when acustimulation was administered perioperatively (versus preoperatively). In conclusion, acustimulation with the Relief Band was most effective in reducing postoperative nausea and vomiting and improving patients'satisfaction with their antiemetic therapy when it was administered after surgery. Sun er al.conducted a systematic review to quantitatively evaluate the efficacy of acupuncture and related techniques as adjunct analgesics for acute postoperative pain management. The authors concluded that perioperative acupuncture might be a useful adjunct for acute postoperative pain management.there are few Literatures about preoperative eletroacupuncture for postoperative pain after total knee arthroplasty, in our hospital, patients who takes the operation of total knee arthroplasty will be received preoperative eletroacupuncture at bilateral points (LI4–LI11, LR3–ST36, PC6–TE5) for 30 min with alternating frequencies of 3 and 15 Hz., postoperative range of motion(ROM)Of knee joint and Hospital for Special Surgery(HSS)score were recorded. two weeks after operation the initiative ROM and the HSS score were improved, so Applying preoperative eletroacupuncture in perioperative period Of knee joint replacement is favorable for alleviating postoperative pain, decreasing narcotic consumption, and promoting early rehabilitation.

Many studies have supported the effectiveness of acupuncture for postoperative pain relief However, the mechanism of acupuncture analgesia remains unclear. Acupuncture theory is based on two conditions:"yin", which is considered feminine, passive, dark, and cold, and "yang", which is masculine, aggressive, bright, and hot, as well as "qi, " which is considered thevitalenergy that flows and cycles throughout the body.The acupuncture theory is to harmonize any imbalance in yin-yang and qi in a human body to restore the body to a healthy condition.Acupuncture is thought to unblock any obstruction to the flow of qi and, thereby, relieves pain.The acupuncture technique that has been most often studied scientifically involves penetrating the skin with thin, solid, metallic needles that are manipulated by the hands or electrical stimulation. Although in the past scepticism has been voiced over the effects claimed for acupuncture, in recent years the effect of acupuncture on different conditions (pain and diseases) has been studied from a Western scientifc perspective, and the results have demonstrated that acupuncture has both physiological and psychological impacts. Needle insertion into the skin and deeper tissues, in addition to subsequent stimulation of the needles, results in aparticular pattern of afferent activity in peripheral nerves, mainly the A-delta and possibly also the C fibres. Acupuncture stimulation has been demonstrated to activate inhibitory systems in the spinal cord, which results in segmental inhibition of the sympathetic outfow and pain pathways, as predicted by the gate control theory. EA releases endogenous opioids and oxytocin, which seem to be essential in the induction of functional changes in different organ systems In this respect, particular interest has been dedicated to β-endorphin-an endogenous opioid with a high affnity for the m receptor. Indeed, evidence suggests that this hypothalamic β-endorphin system plays a central role in mediating the pain-relieving effect of acupuncture.

Furthermore, it has been shown that intense stimulation results in the activation of supraspinal pain inhibitory centres, and this mechanism is denoted diffuse noxious inhibitory controls (DNIC) or counterirritation.

In conclusion, the preoperative eletroacupuncture may be a useful adjunct for postoperative analgesia. Further large, well-designed studies are required to confirm those findings and to answer questions regarding the most efficacious type of acupuncture and optimal timing of administration.and the mechanism of acupuncture analgesia

4. Pain relief by acupuncture

Normal knee is freedom in flexion and extextension, which is limited now, just because of pain due to obstruction of Qi and blood in meridians, even there'stagnation. Where meridians pass, there is available to be treated. Accordingly, we should take local or remote acupoints in meridians where the disease is. Prescription: Yinlingquan (SP9), Yanglingquan (GB34), Neixiyan (EX-LE4), Taichong (LR3), Dachangshu (BL25), Quchi (LI11), Fengchi (GB20), both bilateral acupoints. If the course is long, we can add Zusanli (ST36), Sanyinjiao (SP6). Select 5 to 6 points each, after the arrival 0f Qi, we take reinforcing and reducing movement, needle retention 15min.2 to 3 times per week, 2 weeks as a course of treatment. Acupuncture treatment can be adjusted locally by tendon thinning the blood, promoting blood circulation, eliminating wind, removing obstrution from the meridians and relieving pain. Effective stimulation of acupuncture points receptors, so that pain signals are inhibited, anti-pain, enhance its ability to achieve the balance restored both inside and outside the state of the local meridian, and promote early recovery after surgery.

5. Application and effect of auricular acupoint pressing for analgesia in perioperative period of total knee arthroplasty

The role of Total knee arthroplasty has been widely recognized in the reconstruction of knee joint function and the remission the patient's pain. Effective postoperative analgesia is not just to alleviate the pain of patients, but also to help to do early ambulation, to do active physical therapy, to restore the knee's Range of motion as possible, to prevent deep vein thrombosis or other complications, to shorter hospital stay Time. In addition, effective postoperative analgesia reduces stress response, so that patients with stable internal environment, and can reduce patient anxiety and help patients sleep and rest, to improve the quality of life in patients with short-term.

Acupuncture has been used for more than 2, 000 years in traditional Chinese medicine to treat pain and other ailments. This technique was traditionally thought to work by channeling energy or Qi through body 'meridians' with acupuncture needles.And modern medicine has been trying to figure out the mechanism of acupuncture analgesia. And now various hypotheses about the mechanism of acupuncture analgesia are currently being discussed, e.g., the endogenous opioid system, gate-control mechanism, longterm depression, and diffuse noxious inhibitory controls (DNIC), as well as involvement of different neurotransmitters such as serotonin and norepinephrine, But none of them can explain it completely. Hence, acupuncture-induced analgesia seems to be a complex, multimodal interaction of neuronal and humoral pathways. On the other hand, large randomized controlled trials have proven a clinically relevant effect of acupuncture on pain conditions in the past years.

Auricular acupuncture is defined as 'a form of acupuncture in which needles are placed in various positions of the ear to affect the person. It postulates body correlates on the ear, so a treatment performed upon the ear will have effects reflected on the body part'. The Silk Book, China's earliest medical treatise written approximately 500 B.C, and Nei Jing, the Classic of Medicine, written around 200 B.C, both documented the theory Auricular acupuncture for analgesia.In Traditional Chinese Medical, it was concluded that all meridians converge at the ear.and the relationships of the Auricle, the Meridians, and the Zangfu Organs were very closely. Auricular acupuncture was first introduced into clinical western medicine by Nogier (1972)(Nogier PFM, 1972)., who empirically identified Auricular acupuncture points. The generally accepted view on auricular acupuncture is based on the conjecture that the human body is represented on the auricle in the form of an inverted fetus. It is claimed that this representation is constant, and can be detected by measuring the electrical resistance of the auricular skin and used for diagnostic purposes and/or treatment. Although the morphological structures connecting the specific auricular zones (acupuncture points) with corresponding parts of the body have not yet been identified, the effects of various stimulations applied to these regions have been verified in experimental and clinical studies.

Although no anatomical pathways exist to directly connect inner organs with the ear, a lot of nerve fiber distribution In the ear. The innervation of the central part of auricle (triangular fossa and concha) comes from trigeminal, geniculate and superior vagal ganglions, whereas the peripheral regions receive their innervation mainly by spinal nerves. The central parts of the neurons constituting the auricular branch of the vagal nerve are situated in the superior ganglion of the vagal nerve and nucleus tractus solitarii. Functionally, the stimulation of the inferior concha induced a significant increase in parasympathetic activity. In another study, the stimulation of the sympathetic AA point significantly decreased the stimulus-evoked electrodermal response compared with an AA stimulation to a non-specific point of the helix.. This resembles the design of studies performed by (Usichenko et al, 2005, 2007)where stimulation of the points in the central regions of the auricle was better than sham acupuncture at the non-specific points of the helix for reduction of postoperative analgesic requirement.

Early studies of Auricular acupuncture have demonstrated beneficial effects on both pain and anxiety including pain associated with cancer, knee arthroscopy, and hip fracture and hip arthroplasty. Several recent small studies have suggested that auricular acupuncture alone can relieve pain and anxiety in the prehospital transport phase of hip fracture and reduce acute pain due to a variety of causes in the emergency department setting.. Auricular acupuncture may be effective for the treatment of a variety of types of pain, especially postoperative pain

Auricular acupoint pressing(AAP), Vaccaria seeds be used to press in auricular acupoint, is the most commonly clinically Auricular acupuncture, In our hosptial we observe the effect of AAP for analgesia during perioperative period of total knee joint replacement, Methods: Sixty patients with osteoarthritis of ASA grade I to III scheduled to receive unilateral total knee joint replacement were equally randomized into the AAP group and the control group, 30 in each group. The general anesthesia on all patients was implemented by physicians of an identical group through endotracheal intubation. To the patients in the AAP group, AAP with Vaccaria seed was applied before operation, and the local analgesia on affected limb with acupoint pasting was used after operation. Besides, adm inistering of celecoxib 400 mg on the day before operation, and celecoxib 200 mg twice daily postoperation was given to all patients. When the visual analogue scales(VAS)reached more than 7 points, 0.1 g of bucinnazine hydrochloride was given for supplement Meantime same post-operative training methods were adopted in both groups. The resting VAS pain scores, contentment of sedation, incidence of adverse event, postoperative range of motion (ROM)Of knee joint and Hospital for Special Surgery(HSS) score were recorded Results: The resting VAS pain scores at 6 h and 24 h after operation was 5. 99±0. 67 scores and 4. 26±0. 59 scores in the AAP group respectively, which was significantly lower than that in the control group at the corresponding time (7. 02±0. 85 scores and 4. 92±0. 43 scores, P<0. 01), Through clinical observation we found that the resting VAS pain scores at 6 h and 24 h after operation reach its peak; but it showed insignificant difference between the two groups at 1 h and 48 h after operation (P>0. 05), which regard as the effect of Narcotic for analgesia at 1 h after operation is not eliminate Thoroughly, and Patients has tolerated the pain gradually at 48 h after operation so threshold of pain tolerance Increased, The result is the acute pain of the knee after surgery relieve gradually, After 48 hours after operation, patient's Acute pain was replaced by Chronic Pain that can be relieved by drugs for inflammation and pain, so the intergroup difference of the resting VAS pain scores at 1 h and 48 h after operation was statistically insignificant; sedation contentment in the two groups was similar: incidence of adverse event in the AAP groups seemed lower (4 cases VS. 1 1 cases), but the intergroup difference was statistically insignificant (P>0. 05). The application of postoperative narcotic analgesics and analgesic effects related to the occurrence of adverse reactions is the use of narcotic analgesics was positively correlated ROM before surgery were 75. 630±5. 74 and 75. 43±5. 63 in the two groups respectively, showing no significant difference (P>0. 05), two weeks after operation, the initiative ROM raised to 96. 500±3. 790 and 93. 500±3. 50 and the passive ROM reached 1 07. 80±3. 370 and 1 05. 27±3 250 in the two groups respectively, with statistical significance between them (P<0. 05) HSS score was similar between groups before operation (60. 23±3. 44 scores VS. 61. 70±2. 83 scores, p>0. 05); while it became 86. 97±2. 33 scores and 85. 37±2. 30 scores after operation. showing significant difference between groups(P<0. 05) so we draw the conclusion that Applying auricular acupoint pressing in perioperative period Of knee joint replacement is favorable for alleviating postoperative pain, decreasing narcotic consumption, and promoting early rehabilitation, and it has the advantages of low cost, less complication, simple manipulation and high safety.

After analysis the resting VAS pain scores at each time point, we must consider long enough analgesia for patient and additional analgesia aimed to the Peak pain point when we Select analgesic method. the satisfaction with analgesia in two groups of patients is about 50%, This shows that we must improved our Analgesia in the future, So in the next task we can combined many methods for better Analgesia in Perioperative Period of total knee arthroplasty, such as Auricular Acupoint Pressing, nerve block, intra-articular infusion reserved and so on, as far as Auricular Acupoint Pressing was considered, we prepare to Increase the intensity of the stimulus for better Analgesia through needle-embedding therapy and electric acupuncture in Auricle.

6. References

Albrecht S, le Blond R, Kohler V et al. Cryotherapy as analgesic technique in direct, postoperative treatment following elective joint replacement [J] z Orthop Ihre Grenzgeb, 1997, 135(1): 45-51

Alimi D, Rubino C, Pichard-Leandri E, et al. Analgesic effect of auricular acupuncture for cancer pain: A randomized, blinded, controlled trial. J Clin Oncol 2003;21:4120 – 4126

Bonica JJ. Postoperative pain/Bonica JJ, editor. The management of pain. 2nd ed. Philadelphia: Lea and Febiger, 1990: 461-480.

Bing Z, Villanueva L, Le Bars D. Acupuncture and diffuse noxious inhibitory controls: Naloxone-reversible depression of activities of trigeminal convergent neurons. Neuroscience 1990;37:809-18.

Bo Huijuan, Wang Haiyan, Xu Jianyang, etc. RA rats for experimental electrical pain explain and brainstem NO / NOS changes of [JJ]. Shanghai Journal of Acupuncture and Moxibustion, 2002, 21 (5): 48-50.

Barker R, Kober A, Hoerauf K, et al. Out-of-hospital auricular acupressure in elder patients with hip fracture: A randomized double-blinded trial. Acad Emerg Med 2006; 13: 19-23.

Brander V, Gondek S, Martin E, et al. Pain and depression influence outcome 5 years after knee replacement surgery [JJ]. Clin Orthop Relat Res, 2007, 464: 21-26.

Chen Jin, Liu Guangpu, Zhou Chunyang. Pieces of the hypothalamus and POMC mRNA expression of EP in the role of after-effects of acupuncture analgesia [JJ]. Acupuncture Research, 2004, 29 (1): 5-9.

Chen J, Sandkuhler J. Induction of homosynaptic long-term depression at spinal synapses of sensory a delta-fibers requires activation of metabotropic glutamate receptors. Neuroscience 2000; 98: 141 – 8.

Dorr L D, Chao L. The emotional state of the patient after total hip and knee arthroplasty [JJ] Clin Orthop Relat Res, 2007, 463: 7-12.

Endres HG, Bowing G, Diener HC, et al. Acupuncture for tension-type headache: A multicentre, shamcontrolled, patient- and observer-blinded, randomized trial. J Headache Pain 2007;8:306 – 14.

Fang Zongren, Yu Qin, Li Yanhua. Transmission of peripheral C fibers in acupuncture analgesia in the observation of the effects [JJ]. Acupuncture Research, 1992, 17(1): 48-53.

GiuffreM, Asci J, Arnstein P, et al. Postoperative joint replacement pain: description and op ioid requirement[JJ]. Post Anesth Nurs, 1991, 6 (4) : 239-245.

Goertz CM, Niemtzow R, Burns SM, et al. Auricular acupuncture in the treatment of acute pain syndromes: A pilot study. Mil Med 2006;171:1010 – 1014.

Gao Chengshun, Xiong Junyu, Analgesic strategy after total knee arthroplasty [JJ]. Medicine & Philosophy, 2009, 30(1):49-50.

Gary N. Asher, Daniel E. Jonas, Remy R. et al. Auriculotherapy for Pain Management: A Systematic Review and Meta-Analysis of Randomized Controlled Trials. The Journal of Alternative and Complementary Medicine. October 2010, 16(10): 1097-1108

He Xiaoling, Liu Xiang, Zhu Bing, etc. Strong electro-acupuncture points on the dorsal horn neurons in the central mechanism of the analgesic effect of extensive [JJ]. Acta Physiologica Sinica, 1995, 47 (6): 605-609.

Huang Yong. Najia acupuncture on adjuvant arthritis in rabbits leucine effects of brain endorphins [JJ]. Chinese Clinical Rehabilitation, 2004, 8 (30): 6676-6677.

Han JS, Terenius L. Neurochemical basis of acupuncture analgesia. Annu Rev Pharmacol Toxicol 1982; 22: 193-220.

Hebl JR, Dilger JA, Byer DE et al. A pre-emptive multi-modal pathway featuring peripheral nerve block improves perioperative outcomes after major orthopedic surgery [JJ]. Reg Anesth Pain Med, 2008, 33(6): 510-517.

Haake M, Muller HH, Schade-Brittinger C, et al. German Acupuncture Trials (GERAC) for chronic low back pain: Randomized, multicenter, blinded, parallelgroup trial with 3 groups. Arch Intern Med 2007; 167:1892 - 8.

Jiang Li, Zhao Canghuan. From a psychological point of view of acupuncture analgesia [J]. Liaoning Journal of Traditional Chinese Medicine, 2007, 34 (9): 1240-1241.

Jonas WB. Mosby's Dictionary of Complementary and Alternative Medicine. St Louis US: Elsevier Mosby, 2005.

Liu Xiang. Cerebral cortex and subcortical nuclei of the raphe nucleus of control and their role in acupuncture analgesia [J] Acupuncture Research, 1986, 21(2):4-10.

Lu Fang, Tang Jinshi, Yuan Bin, etc. Bilateral damage to the ventrolateral orbital cortex on the rat tail flick reflex inhibition of EA's influence [J]. Acupuncture Research, 1996, 21 (2): 39-42.

Liu Xiang, Huang Pingbo, Jiang Wuchun. Capsaicin blocked nerve C fiber ranked overall effect and its impact on EA "Zusanli" analgesic effect [J]. Acupuncture Research, 1997, 22(4): 295-303.

Liang Fanrong, Luo Rong, Liu Yuxing, etc. The experimental study of Effect of electroacupuncture analgesia and inflammation after partial 5-HT, NE, DA content [J]. Chinese Journal of Basic Medicine in Traditional Chinese Medicine, 2001, 7 (1): 52-55.

Nogier PFM. Traite´ d' auriculotherapie. Moulinle´s-Metz: Maisonneuve; 1972.

NaliniVadivelu, ;SukanyaMitra, DeepakNarayan, RecentAdvances in Postoperative Pain Management, YALE JOURNALOF BIOLOGYAND MEDICINE, 2010, 83, pp.11-25.

Peuker ET, Filler TJ. The nerve supply of the human auricle. Clinical Anatomy 2002; 15: 35-7.

Skinner HB. Multimodal acute pain management[J]. Am J Orthop, 2004, 33 (5 Supp l) : 5-9.

Saito N, Horiuchi H, Kobayashi S, et al.. Continuous local cooling for pain relief following total hip arthroplasty[J] J Arthroplasty, 2004, 19 (3): 334-337.

Scharf HP, Mansmann U, Streitberger K, et al. Acupuncture and knee osteoarthritis: A three-armed randomized trial. Ann Intern Med 2006;145

Tang Jinshi, Yuan Bin. A new discovery of pain modulation pathway[J]. Journal of Xi'an Jiaotong University(Medical Sciences), 2002, 23(4):329-332.

Tian Jinhua, Wang Xiaomin, Han Jisheng. Nitric oxide and pain modulation [J]. Progress in Physiological Sciences, 1996, 27(2):161-164.

Usichenko TI, Hermsen M, Witstruck T, et al. Auricular acupuncture for pain relief after ambulatory knee arthroscopy. Evidence Based Complementary and Alternative Medicine 2005; 2: 185 - 9.

Usichenko TI, Kuchling S, Witstruck T, et al. Auricular acupuncture for pain relief after ambulatory knee surgery: a randomized trial. Canadian Medical Association Journal 2007; 176: 179 - 83.

White R H, Henderson M C. Risk factors for venous thromboembolism after total hip and knee replacement surgery [J] Curr Opin Pulm Med, 2002, 8(5): 365-37L

Wu c L, Naqibuddin M, Rowlingson A J et al. The effect of pain on health-related quality of life in the immediate postoperative period [J] Anesth Analg, 2003, 97 (4): 1078-1085

Wang Yuexiu, Yuan Bin, Tang Jinshi. Central thalamic nucleus and under the front cover before the district were involved in mediating the nuclear strong and weak electroacupuncture analgesic effect of acupuncture [J]. Chinese Journal of Neuroscience, 1999, 15 (2): 125-130.

Wang Hongbei, Dong Xiaotong, Wang Shuangkun, etc. Different frequencies of electroacupuncture adjuvant arthritis in rats with acute pain and tissue reaction of P-endorphin content of the belly [J]. Chinese Acupuncture & Moxibustion, 1998, 18 (3): 163-166.

Wang Shengxu, Lai Xinsheng, He Haitang, etc. EA Jiaji on adjuvant arthritis in rats before spinal cord dynorphin mRNA expression in the belly yuan [J]. Chinese Journal of Traditional Medical Science and Technology, 1999, 6(10): 1-4.

Wang Shengxu, Hong Jun, Zhou Yilin, etc. EA Jiaji on adjuvant arthritis in rat peripheral blood monoamine content of the material[J]. Chinese Journal of Traditional Medical Science and Technology, 2000, 7(5):273-275.

Wang Shengxu, Hong Jun, Lai Xinsheng, etc. EA Jiaji on adjuvant arthritis in rats with spinal cord effects of substance P immunohistochemical study [J]. Chinese Journal of Traditional Medical Science and Technology, 2000, 7(3): 131-132.

Wang Shengxu, Hong Jun, Lai Xinsheng. EA Jiaji on adjuvant arthritis in rats with spinal cord content of monoamine neurotransmitters [J]. Chinese Journal of Traditional Medical Science and Technology, 2001, 80:1-3.

Wu CL, Naqibuddin M, Rowlingson AJ, et al. The effect of pain on health-related quality of life in the immediate postoperative period [J]. Anesth Analg, 2003, 97 (4): 1078-1085

Xun Rong, Guan Xinmin, Wang Caiyuan. Capsaicin treatment on rat sciatic nerve pain off and analgesic effect of EA[J]. Acupuncture Research, 1993, 18(4):280-284

Yin Xiaolei, Li Dan, Advances in postoperative analgesia [J]. People's Military Surgeon, 2004, 47 (4): 243-245.

Yang Jie, Tang Jinshi, Yuan Bin, etc. Rat hypothalamic neurons under the center's response to acupuncture [J]. Chinese Journal of Pain Medicine, 1997, 3(4): 223-227.

Yang Jiebin, Song Kaiyuan, Liang Fanrong, etc. Different acupuncture therapy on rat adjuvant arthritis of peripheral mechanism of analgesia[J]. Chinese Acupuncture & Moxibustion, 1999, 18(6):362-366.

Y. Sun, T. J. Gan, J. W. Dubose and A. S. Habib Acupuncture and related techniques for postoperative pain: asystematic review of randomized controlled trials British Journal of Anaesthesia 2008, 101 (2): 151 – 60

ZhangY Q, Tang J S, Yuan B, et al. Effect of the alamicnucleussubme diu sle sionso nt heta ilfli ckr eflexin hibitione vokedb yh indli mbelec trical st imulationi nt her at [J].NeuroR eport, 1995, 6(9): 1237-1240.

Zhao Canghuan. Electricity for local inflammation in adjuvant arthritis in rats the effects of opioid peptide gene expression[J]. Journal of Jinan University（Natural Science & Medicine Edition）, 1997, 18(5): 158-161.

Zhao Canghuan, Zhou Jun. Inflammation of the EP and LEK local injection of anti-serum components on the effect of electroacupuncture analgesia [J]. Shaanxi Journal of Traditional Chinese Medicine, 2002, 23(6): 569-570.

A Comparison Study on Arterial Blood Pressure and Pulse Data of Condenser Microphone[*]

Yin-Yi Han[1], Yih-Nen Jeng[2], Si-Chen Lee[3] and Hao-Jian Hung[4]
[1]Department of Trauma, National Taiwan University Hospital,
Graduate institute of Electrical Engineering, National Taiwan University,
[2]Department of Aeronautics and Astronautics, National Cheng-Kung University,
[3]Department of Electrical Engineering, National Taiwan University,
[4]Department of Aeronautics and Astronautics, National Cheng-Kung University,
Taiwan

1. Introduction

Recently, [Wang et al. 1989; Young et al. 1989, 1992; Jan et al, 2003; Wang Lin et al, 2004; Kuo et al, 2004; and Hsu et al. 2006] developed the resonance theory that each arterial bed in the vascular system is oscillated by the pressure waves at its own resonant frequency. They reported that ligating the renal, gastric, splenic or superior mesenteric artery of Wistar rats for a short duration could cause specific changes to the individual harmonics. They also showed that the ligation effects of different systems were linearly additive: as the renal artery and the superior mesenteric artery were simultaneously ligated, the change in the pulse spectrum was similar to the direct addition of two spectra resulting from the two individual ligations. They came to two important conclusions: First, the organ spectra can be used as parameters to elucidate the physical status of the specific vascular beds. Specifically, the magnitude of a harmonic mode reflects the amount of blood spent by the corresponding organ. Second, as the physical properties of a specific arterial bed change, the amplitude of the corresponding resonant mode changes more than that of the others. However, the corresponding resonant frequency will be approximately maintained by the heart rate control system to minimize the energy loss [Jan et al. 2003]. Most of their experimental data used pressure transducers to collect tail arteries of Wistar rats.

Based on this theory, Yu and Wang developed an artery blood pressure pulse acquisition system to take the wrist arterial blood pulse pressure data via a commercial microphone [Yu & Wang, 2006]. Unlike the experimental data of Wang et al., the sensor of the sonocardiography system of Yu and Wang are non-invasive and were more convenient to collect data than most existing systems. However, the interested frequency range of the wrist pulse data of the traditional Chinese medicine is lower than the announced range of most commercial microphone, say 20-20kHz. In [Jeng & Lee, 2008; Jeng, et al., 2011], it was proven that, if the acoustic signal source, pressure waves and small air cell containing the diaphragm of the electret condenser microphone are properly confined to a small air

---

[*] Project 2009101017D under the regulation of National Taiwan University Hospital, Research Ethics Committee A.

chamber, the lower bound of the effectively frequency response can be as low as 0.5Hz. The environment of signal confinement is equivalent to the situation that one firmly presses the microphone to the measured skin. In other words, the system using an electret condenser microphone is a potential tool to re-study the human organ-meridians which had achieved great achievement in the traditional Chinese medicine.

The above discussions confirm the fact that the arterial signals picked up by the sonocardiography system are closely related to the human organ-meridians. An interested problem is whether the microphone arterial pulse data also closely relates to the modern medicine data such as the well known invasive ABP and ECG. The ECG and ABP are the two commonly employed physiological parameters to monitor patients in the setting of critical illness [Civetta et al. 1992 & Marino 2007]. They offer the basic information of how the circulatory system performs in complex clinical conditions.

In order to look into complicated information embedded in signals of microphone's arterial pressure, ABP and ECG, both the FFT [Brigham, 1998] and time-frequency transform should be simultaneously used [Jeng & Lee, 2008; Jeng, et al., 2011]. The FFT provides a spectral parameter representation and the time frequency transform even give us the possibility of revolving the temporal varied amplitude and frequency of a wave component. In this study the Gabor transform will be employed.

In some sense, the ECG data reflects the input command, whereas the ABP signal reflects the corresponding vascular response. In case of homeostasis, the circulatory system should behave as a linear transfer function in the spectral band of the heart beat mode that the variation of ABP should be highly correlated with that of ECG. When the system is not properly functioning, the correlation may be violated such that the person may have healthy problem. From this view point, the correlation between variation of ECG and ABP can be a potential biomarker of human health assessment. However, continuous ABP data is usually only conveyed in critically ill patient with invasive intra-arterial measurement. Being non-invasive and more easily applicable, microphone pressure sensor is an alternative choice to get the continuous pulse signals. If we can prove that the microphone arterial signal's heart rate mode can be used to provide the index, the preventive medicine would become a practical issue for the general population. Moreover, the connection between the ancient Chinese and modern medicines will become more solid in near future.

2. Data and method

2.1 Theoretical development
Because the time series picked up by the microphone system, ECG or ABP may involve drift and/or trend, it frequently involves a monotonic non-periodic part. Therefore, a time series data string, $y_j = y(t_j), j = 0,1,2..., J$, can be written in the following form [Jeng et al. 2009]:

$$y_j = \sum_{l=0}^{J-1} [c_l \cos \frac{2\pi t_j}{\lambda_l} + d_l \sin \frac{2\pi t_j}{\lambda_l}] + \sum_{n=0}^{N} a_n t_j^n, \quad 0 < j < J-1 \qquad (1)$$

where $t_{j+1} - t_j = \Delta t$ = constant, l is the mode index, and $\lambda_l = J\Delta t / l$ is the wavelength of the l-th mode, the second summation represents the non-sinusoidal drift and/or trend and N represents the largest power for which $a_n \rightarrow 0$ for all $n > N$. For most engineering applications, $N = 250$ is a reasonable value. The non-sinusoidal trend is interpreted as the sum of monotonic parts and all the Fourier modes whose wavelengths are longer than the data span $T = J\Delta t$. This study uses the iterative Gaussian smoothing method in the spectral domain to serve as a high-passed filter. It can be proven the resulting response takes the following form [Jeng et al. 2008, 2009, 2011]:

$$y'_{j,m} \approx \sum_{l=0}^{J}[1-\exp[-2\pi^2\sigma^2 / \lambda^2]^m \left[c_l \cos\frac{2\pi t_j}{\lambda_l} + d_l \sin\frac{2\pi t_j}{\lambda_l} \right] + O(\Delta t^2)$$

$$\overline{y}_j^m = y_j - y'_{j,m}$$

(2)

where $y'_{j,m}$ and $\overline{y}_j^m$ represent smooth and high frequency responses after applying the iterative Gaussian smoothing method for m cycles and $[1-\exp[-2\pi^2\sigma^2/\lambda_l^2]^m$ represents the attenuation factor, in which σ is the smoothing factor of the Gaussian smoothing method and $m>N/2$. In this study, the iteration parameter m and smoothing factor σ use the value of 127 and 0.8seconds, respectively. These parameters means that the filter's transition zone is $\lambda_2/\lambda_1=2$ and $\lambda_1 \approx \sigma/0.772 \approx 1.036$seconds. More specifically, all wave modes of y'_m with wavelength $\lambda \leq 1.036$seconds are almost the same as that of original data and those wave modes with wavelength $\lambda \leq 2.072$seconds are removed. Now the trend is ultimately removed. Because this result is principally derived by assuming the data span running from $-\infty$ to ∞, small errors are thus induced by the missing data beyond the two ends. Next, the zero crossing points around the two ends can be located by a search procedure and interpolation formula. After dropping the data segments beyond the two zeros, a monotonic cubic interpolation [Huynh, 1993;Jeng et al. 2009, 2011] is used to redistribute the data into uniform spacing whose points equal an integer power of 2. Subsequently, the odd function mapping is used to double the data span. Finally, the FFT [Brigham, 1998] will generate a Fourier sine spectrum. This spectrum reflects many details in the low frequency region because the trend has already been removed and all the required periodic conditions are ensured by the odd function mapping.

In this study, the following Gabor wavelet transform using the Gaussian window (with a given window width a on the time domain) is used for the sinusoidal data y'_m :

$$G(f,\tau) = \frac{1}{\sqrt{a}}\int_0^T y'_m(t)e^{-2i\pi f(t-\tau)}e^{-(t-\tau)^2/(2a^2)}dt$$

(3)

in which τ denotes the central time instant of the Gaussian window and f is the central frequency index on spectral domain. By scanning both f and τ over the desired range of time-frequency domain, the desired two-dimensional Gabor wavelet coefficient plot or the spectrogram can be obtained. It can be proven it is about equal to the following form [Jeng et al. 2009, 2011]:

$$G(f,\tau) \approx \sqrt{\frac{a\pi}{2}}\sum_{l=1}^{J-1}\{[d_l-ie_l]e^{i2\pi f_l\tau}\exp[-2a^2\pi^2(f_l - f)^2]\}$$

(4)

where $d_l \approx (1-2\pi^2\sigma^2 / \lambda_l^2)^m b_l$ and $e_l \approx (1-2\pi^2\sigma^2 / \lambda_l^2)^m c_l$ are Fourier spectrum of y'_m. These relations indicate the wavelet coefficient is just an inverse FFT of a finite spectrum band specified by an associated Gaussian window whose window width is $1/(2a\pi)$ and is centered at the frequency of f. For the sake of completeness, the procedures are summarized below [Jeng et al. 2009, 2011].

1. Use the iterative Gaussian smoothing method to remove the non-sinusoidal part and a fraction of several lowest modes whose wavelengths are ranged from λ_L to T, where $T=J\Delta t$ is the data length.
2. Find the Fourier sine spectrum : find the zero around the two ends; discard data segments beyond the zeros; redistribute the data via a proper interpolation method so that the data point is an integer power of 2 (= 2**k > 2L, where L denotes the original data size); make an odd function mapping with respect to one end; employ in an FFT.
3. Choose the frequency resolution $f_i = f_0 + i\Delta f$ and $a = 2c \,/\, \Delta f$ to evaluate the band-pass limited spectrum via the Gaussian window with window width c, where f_0 is the lowest frequency employed to plot the spectrogram and c is an user specified parameter (e.g. $c =1.5$).
4. Find the inverse FFT of the band-pass limited spectrum, which is the real part of the spectrogram coefficient corresponding to the f_i mode. The corresponding amplitude distribution with respect to time is then evaluated by applying the Hilbert transform.
5. Scan all f_i s and plot the spectrogram.

Note that the resulting wavelet coefficients (spectrograms) are subject to the blur effect of the uncertainty principle [Goswami & Chan, 1999; Mallat, 1999; Jeng et al. 2009, 2011]. At most one obtains the best resolution with certain compromise between the temporal and spectral scales. In practical application, an approximate optimal resolution can be achieved via a few trial and error procedures by varying the parameter c in the third step.

A careful inspection upon Eq.(2) reveals that one can simultaneously remove the trend and obtain the high frequency spectrum by merely calculating in the spectral domain. Moreover, one can further obtain a single mode or a band-pass-limited spectrum by imposing a suitable window upon the spectrum of the high frequency part.

In this study, the relation between the microphone pulse data, ECG, and ABP is assumed to be determined by the cross-correlation of two wave components of the heart rate mode. The following familiar method directly calculates the cross-correlation coefficient [Bendat & Piersol 2000] between two wave components $y_1(t)$ and $y_2(t)$ is employed.

$$c = \frac{\int_{t_0}^{t_f} y_1(t)y_2(t)dt}{\left[\int_{t_0}^{t_f} y_1^{\,2}(t)dt\int_{t_0}^{t_f} y_2^{\,2}dt\right]^{1/2}} \tag{5}$$

where t_0 and t_f are the initial and final instances of the two wave components. The associated time series wave component, say $y_1(t)$ or $y_2(t)$, is obtained by the inverse FFT algorithm of the spectral band. For convenience, only two Fourier modes are considered here.

In order to eliminate the phase lag induced by the pressure wave propagation along the artery wall, one of the two wave components will be shifted, say $y_1(t \pm \tau)$ or $y_2(t \pm \tau)$. The parameter τ is the amount of time shift which achieves the maximum absolute value of c in Eq.(5). For a person not in critical state, his heart beat modes of ECG and ABP should be highly correlated in this sense.

For a patient in an intensive care unit, the modern medicine provides many effective supports and treatments. He may still survive even if his heart beat modes of ECG and ABP are not correlated. The reason is Eq.(5) principally depends on the phase lag between these modes. With the strong support of the intensive care unit, it seems that the correlation between the envelopes of these ECG and ABP modes is also an important index for such a patient. The envelopes, which represent the energy or amplitude of these modes, are believed to be roughly reflected by the shapes of corresponding wave components in spectrograms of amplitude [Jeng & Cheng, 2007].

According to the above discussions, in addition to Eq.(5), a partial information of the cross-correlation between two sinusoidal data strings is roughly considered to be the similarity of wave components in the spectrograms of amplitude. It is clearly that, as two wave components are partially correlated, the phase lag may or may not occur. If the phase lag is insignificant, it is certain that $|c| \geq 0.6$. If a large phase lag exists between two wave components with partial energy correlation, their correlation coefficient calculated by Eq.(5) may be low, say $|c| < 0.5$. To explain this state, consider the correlation between the heart rate modes of ECG and ABP of a patient as an example. Suppose their temporal amplitude and frequency distributions are similar so that energies of their corresponding wave components are correlated. The command of the heart (ECG) is transferred to the point of measuring the wrist pulse (ABP) via the pressure wave propagation through a series of vascular tubes. Due the some reasons, however, the wave propagation speed is not homogeneous and not invariant from one location to another. Thus, the periodicity of the heart rate is distorted at the ABP measuring point and the phase lag occurs. Although this stage is not perfect, the entire circulation system still partially functioned.

2.2 Data acquisition

In this study, the ECG signals were obtained from the three-lead ECG recording device. The ABP signals were conveyed from an invasive arterial-line system which involves an insertion of an arterial catheter connecting to a conducting tube filled with properly pressured fluid (see Fig.1). The mechanical signals were then transformed to the electrical ones with a midway pressure transducer. Both ECG and ABP data were transferred back to the Philips MP60 module which was the physiological signal monitoring system used in our study. The analog signals were output to the data acquisition card where they would be converted to the digital signals with a sampling rate of 500Hz and then forwarded to the portable computer for further analysis.

In order to achieve a stable sensitivity in response to the tiny wrist arterial pressure data, a commercial electret condenser microphone is employed, whose instructions are 20-20,000 Hz, 100mw, 32 Ω 105db sound pressure level sensitivity at 1kZ ±2 %. The experimental facilities include a digital audio board (Onkyo Inc. SE-150 PCI, SN ratio 100dB, 0.3-44KHz, sampling rate 32-192KHz). Before the wrist artery with a sampling rate of 500Hz was acquired, the measuring point should be carefully located by human finger so as to make sure that the pulse signal is prominent. The schematic diagram is shown in Fig.2a where the front face with the actuating diaphragm of microphone (Figs.2b and 2c) was firmly attached to the measuring point.

The data of six different patients in the intensive care unit of a hospital in Taiwan were included in our study. The ECG, ABP, and microphone data were in all cases successfully and simultaneously recorded in the same sampling rate. During the period of acquiring data, the ABP data was taken from the left wrist while the microphone data from the right wrist.

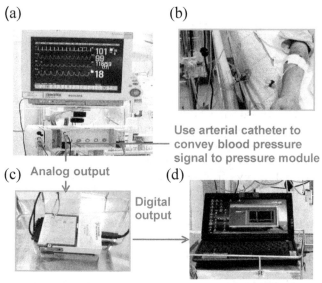

Fig. 1. Experimental instruments for the signal acquisition. (a) physiological signal monitoring system, Philips MP60, and pressure module; (b) invasive ABP monitoring system including an arterial catheter connecting to a conducting tube filled with fluid; (c) data acquisition card; (d) portable computer for displaying and storing the vital signs.

Although the direct invasive arterial-line system applied here provides the advantage of continuous and real-time monitoring, it may introduce additional signal damping, especially when the pressure conducting tube is long [Marino, 2007]. The inertia of the medium within the tube would inevitably remove most high frequency Fourier modes. Nevertheless, it is the currently available method to collect a continuous ABP signal during surgery.

Principally speaking, an electret condenser microphone uses the rate change of capacity to collect pressure signal so that it picks up the motion signal of the pulse. In other words, the microphone data reflect variations of pulse pressure rather than the pressure itself. In Ref.[Yu and Wang, 2006; Jeng & Lee, 2008], this signal had been successfully linked to the Wang pulse spectrum theory. However, in order to study the relation between ABP and microphone signal, the latter will be integrated once so that they have the same base.

3. Results and discussions

Consider the case of Fig. 7 of [Jeng & Lee, 2008] that the person had slight spleen disease as an example. Figure 3.1a plots the data before and after performing the integration once and their corresponding spectra are shown in Fig.3b. These figures indicate that the integration significantly smears the irregularity and rendering the fast attenuation of mode amplitude as the mode index increases. For the sake of clarity, their corresponding spectrograms of amplitudes are plotted in Fig.4a and 4b, respectively, in which the amplitude is transformed to be $\log_{10}(1+amp)$ to reveal the detailed information. According to the arterial wave theory [Wang et al. 1989; Young et al. 1989, 1992; Jan et al, 2003; Wang Lin et al, 2004; Kuo et al, 2004; and Hsu et al. 2006] the fourth mode reflects the healthy condition of the spleen. The significant amplitude and frequency variations of the spleen mode of both figures provided by microphone system indicate that the person had better to see a doctor. In other words, the integration of the microphone arterial signal does not much alter its capability of resolving the detailed information.

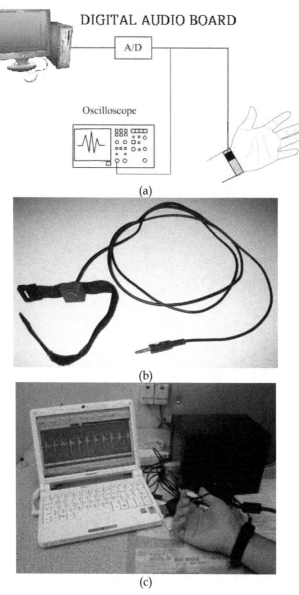

(a)

(b)

(c)

Fig. 2. An example of the sonocardiography system: (a) schematic diagram; (b) the microphone; and (c) an example of acquiring pulse data.

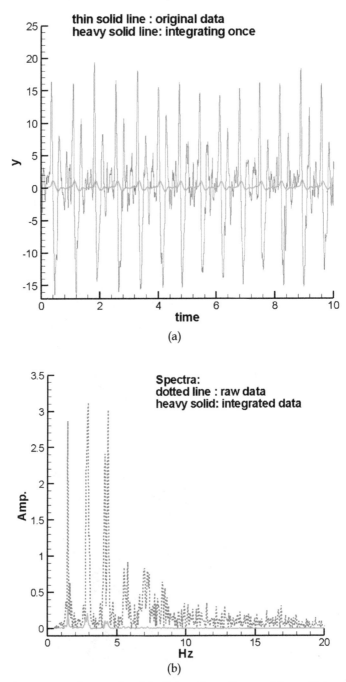

Fig. 3. Data and spectrum of a people with slight spleen disease: (a) raw (thin solid line) and integrated (heavy solid line) data; (b) spectrum of the raw and integrated data.

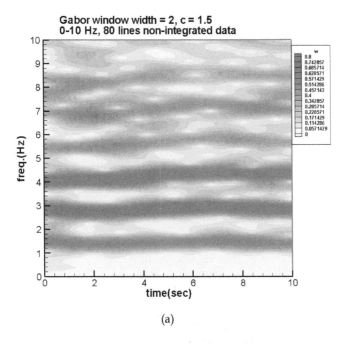

(a)

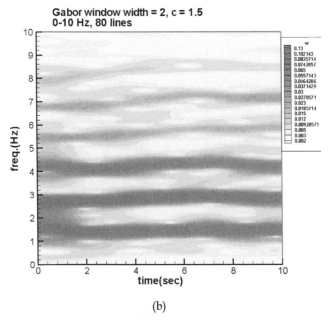

(b)

Fig. 4. Three-dimensional spectrograms: (a) raw data; and (b) integrated data.

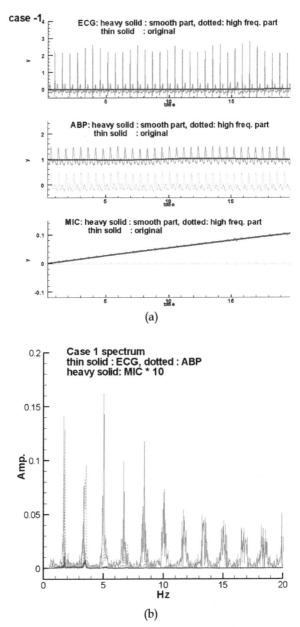

Fig. 5. The data and spectra of the first test case: (a) raw data; (b) spectrum in which the microphone's spectrum is enlarged 10 times.

In this study, data of six test cases are examined. All of them survived. However, the third case stayed in the hospital for one year after data collection. They are separately discussed below.

The first one is a case of head injury with epidural hematoma resulted from a car accident. His raw data are shown in Fig.5a, in which the ECG, ABP and microphone data are plotted from top to bottom, respectively. He was in comatose state with ventilator use while the data was collected. As the governing center had some problems, the output command of the heart rate control system, say the envelope of his ECG, is obviously variable so as to keep a highly adaptive state as shown in Fig.5a. According to the wave theory [Wang et al. 1989; Young et al. 1989, 1992; Jan et al, 2003; Wang Lin et al, 2004; Kuo et al, 2004; and Hsu et al. 2006] and ancient Chinese medicine, the fourth (lung mode) and sixth harmonic (gall mode) are closely related to the circulatory homeostasis of lung and brain, respectively. The spectrograms of Figs.6b and 6c show that the amplitude and frequency of the sixth mode are variable. However, since the steady mechanical ventilator use under sedation provides a smooth breathing pattern, the fourth mode is slightly more stable than the sixth mode.

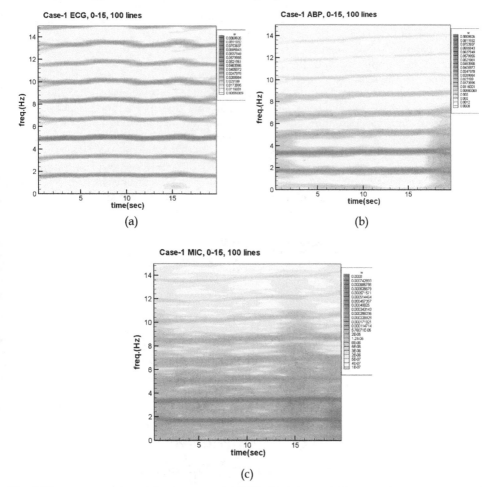

Fig. 6. The spectrograms of the first case: (a) ECG; (b) ABP; and (c) microphone wrist arterial signal.

The cross-correlations between three signals are plotted in Fig.7a through 7c, which are ECG, ABP, and microphone from top to bottom. Note that the time series of the three signals are measured at different points. Therefore, they should have certain phase differences between one another. Because the wave propagation speed distribution through the circulation system is not known, we shift the time scale of one of the wave components so as to attain a maximum absolute value of cross correlation coefficients. The shifted amounts are marked on the figures as shown. It seems that, around the heart rate mode of 1.7Hz, the ECG and ABP are almost totally correlated. In fact, the patient finally recovered after one month. It is interested to see that the correlations of both ECG and ABP with respect to the microphone signal are very high too.

It is interesting to see that the color distributions (represent the amplitude distribution) and wavy shapes (represent the frequency variation) of the fundamental and harmonics of Fig.7a are not similar to those of Fig.7b and 7c, respectively. Nevertheless, their differences of the heart beat wave component are not significant so that their cross-correlation coefficients are still very high and vital signs of the patient are stable.

A careful comparison between the sixth mode of Fig.6c and the fourth mode of Fig.5b reveals that the amplitude and frequency variations of the latter are obviously more complicated than those of the former. The former is corresponding to the signal of emergent case while the latter is not. This means that the behavior of the spectrum of the organ-meridian in emergency is much less sensitive than that does not in serious trouble. The reason is that, in critical situation, the adaptive capability of the blood circulation system concentrates on how to survive so that it takes care of the entire organ-meridians simultaneously. On the other hand, when only one organ is in trouble, the circulation system focuses on supporting this specific target. This difference occurs in all the rest test cases. In other words, both the wave theory of Wang et al. and ancient Chinese organ-meridian technology are suitable for most people before they face emergent health problems and are closely related to the preventive medicine.

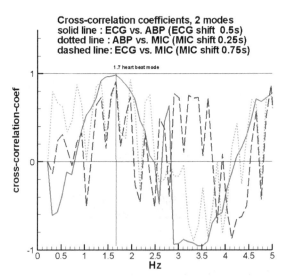

Fig. 7. The cross-correlation coefficients around the heart rate mode of the first test case.

The second one is a case of liver laceration resulted from a car accident. When the data was collected, the patient was in a stable hemodynamic state and non-operative management was applied. The corresponding raw data and spectra are shown in Figs.8a and 8b, respectively. It is seen that the spectral band around the fundamental (heart) and harmonics

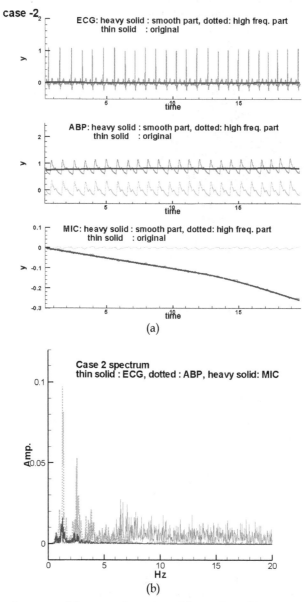

(a)

(b)

Fig. 8. The data and spectra of the second test case: (a) raw data; (b) spectrum in which the microphone's spectrum is enlarged 10 times.

seriously scattered. All the corresponding spectrograms of ECG, ABP and microphone signals exhibit significant variations of both amplitude and frequencies. It seems that the spectral scattering of a wave component is corresponding to the variation of one or two of the amplitude and frequency. The degrees of these dominant modes' variations are not less than the first harmonic (live mode). It seems that the injury of the major organ, liver, brought great impact on the operation of other systems, and the adaptation of the entire system was switched on. Fortunately, the situation is not serious enough to become chaos so that we can still trace every mode.

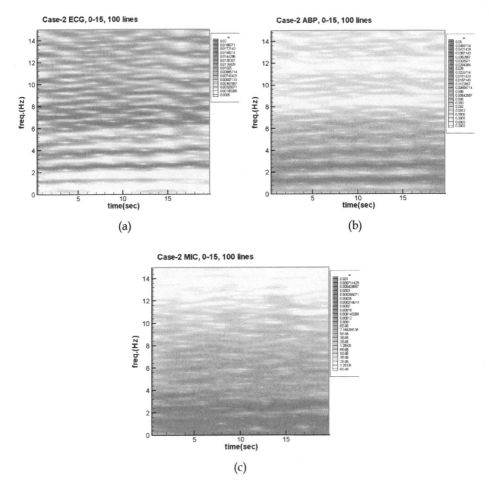

Fig. 9. The spectrograms of the second case: (a) ECG; (b) ABP; and (c) microphone wrist arterial signal.

The cross correlation coefficients are shown in Fig.10. The correlations of ECG-ABP and ABP-microphone are moderately high (about 0.7 and 0.6 respectively). The ECG and microphone signal is in highly negative correlation (-0.9). Now the color distributions and wavy shapes of most organ meridians shown in the three spectrograms are similar to each other such that they are also partially correlated. Therefore, the patient's circulation system is healthy. This explanation was confirmed by the record that the patient had recovered after one month.

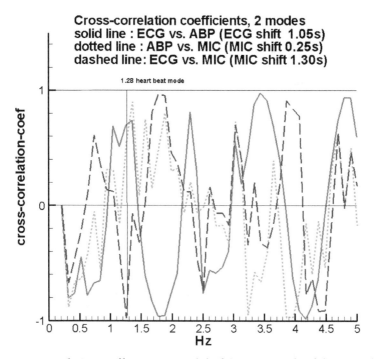

Fig. 10. The cross-correlation coefficients around the heart rate mode of the second test case.

The third test case suffered from serious electric shock and had cardiopulmonary resuscitation right before onto the ambulance. Though the vital signs resumed, he remained in comatose state with ventilator support while the data was collected. Unfortunately, the case had prolonged hospitalization for one year after that. The raw data and spectra are shown in Figs.11. Like the spectra shown in Fig.11b, spectrograms of Figs.12a through 12c are regular and do not have much amplitude variation. It seems that the coma had suppressed the system adaptation. Moreover, the similarity of color distribution and wavy shape of every organ meridian indicates that the three data are partially correlated too. Moreover, Fig.13 shows that all the correlation coefficients of the heart rate mode are very high as shown. In spite of the fact that the patient can not completely recover for a long time, the highly correlated state indicates that vital signs are stable.

The next case got right frontal parietal and temporal subdural hematoma after falling down. She also had the history of old stroke. The corresponding raw data and spectra are plotted in Figs.14a and 14b, respectively. From these signal we can not have much information. From the resulting spectrograms, it is obviously that the gall mode (related to brain organ-meridian) has obvious variations of both amplitude and frequency. Consequently, the second and still higher harmonics are all affected too.

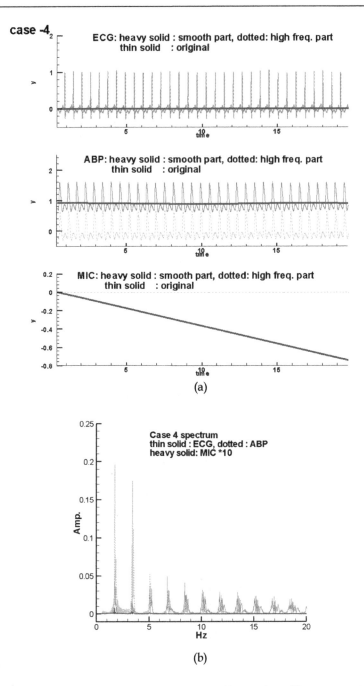

(a)

(b)

Fig. 11. The data and spectra of the third test case: (a) raw data; (b) spectrum in which the microphone's spectrum is enlarged 10 times.

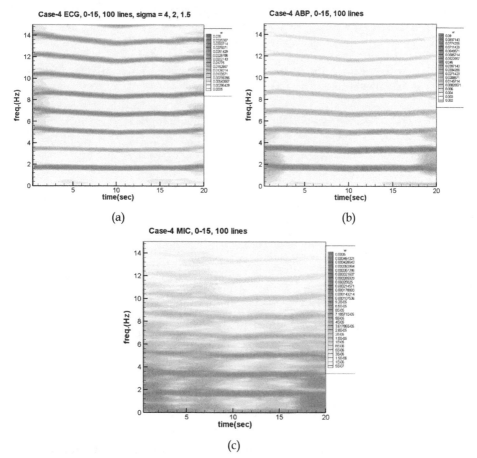

Fig. 12. The spectrograms of the third case: (a) ECG; (b) ABP; and (c) microphone wrist arterial signal.

The cross correlation between the ECG and ABP are very high (about 0.9 as shown in Fig.15). On the other hand, signals of ABP-microphone and ECG-microphone have negative correlations of about -0.6. The reason may be cause by the weak wrist pulse signal of the patient. Nevertheless, it seems that the system adaptation of the patient worked very well so that mode wave components gradually fluctuated as shown. These fluctuations are similarly existed in the three spectrograms of Figs.14a-14c which show that their energies are partially correlated. These correlations reflect the high possibility of recover which is verified by the fact that the patient had recovered after one month.

The fifth test case was suffered from a cervical vertebra injury after falling down and received the support of the endotracheal intubation. At the instant of measuring data, the patient lost consciousness and was quadriplegia. His raw data and spectra are shown in Figs.17a and 17b, respectively. The resulting spectrograms (Figs.18a-18c) show that both fundamental mode and harmonics have obvious amplitude and frequency fluctuations. His gall modes even have jumps at the instances of the tenth and fifteenth second as shown. It indicates his self-protection system was in the adaptive state and tried to recover his health. In Fig.19, it is seen the ECG, ABP, and microphone signal have very high correlation between one another such that his circulation worked very well. The partial correlations among their energy are also reflected by the similarity between their organ meridians' amplitude and frequency distributions. These conclusions have the strong evident that he finally recovered after six months.

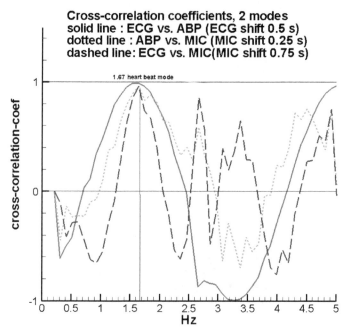

Fig. 13. The cross-correlation coefficients around the heart rate mode of the third test case.

The last test case got severe head injury with intracranial hemorrhage, subdural hematoma and subarachnoid hemorrhage. The raw data and spectra are shown in Figs.20a and 20b, respectively. Envelopes of the ECG and APP raw data have obvious oscillations as shown. The corresponding spectrograms of Figs.21a through 21b show that his circulation system tried to adapt itself. The three gall modes has abnormal jump in the interval of 5-7 second as shown. In this case, the heart rate modes of ABP and microphone signal are highly correlated (correlation coefficient is about 0.9 in Fig.22). Figure 22 shows that his cross-correlation coefficients of ECG-ABP and ECG-microphone are about 0.3 and 0.1, respectively. Obviously, the phase lags are serious between these two signals. That indicates he was in a life-threatening situation at that time. Fortunately, the patient has partial correlation between three data because his amplitude and frequency fluctuations of all the organ meridian modes of three spectrograms are similar to one another. He recovered gradually and was transferred to the general ward within one month. Recently, he returned to the clinic for the treatment of epilepsy, a neurological sequel of the previous head injury. That means his neural control system is impaired. Although his circulation system has phase lag problems, the overall response is not too bad so that he finally recovered under the proper supports and treatments in the intensive care unit. These messages indicate that he effectively struggled for his life during the period in the intensity care unit.

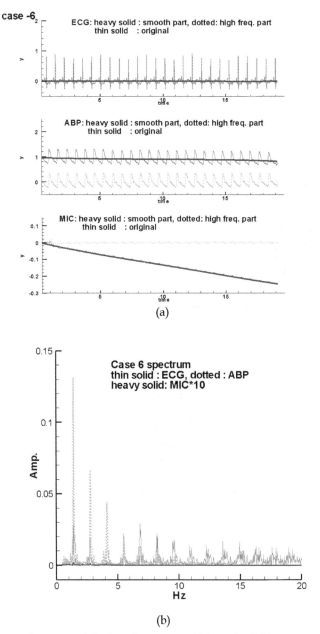

(a)

(b)

Fig. 14. The data and spectra of the fourth test case: (a) raw data; (b) spectrum in which the microphone's spectrum is enlarged 10 times.

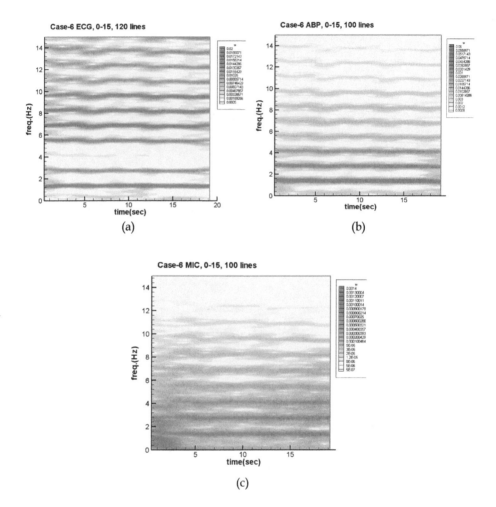

Fig. 15. The spectrograms of the fourth case: (a) ECG; (b) ABP; and (c) microphone wrist arterial signal.

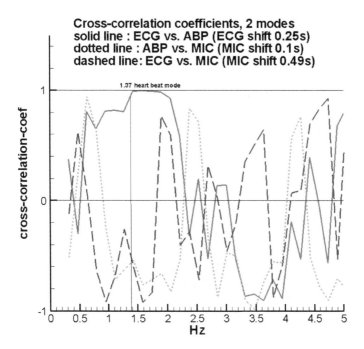

Fig. 16. The cross-correlation coefficients around the heart rate mode of the fourth test case.

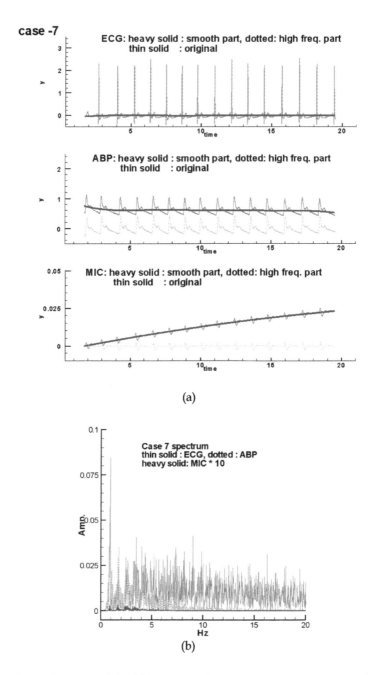

Fig. 17. The data and spectra of the fifth test case: (a) raw data; (b) spectrum in which the microphone's spectrum is enlarged 10 times.

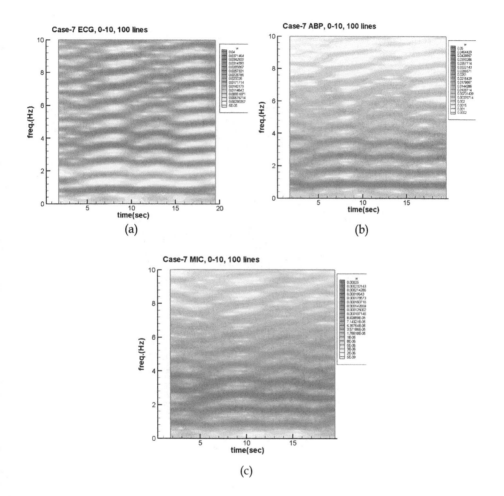

Fig. 18. The spectrograms of the fifth case: (a) ECG; (b) ABP; and (c) microphone wrist arterial signal.

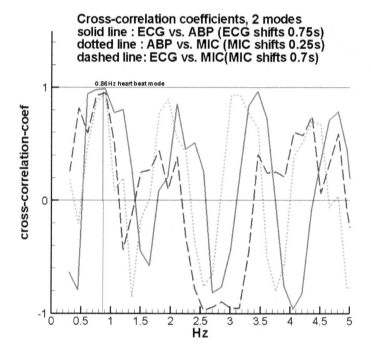

Fig. 19. The cross-correlation coefficients around the heart rate mode of the fifth test case.

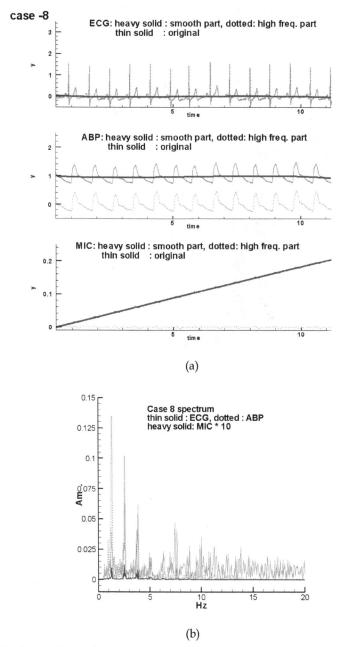

Fig. 20. The data of the sixth test case, fell down, bilateral temporal bone fractures extends into the right middle ear cavity: (a) raw data; (b) spectrum in which the microphone's spectrum is enlarged 10 times.

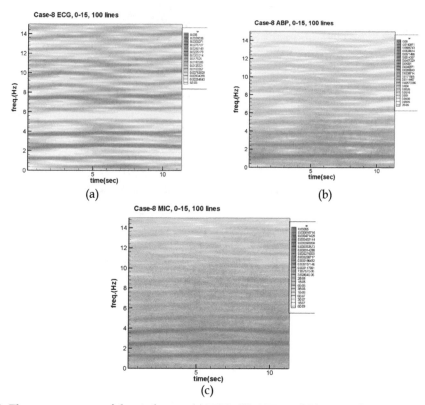

Fig. 21. The spectrograms of the sixth case: (a) ECG; (b) ABP; and (c) microphone wrist arterial signal.

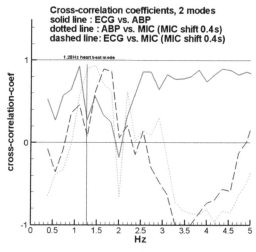

Fig. 22. The cross-correlation coefficients around the heart rate mode of the sixth test case.

In summary, several consistent points of the above discussions are listed below.

1. The heart modes of microphone signal and ABP are correlated. It indicates the possibility that the electret condenser microphone system is a potential tool to be an alternative of ABP system. Since the microphone is a non-invasive sensor and closely related to the ancient Chinese medicine, it can be equipped with simple ECG system to become a valuable tool of clinic and preventive medicine.

2. The cross-correlations between ECG, ABP and microphone can be examined either by the directly calculating the coefficient among time domain heart rate components or by checking the similarity of every organ meridian's shape and color variations with respect to time in their spectrograms. All the test cases show that the heart rate modes of ECG and ABP are correlated. The followed up records show that all these patients remain alive under the effective treatments of the intensive care unit.

3. In critical cases, the wave theory of Wang et al. about single organ meridian still works but is not prominent as in the less emergent situations.

4. When the state is not critical, all the organ-meridians fluctuate which reflect the adaptation of the blood circulation system to struggle for survive.

Since the sample size is too small to achieve a statistical level, further studies will be done to enrich the data base so as to make these facts become useful.

4. Conclusions

The precise post processing algorithm combining the trend removal, Fourier transform and modified Gabor transform provides a tool to look into details of ECG, ABP, and microphone data of wrist arterial signal. The heart modes of all the microphone signals are correlated with ABP. In other words, the non-invasive acoustic sensor can also be a potential tool to monitor human healthy state. The cross correlation coefficient between heart beat modes of ECG and ABP seems to be a possible index of human vital sign. In summary, the microphone system is a potential tool to effectively construct a bridge among ancient and modern medicine and modern technologies.

5. References

Bendat, J. S. & Piersol, A. G.. (2000). *Random Data Analysis and Measurement Procedures*, 3rd ed., John Wiley & Sons, New York, Chapters 10 & 11, pp.349-456.

Brigham, E.O. (1998). *The Fast Fourier Transform and Its Applications*; Prentice Hall: Englewood Cliffs, NJ, USA.

Civetta, J. M.; Taylor, R. W. & Kirby, R. R. (1996). *Critical Care*. 3rd ed., Lippincott-Raven, Ch. 16 & 26, pp. 227-245, 368-372

Goswami, J. C., & Chan, A. K. (1999). *Fundamentals of Wavelets, Theory, Algorithms, and Applications*, John Wiley & Sons, New York.

Hsu, T. L.; Chao, P. T., Hsiu, H., Wang, W. K., Li, S. P. & Lin Wang Y. Y. (2006). Organ-Specific Ligation-Induced Changes in Harmonic Components of the Pulse Spectrum and Regional Vasoconstrictor Selectivity in Wistar Rats, *Experimental Physiology*, vol. 91, no.1, pp.163-170, 2006.

Huynh, H.T. (1993). Accurate monotone cubic interpolation. *SIAM. J. Numer. Anal.* Vol.30, pp.57-100

Jan, M. Y.; Hsiu, H., Hsu, T. L., Wang, W. K., & Wang, Y. Y. (2003). The Physical Conditions of Different Organs Are Reflected Specifically in the Pressure Pulse Spectrum of the Peripheral Arterial, *Cardiovascular Engineering: An Int. J.,* vol. 3. no.1, pp.21-29.

Jeng, Y. N. & Lee, S. Y.. (2008). Qualitative Frequency Response Calibration of Sonocardiography System to Sense Wrist Pulse, *The 7th Asian-Pacific Conference on Medical and Biological Engineering,* APCMBE 2008 March 21-26, 2008, Beijing, China, paper no. T22. No.5-15.

Jeng, Y. N. and Cheng, Y. C. (2007). A First Study of Speech Processing via a Novel Mode Decomposition Basing on the Fourier Sine Spectrum and Spectrogram, *Proc. IEEE 2007 TENCON,* 10/30~11/2 Taipei, Taiwan, WeSP-01 section, paper no.00079.

Jeng, Y. N.; Yang, T. M. & Lee, S. Y. (2011). Response Identification in the Extremely Low Frequency Region of an Electret Condenser Microphone, *Sensors,* vol.11, pp.623-637; doi:10.3390/s110100623.

Jeng, Y.N.; Huang, P.G. & Cheng, Y.C. (2008). Decomposition of one-dimensional waveform using iterative Gaussian diffusive filtering methods. *Proc. R. Soc. Lond. A* 2008, 464, 1673-1695.

Jeng, Y.N.; Yang, T.M. & Wu, C.H. (2009) Low Frequency Analysis of Acoustic and Vibration Data of a Remote Control Electronic Helicopter. *Proceeding of 47th AIAA Aerospace Sciences Meeting.* Orlando, FL, USA, January 2009; pp. 5-8.

Kuo, Y. C. Kuo; Chiu, T. Y., Jan, M. Y., Bau, J. G., Li, S. P., Wang, W. K. & Wang, Y. Y. (2004). Losing Harmonic Stability of Arterial Pulse in Terminally Ill Patients, Clinical Methods and Pharmachology, *Blood Pressure Monitoring,* vol. 9. no. 5, pp.255-258, Oct. 2004.

Mallat, S. G. (1999). *A Wavelet Tour of Signal Processing.* Academic Press, New York.

Marino, P. L. (2007). *The ICU book.* 3rd ed., Lippincott Willian & Wilkins, Ch 8 & 12, pp.151-159, 211-230.

Wang Lin, Y. Y.; Jan, M. Y., Shyu, C. S., Jiang, C. A. & Wang, W. K. (2004). The Natural Frequencies of the Arterial System and Their Relation to the Heart Rate," *IEEE Trans. Biomed. Eng.,* vol. 51. no.1, Jan. 2004, pp. 193-195.

Wang, W. K.; Lo, Y. Y., Chiang, Y., Hsu, T. L. & Wang Lin Y. Y (1989). Resonance of Organs with the Heart, *Biomedical Engineering – An International Symposium,* ed. Young, W. J., Hemisphere, Washington, DC. USA, pp.259-268.

Young, S. T.; Wang, W. K., Chang, L. S. & Kuo, T. S. (1992). The Filter properties of the Arterial Beds of Organs in Rats, *Acta Physiol Scand.,* vol. 145, pp.401-406.

Young, S. T.; Wang, W. K., Chang, L. S., & Kuo, T. S. (1989). Specific Frequency Properties of the Renal and the Superior Mesenteric Arterial Beds in Rats, *Cardiovas Res.* Vol. 23, pp.265-467.

Yu, F. M. & Wang, S. C. (2006). Design of a Sonocardiography System and Its Application in the Diagnostic of the Cardiovascular Disease, *Proceedings of 2006 TSB conference,* Taiwan, Paper No. TSB2006-O-205, pp.16, Dec. 2006.

Permissions

The contributors of this book come from diverse backgrounds, making this book a truly international effort. This book will bring forth new frontiers with its revolutionizing research information and detailed analysis of the nascent developments around the world.

We would like to thank Prof. Kuang Haixue, for lending his expertise to make the book truly unique. He has played a crucial role in the development of this book. Without his invaluable contribution this book wouldn't have been possible. He has made vital efforts to compile up to date information on the varied aspects of this subject to make this book a valuable addition to the collection of many professionals and students.

This book was conceptualized with the vision of imparting up-to-date information and advanced data in this field. To ensure the same, a matchless editorial board was set up. Every individual on the board went through rigorous rounds of assessment to prove their worth. After which they invested a large part of their time researching and compiling the most relevant data for our readers. Conferences and sessions were held from time to time between the editorial board and the contributing authors to present the data in the most comprehensible form. The editorial team has worked tirelessly to provide valuable and valid information to help people across the globe.

Every chapter published in this book has been scrutinized by our experts. Their significance has been extensively debated. The topics covered herein carry significant findings which will fuel the growth of the discipline. They may even be implemented as practical applications or may be referred to as a beginning point for another development. Chapters in this book were first published by InTech; hereby published with permission under the Creative Commons Attribution License or equivalent.

The editorial board has been involved in producing this book since its inception. They have spent rigorous hours researching and exploring the diverse topics which have resulted in the successful publishing of this book. They have passed on their knowledge of decades through this book. To expedite this challenging task, the publisher supported the team at every step. A small team of assistant editors was also appointed to further simplify the editing procedure and attain best results for the readers.

Our editorial team has been hand-picked from every corner of the world. Their multi-ethnicity adds dynamic inputs to the discussions which result in innovative outcomes. These outcomes are then further discussed with the researchers and contributors who give their valuable feedback and opinion regarding the same. The feedback is then collaborated with the researches and they are edited in a comprehensive manner to aid the understanding of the subject.

Apart from the editorial board, the designing team has also invested a significant amount of their time in understanding the subject and creating the most relevant covers. They scrutinized every image to scout for the most suitable representation of the subject and create an appropriate cover for the book.

The publishing team has been involved in this book since its early stages. They were actively engaged in every process, be it collecting the data, connecting with the contributors or procuring relevant information. The team has been an ardent support to the editorial, designing and production team. Their endless efforts to recruit the best for this project, has resulted in the accomplishment of this book. They are a veteran in the field of academics and their pool of knowledge is as vast as their experience in printing. Their expertise and guidance has proved useful at every step. Their uncompromising quality standards have made this book an exceptional effort. Their encouragement from time to time has been an inspiration for everyone.

The publisher and the editorial board hope that this book will prove to be a valuable piece of knowledge for researchers, students, practitioners and scholars across the globe.

List of Contributors

Haixue Kuang
Key Laboratory of Chinese Materia Medica (Heilongjiang University of Chinese Medicine), Ministry of Education, Harbin, China

Stefan Jaeger
National Library of Medicine, United States

Haixue Kuang, Yanyan Wang, Qiuhong Wang, Bingyou Yang and Yonggang Xia
Key Laboratory of Chinese Materia Medica (Heilongjiang University of Chinese Medicine), Ministry of Education, Harbin, China

Yasuyo Hijikata
Toyodo Hijikata Clinic, Japan

Xing-Tai Li
College of Life Science, Dalian Nationalities University, Dalian, China

Jia Zhao
Norman Bethune College of Medicine, Jilin University, Changchun, China

Qingli Li
Key Laboratory of Polor Materials and Devices, East China Normal University, China

Renquan Liu and Guoyong Chen
Beijing University of Chinese Medicine, Beijing, China

Yuhao Zhao
School of Traditional Chinese, Medicine, Capital Medical University, Beijing, China

Chenghe Shi
Department of TCM,Peking University Third Hospital, Beijing, P.R. China

Arthur de Sá Ferreira
Centro Universitário Augusto Motta, Brazil

Wendy Wong and Cindy Lam Lo Kuen
Department of Family Medicine and Primary Care, LKS Faculty of Medicine, Hong Kong

Daniel Fong Yee Tak
Department of Nursing Studies, LKS Faculty of Medicine, The University of Hong Kong, Hong Kong

Jonathan Sham Shun Tong
Department of Clinical Oncology, LKS Faculty of Medicine, Hong Kong

Bang Jian He and Peijian Tong
Zhejiang Traditional Chinese Medicine University, China

Yin-Yi Han
Department of Trauma, National Taiwan University Hospital, Graduate institute of Electrical Engineering, National Taiwan University, Taiwan

Hao-Jian Hung
Department of Aeronautics and Astronautics, National Cheng-Kung University, Taiwan

Si-Chen Lee
Department of Electrical Engineering, National Taiwan University, Taiwan

Yih-Nen Jeng
Department of Aeronautics and Astronautics, National Cheng-Kung University, Taiwan

Printed in the USA
CPSIA information can be obtained
at www.ICGtesting.com
JSHW011430221024
72173JS00004B/738